Transitions
IN DYING AND
BEREAVEMENT

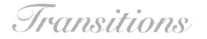
in Dying and Bereavement

A Psychosocial Guide For Hospice and Palliative Care

by

Victoria Hospice Society

and

Moira Cairns
Marney Thompson
Wendy Wainwright

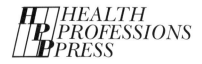
HEALTH PROFESSIONS PRESS

Baltimore • London • Winnipeg • Sydney

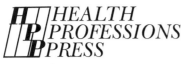

Health Professions Press, Inc.
Post Office Box 10624
Baltimore, Maryland 21285-0624
www.healthpropress.com

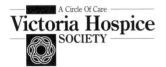

Typeset by Auburn Associates, Inc., Baltimore, Maryland.
Manufactured in the United States of America by
Versa Press, East Peoria, Illinois.

The individuals and situations described in this book are based on the authors' actual experiences. In all instances, names have been changed; in some instances, identifying details have been altered to protect confidentiality.

Photograph on page 254 used by permission of Moira Cairns.
Photograph on page 170 used by permission of John Glinn.
Photographs on the cover and pages xii, 134, 214, and 286 used by permission of Rosemary Neering.
Photographs on pages 22, 46, 92, 328, and 364 used by permission of Susan Schmitt.

The poem on page 194 and the quotation on page 231 are from *The Prophet* by Kahlil Gibran, copyright 1923 by Kahlil Gibran and renewed 1951 by Administrators C.T.A. of Kahlil Gibran Estate and Mary G. Gibran. Used by permission of Alfred A. Knopf, a division of Random House, Inc.

"Late Love" by Judith Viorst (p. 373). From *Suddenly Sixty and Other Shocks of Later Life*. Published by Simon & Schuster. Copyright © 2000 by Judith Viorst. Reprinted by permission of Lescher & Lescher, Ltd. All rights reserved.

Excerpt on p. 354 from *High Tide in Tucson: Essays from Now or Never* by Barbara Kingsolver. Copyright © 1995 by Barbara Kingsolver. Reprinted by permission of HarperCollins Publishers Inc.

The definitions on pages 182 and 221 are reprinted by permission of Oxford University Press.

Library of Congress Cataloging-in-Publication Data
Victoria Hospice Society
    Transitions in dying and bereavement : a psychosocial guide for hospice and palliative care / by Victoria
    Hospice Society, Moira Cairns, Marney Thompson, Wendy Wainwright.
        p.   cm.
        Includes bibliographical references and index.
        ISBN 1-87881-292-0
        1. Hospice care—Social aspects. 2. Hospice care—Psychological aspects.
3. Palliative treatment—Psychological aspects. 4. Palliative treatment—Social aspects.
5. Grief therapy—Psychological aspects. 6. Grief therapy—Social aspects. I. Moira
Cairns. II. Marney Thompson. III. Wendy Wainwright. IV. Title.

R726.8 .C336 2003
362.1/756 21   2003049912

British Library Cataloguing in Publication data are available from the British Library.

Contents

Victoria Hospice Society, 1952 Bay Street, Victoria, British Columbia, CANADA, V8R 1J8. Providing quality end-of-life care, and teaching others how to provide that care, has been a Victoria Hospice Society (VHS) tradition since the organization was founded in 1980 in Victoria, British Columbia. As well as caring for those facing advanced illness, death, and bereavement, Victoria Hospice staff are also involved in provincial and national initiatives dedicated to palliative care training, research, and advocacy. In 1999, the Victoria Hospice Learning Centre for Palliative Care was formally established to work in partnership with other health care and academic organizations to advance excellence in palliative care.

The Victoria Hospice program of care includes a 17-bed palliative care inpatient unit, a Palliative Response Team that provides 24-hour crisis support to patients and families at home, a comprehensive bereavement program, and clinical consultation services to patients in other health care facilities. Victoria Hospice palliative care courses and publications, such as the textbook *Medical Care of the Dying* (1998), are valuable resources to professional care providers throughout North America. For more information, visit the Victoria Hospice website at www.victoriahospice.org.

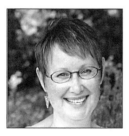

Moira Cairns, B.A., R.S.W., has worked in the counseling field since 1977. She served as a hospital social worker, hospice counselor, branch administrator, and development officer for palliative care in Wales, and is now the bereavement coordinator for the VHS. She has a bachelor's degree in psychology and is a certified social worker. Ms. Cairns is an experienced author, conference presenter, and workshop trainer on palliative care and bereavement.

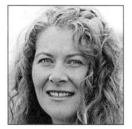

Marney Thompson, M.A., worked at the VHS as a volunteer, then as a group facilitator, and has worked as a counselor since 1990. She has a bachelor's degree in child and youth care and a master's degree in human and social development. An experienced conference presenter on psychosocial palliative topics, she is also the author of various publications on bereavement published by the VHS.

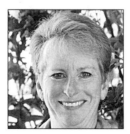

Wendy Wainwright, M.Ed., has worked with the VHS since 1983 as a community counselor, as a bereavement coordinator, and now as the manager of counseling services. She has a bachelor's degree in sociology and a master's of education in counseling psychology. She has developed staff and volunteer training programs for VHS and educational materials for patients, families, and professionals. Ms. Wainwright is president of the British Columbia Hospice Palliative Care Association and is the author of numerous professional journal articles on counseling activities, child and parent support groups, and young people and death.

Contributors

The following individuals provided essays, photographs, insights, and support for this project.

Angela Anscombe

Michael Boyle

Dr. Deb Braithwaite

Rachelle Campbell

Elizabeth Causton

Ruby Chapman

David Cheperdak

James Dolan

Dr. Michael Downing

Ed Founger

John Glinn

Pauline Johnson

Eve Joseph

Barb Landell

Dan Maloney

Lucie Mattar

Katherine Murray

Rosemary Neering

Eileen O'Donnell

Adaline O'Gorman

Brenda Pengelly

Christine Piercy

Caelin Rose

Jerry Rothstein

Eileen Rutherford

Jill Sartorio

Mairi Scanlan

Susan Schmitt

Dr. Ruth Simkin

Betty Vining

Rae Westcott

Allyson Whiteman

Helen Wong

Marjorie Woodroffe

Acknowledgments

So many people have helped and sustained us in the writing of this book. First and always, we are grateful to the thousands of patients and families who have taught us over the years through their generosity, pain, humor, and courage.

We thank our team at Victoria Hospice Society and colleagues at the British Columbia Cancer Agency, in particular Michael Boyle and Helen Wong, patient and family counselors. We also thank social work and counseling colleagues who are working in hospice and palliative care in British Columbia, Canada, and around the world. We are especially grateful to those who read chapters and commented on them and to those who stood in for us in clinical and management roles while we were writing. The faith and support of Victoria Hospice Executive Director Dave Cheperdak and the rest of the Victoria Hospice management team as well as our society and foundation boards inspired us and made our task possible. We much appreciate the time and energy that Victoria Hospice Medical Director Dr. Michael Downing expended on the project.

We extend our gratitude to consulting editor Rosemary Neering for encouraging us as writers and guiding us through the process of creating a book and to Brenda Pengelly and Judy Martell of the Victoria Hospice Learning Centre for Palliative Care for their support, advocacy, and assistance.

The scope of this guide has been broadened and deepened by the contributors who the reader will meet within its pages. We thank them for their time and wisdom—and for their willingness to share both. We also express our appreciation to those who contributed the photographs that help us symbolize the transitions of the journey through dying and bereavement.

We thank the many students, volunteers, colleagues, and others who have listened to us, challenged us, and supported us as our thoughts about this book developed.

And thank you especially to our own families, who saw us through the difficult challenges and celebrated the good times with us.

*   *   *

Victoria Hospice Society gratefully acknowledges the generous financial support of donors in making the development of this book possible. In particular we extend our appreciation to the following donors for their support and commitment to this important project:

> The Allen and Loreen Vandekerkhove Family Foundation
> John B. Miller Family
> The Victoria Foundation
> Victoria Hospice and Palliative Care Foundation

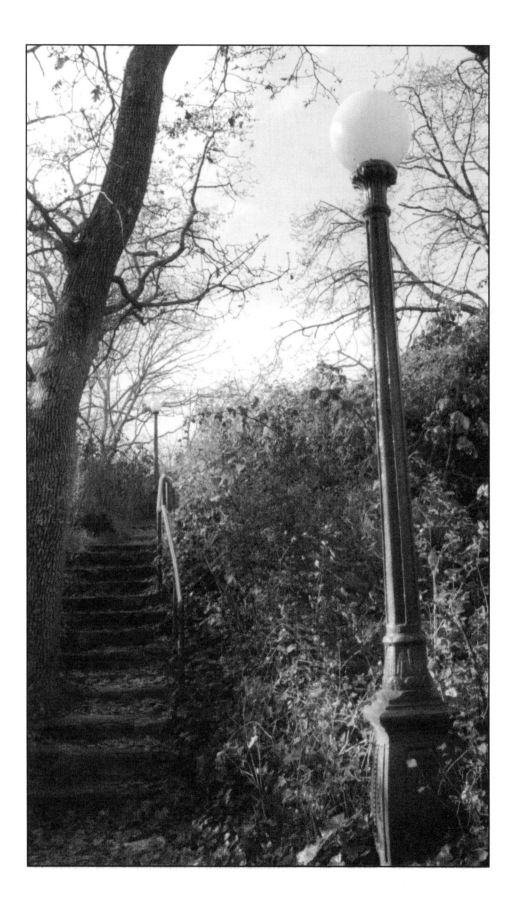

Signposts

PRINCIPLES, VALUES, AND ASSUMPTIONS

After a particularly long and difficult meeting with a patient, Mr. Perryman, and his family, the counselor sat down next to a colleague feeling drained and upset. The colleague asked what was wrong. The counselor explained that she had expected to meet with the man and his family to decide whether he would stay at the hospice or go home to die. Instead, she discovered that before they were able to make any plans, they really needed to talk openly with each other about some unresolved issues; namely, the circumstances surrounding how Mr. Perryman's mother had died 14 years earlier. Apparently, her death had been so disturbing and painful for the family that any discussion about Mr. Perryman's death was being avoided, making the meeting with the counselor very difficult.

"Oh, so that's what you do," exclaimed the colleague. "I thought you just sat at the bedside and held the patient's hand."

As we reflect on what palliative and bereavement counselors actually do, several questions come to mind. What are their aims, and how do they accomplish these aims? How can they work as a team with nurses, physicians, other professionals, and volunteers? How can this team work together with terminally ill or bereaved individuals to improve the overall quality of the service? This book attempts to answer these questions by examining, in theory and in concrete detail, the psychosocial care of individuals who are dying and bereaved. The term *psychosocial* encompasses the "emotional, intellectual, spiritual, interpersonal, social, cultural and economic dimensions" of dying and bereavement (Bates et al., 1993, p. 29). This book identifies the key transitions that most dying patients and their families face and describes the interventions that are most likely to help. The authors believe it is possible to identify and anticipate common experiences and still remain open to the awesome mystery of this work, the varying disease processes, and the unique and exceptional people involved.

Although many materials provide information about the medical care of those who are seriously ill and dying, or about bereavement, resources that focus on psychosocial aspects of care from diagnosis through bereavement are scarce. The goal of this book is to improve overall care by making psychosocial aspects more identifiable and predictable. This information can be used by newcomers to the field and by experienced practitioners alike.

WHAT BRINGS PEOPLE TO THIS WORK?

People who work in hospice palliative care inevitably face well-meaning, incredulous, or concerned friends and family members who ask the question, "Why [or how] do you do it?" Hospice workers may even ask themselves the same question. For some health care providers, the answers change over time as does the ability to ask and answer this question. Following are the reflections of counselors working in hospice palliative care. The time periods in parentheses indicate years of experience in the field.

Barb Landell (1 year)

The experience of my mother's death and my subsequent bereavement was a transformative process. Now, I come from a place of acceptance of death and know that the pain of grieving is okay. I like to express compassion and caring. I find it meaningful to work in a team and to be involved in profound experiences with what is real, death and loss.

Mairi Scanlan (5 years)

Hospice work was a natural progression from what I was already doing as a social worker in an acquired immunodeficiency syndrome (AIDS) organization. When I was working in the AIDS organization, working with the palliative people felt right. I felt more involved, more buzzed with the people who were dying. I felt entrusted with the stories of these guys, like a repository of their stories. Getting to know who people really are is a tremendous honor.

Pauline Johnson (8 years)

A common thread in my life and work has been grief related to loss, change, and aging. I came to Victoria Hospice looking for an exchange of skills. I wanted a tangible experience to help me to better understand loss and change and I offered my skills and experience in return. I intended to be a volunteer but quickly became an employee.

Caelin Rose (10 years)

Previously, I had worked as a paramedic and after focusing on the physical and medical parts of death I became curious about the spiritual side. When I was working on a degree in counseling psychology, I did a practicum at Hospice. I wanted to sit in the great unknown and get to know more about myself through it.

Allyson Whiteman (11 years)

I started out as a practicum student. I remember I had a curiosity about death, dying, and grief. As a child, my grandparents died, and I was protected from it. As an adult I wanted to learn about grief in a different way. I was fearful and excited knowing that my beliefs about life would be challenged. But I also believe that death and grief give us an opportunity to realize what we're capable of. As a counselor I love to see people heal.

WHO WE ARE: VICTORIA HOSPICE SOCIETY

This book was shaped in large part by our counseling practice at the Victoria Hospice Society in Victoria, on the west coast of Canada. It is a relatively large hospice, palliative care, and bereavement program in a community of approximately

330,000. Founded in 1980, Victoria Hospice has a staff of approximately 100 full-time, part-time, and casual (on-call) professionals (filling 55 full-time positions) and more than 500 volunteers.

The three main authors of this book collectively share more than 45 years of experience as palliative and bereavement counselors with Victoria Hospice. Moira Cairns is a social worker and currently coordinates an extensive bereavement program. Marney Thompson has a background in child and youth care and works with the palliative crisis response team. Wendy Wainwright has a social work and counseling psychology background and is Manager of the counseling and bereavement services.

This book, however, was forged through the collective wisdom and experience of all the social workers and counselors who have worked at Victoria Hospice since 1980. They have challenged, supported, and mentored one another. They have questioned their own practice, developed new programs and materials, and taught workshops, always looking for ways to improve care. Many of them have worked closely with the authors throughout the development, writing, and review of the book.

The counseling department is composed of men and women who represent a diverse spectrum of counseling approaches and life experience. Counseling services include pre-death counseling for patients and families on the inpatient unit and in the community and bereavement counseling with individuals and groups. Furthermore, these counselors provide psychosocial support to the entire hospice team and others in our community who care for seriously ill, dying, and bereaved individuals. Many have become educators and consultants throughout British Columbia and Canada, and several are involved in research about the impact of counseling interventions in hospice and palliative care.

The experience and expertise of this team has grown from our work with the more than 800 patients and 1,800 family members registered with Victoria Hospice each year. Of this population, approximately 81% of patients have cancer, 6% have diseases of the circulatory system (e.g., heart disease), 3% have respiratory system problems (e.g., chronic obstructive pulmonary disease), 2% have problems related to the nervous system (e.g., Alzheimer's disease, amyotrophic lateral sclerosis), and 8% have other diseases (e.g., end-stage renal disease, AIDS, hepatitis). Approximately half of the patients die in the hospice and half die at home, although some die in acute care or long-term care facilities.

Our partnership with counseling, social work, and other professional colleagues, as well as organizations including the British Columbia (BC) Cancer Agency, AIDS Vancouver Island, Amyotrophic Lateral Sclerosis (ALS) Society, and Vancouver Island Health Authority, enhance both our practice and the writing of this book.

THE PRINCIPLES OF HOSPICE, PALLIATIVE, AND END-OF-LIFE CARE

"Everything can be taken from a man but one thing: the last of the human freedoms—to choose one's own way."

—*Viktor Frankl*
(Cotter, 1999, p. 23)

Hospice and palliative care should ensure that dying patients and their families receive the best and most appropriate care possible. Underlying this principle is the quote expressed by psychotherapist and Holocaust survivor Viktor Frankl: "The last of the human freedoms is the freedom to choose one's own way." In the context of hospice palliative care, one's own way would be to die and to mourn in a way that is congruent with how one has lived.

The focus of hospice palliative care is to relieve suffering and improve the quality of living and dying. This kind of care is appropriate for any patient and/or family living with a life-threatening illness

- Due to any diagnosis
- With any prognosis
- Regardless of age

Hospice and palliative care aims to address

- Physical, emotional, psychological, social, spiritual, and practical concerns
- Preparation for, and management of, self-determined life closure and the dying process
- Loss, grief, and bereavement

Hospice palliative care may complement and enhance acute treatment, or it may become the total focus of care (Canadian Hospice Palliative Care Association [CHPCA], 2002).

CORE VALUES OF HOSPICE PALLIATIVE CARE

This book is written under the assumption that hospice and palliative care are most effectively delivered by an interdisciplinary team that "typically includes one or more physicians, nurses, social workers/psychologists, spiritual advisers, pharmacists, personal support workers and volunteers and may also include physiotherapists, dieticians, occupational, recreational, and integrative therapists, and others " (CHPCA, 2002). As part of the interdisciplinary team, counselors and other psychosocial care providers focus on the aspects of illness, death, and bereavement that lie beyond the physical. They recognize the social context that people bring to this journey—a lifetime of experiences, with particular hopes and fears and their own ways of coping with stress or problems (Price, 2001; Sheldon, 2001).

Psychosocial care encompasses a view that acknowledges the wholeness and integrity of each person and family. Working within a medical environment, which may or may not support holistic care, it is important that psychosocial professionals have ways to formalize their particular perspective and approach to care. The counseling team at Victoria Hospice finds their values effectively reflected in the 12 foundation values set out by CHPCA:

1.   Each person has intrinsic worth as an autonomous and unique individual.

2.   Both life and the natural process of death have value; both provide opportunities for personal and spiritual growth.

3.   Patients and families must have their suffering, expectations, and concerns addressed.

4.   Care is guided by quality of life as defined by the individual.

5.   Caregivers enter into a therapeutic relationship with patients and families that respects dignity and integrity.

6.   The patient decides with whom information is shared.

7.   The patient participates in informed decision-making.

8.   Care is patient-centered and family-focused.

9.   All aspects of care are provided in a manner that is sensitive to the patient's and family's personal, cultural, and religious values, beliefs, and practices; developmental state; and preparedness to deal with the dying process.

10. Care is provided only when the patient is prepared to accept it.

11. A unified response to suffering strengthens communities.

12. Access to hospice palliative care is assured to everyone without discrimination.

USING THIS BOOK

This book is structured to mirror the transitions that occur as patients and families follow the journey from diagnosis to death and through bereavement. It identifies significant transitions, defines the psychosocial issues that each patient and family may face, and suggests interventions that can be used by those who work with these individuals. When health care providers, patients, and families have prior knowledge of what to expect, everyone can better anticipate the journey and thereby allay their sense of anxiety, fear, and powerlessness. To achieve this goal,

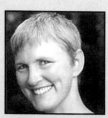

Katherine Murray, R.N., B.Sc.N., is a nurse on the Victoria Hospice Palliative Response Team, a home care nurse, and an educator of nurses and home support workers in the care of dying individuals.

In My Own Voice
The Journey

Katherine Murray

The adventures of life provide us with great lessons as we care for people who are dying. Several years ago, my family prepared to head on a journey. It was time to pack our bags, rent our home, and head out. Because we are seven (five children, Ted, and myself), the planning seemed especially large, and the journey seemed more awesome than if I were traveling alone.

We determined to head south into Mexico and Central America. We bought a tape to learn Spanish and eventually mastered a grand total of four words! We began to ask questions and search the literature. We heard many scary things—we heard of robberies, murders, and kidnapping. One person confided that he was not sure we would all come home alive. That was very unnerving. It took courage to do the final packing.

Eventually, one drizzly, west coast day, leaving our comfort zone behind, we headed south into uncharted territories. We lived in four different communities in Mexico and traveled through Guatemala. We lived amongst the people. We broke tortillas with them, heard their stories, and saw their struggles. We learned to speak their language and appreciated the warmth and kindness that we were shown. We grew closer as a family and stronger in ourselves. Our dreams and goals were reached, and the journey was all that we needed and wanted it to be.

As I prepared to teach a palliative care workshop, I contemplated the parallels between the journey that we went on and the journey of dying. We needed to talk to people who had some ideas, some facts, about the territory we would be passing through; people who were not encumbered by fears based on imaginary dangers and unsubstantiated stories. Dying people also need to be able to talk with someone who is acquainted with their territory. They need to be cared for by people who have experience and knowledge about the myths and realities of dying. They don't need the sensationalism of dying, the Hollywood version, the news hour massacres, the stories of painful, traumatic deaths that suggest that euthanasia is the only comfortable option. They need someone who has addressed their own fears, understands the challenges, and knows the resources available for the journey toward death.

We sought information and heard much advice on where to go, where to stay, and what to see. In our journey, we focused on what was important to us. We met wonderful travelers whose focus was very different. And so it should be. Each journey needs to be unique to provide for the diversity of individual goals.

When dying people are journeying, they too may want to collect information. Some people want minute details. Others want only basic information. Some may read voraciously or talk voraciously, or both. They do not want someone to tell them what, when, and how to do their dying! As members of the health care team, we should listen, help a person identify what information is wanted, and then offer information and options.

In order not to interfere with a dying person's journey, it is essential that we realize our own biases, preferences, and agendas as a way of separating our journey from theirs. It is imperative that we do not attempt to send an individual on our personal journey, but rather, assist them on theirs.

While in Mexico and Guatemala, we had two rough experiences and needed a safe place to regroup and to build up the strength and courage to move on again. We appreciated the good will of people who responded with generosity and kindness when they saw us hurt and distressed and who offered us a refuge from the storm.

In the old days, hospice was a place of refuge—a place where the weary traveler could stop and obtain food and shelter, where the sick could go to recover or to die. What we want to create is this kind of safe, secure place—where a dying person can find the courage to open doors that are difficult to open, where he or she is safe to walk the walk to death, where there is someone who is not afraid to listen and will not need to silence the fears if and when they are expressed, where quiet companioning can nurture when words are no longer needed or when English is no longer the language spoken.

Our journey south was rich in and of itself. The lessons from that adventure continue to teach me in my work as a hospice nurse and educator.

the information within this book is organized around two frameworks or models. These provide the context for understanding the psychosocial issues and needs that patients and families encounter as they move from a diagnosis of life-threatening illness, through death, and into bereavement.

The first framework is tied to a functional tool, used predominantly by medicine and nursing, known as the Palliative Performance Scale version 2 (PPSv2) (Victoria Hospice Society, 2003). The PPSv2 is used throughout the book as a guide to key psychosocial issues that frequently occur at particular transitions in a patient's disease process. Linking psychosocial issues to major PPS transitions provides a simple and effective way for people to orient themselves quickly to a patient's and family's concerns, improve communication among health care providers, and identify relevant psychosocial interventions.

Following a death, the journey taken by bereaved loved ones is also tied to a model of grief based on phases, which similarly improves communication and care.

This book may be used as a reference or clinical handbook. It is divided into ten chapters that encompass patients' and families' journeys through 1) diagnosis, treatment, and recurrence; 2) palliative care; and 3) bereavement. Information about children is in Chapters 2, 4, and 8. This is not intended to compartmentalize children's concerns, but to keep the information accessible. Each chapter contains the following sections:

- **Case Study:** provides a snapshot of one patient and his or her family at the transition that the chapter discusses. Sections of the case study are used to give added focus to key considerations within the chapter.

- **Key Considerations:** identifies significant psychosocial issues within each of the transitions. Although some issues are apparent at more than one transition, they will be attached or found at the PPS level in which they are most critical.

- **Assessment Questions and Interventions:** provides templates that can be adapted to fit each patient/family context. Basic components include 1) listen and reflect back what is heard, 2) communicate understanding, 3) normalize through context, and 4) identify strengths.

- **Our Experience:** presents the perspective of counselors and others who provide psychosocial care to patients, families, and other team members at this transition.

- **Team Issues:** presents some of the major challenges or difficulties that commonly confront health care providers in their work with patients, families, and each other.

- **Summary:** places the transition in each chapter into the perspective of the Palliative Performance Scale or Phases Model of Grief.

- **Reflective Activity:** offers activities and exercises that may be used for teaching or team building to stimulate thought and introspection and help the readers integrate the information into their knowledge and practice.

- **Resources:** provides suggested articles, books, web sites, and other resources that the reader can consult for further information.

- **References:** lists specific references for quotes or other references used within the chapter.

In addition, a number of special features appear throughout the book, including:

- **Perspective:** tackles overarching topics that have broad application across all or most of the transitions and are strategically placed between chapters.

- **In My Own Voice:** inserts the views or insights of individuals other than the main authors.

- **Focus On:** covers issues and areas that are controversial, elicit a wide range of views, or are difficult to deal with.

- **Sidebars:** contains peripheral but important insights that add depth to material discussed in the main text.

This book is intended to convey a deep commitment to and belief in the value and efficacy of psychosocial care for dying and bereaved people. The personal stories, expertise, and insights presented may inform or inspire others to develop high standards of psychosocial care. We hope that by identifying the particular issues that patients and families may face at certain transitions, a framework for what is predictable and typical will emerge. From this framework, a common language can develop that supports examination and understanding of the psychosocial aspects of patient and family care among those providing palliative and bereavement care.

REFLECTIVE ACTIVITY

The purpose of this activity is to increase awareness and insight into the highly personal, often surprising ways that people become involved in hospice palliative care. This activity may help to build rapport and increase understanding within groups of health care providers, volunteers, and others.

"The nature of dying is not medical; it is experiential. Dying is fundamentally a personal experience, not a set of medical problems to be solved."

—Ira Byock (1997)

At a staff meeting, retreat, or training session, form small groups or pairs and ask each other these questions:

- "What brought you to this work/organization?"
- "What impact does this work have on your life?"
- "How would your friends or family say this work has changed you?"

REFERENCES

Anderson, F., Casorso, L., Downing, G.M., Hill, J., & Lerch, N. (1996). Palliative Performance Scale: A new tool. *Journal of Palliative Care, 12*(1), 5–11.

Bates, T., Connor, C., Connor, S., Corr, D., Gjertsen, E., Head, D., et al. (1993). A statement of assumptions and principles concerning psychological care of dying persons and their families. *Journal of Palliative Care, 9*(3), 29–32.

Byock, I. (1997). *Dying well: The prospect of growth at the end of life.* New York: Riverhead Books.

The Canadian Hospice Palliative Care Association (CHPCA). (2002). *A model to guide hospice palliative care: Based on national principles and norms of practice.* Available at http://www.chpca.net.

Cotter, A. (1999). *From this moment on: A guide for those recently diagnosed with cancer.* New York: Random House.

Price, S. (2001). Has something changed? Social work, pastoral care, spiritual counseling and palliative care. *Progress in Palliative Care, 9*(6), 244–246.

Sheldon, F.M. (2001). Social work in palliative care: Counseling and communicating. *Progress in Palliative Care, 9*(6), 242–243.

Victoria Hospice Society. (2003). *Palliative Performance Scale Version 2 (PPSv2).* Available at http://www.victoriahospice.org/pdfs/PPSv2.pdf.

SUPPORT FOR THE HOSPICE PALLIATIVE CARE TEAM

"Our work and our privilege is to assist and accompany others into the discovery of their own intrinsic wholeness existing behind illness, even when death is close at hand or when one faces living with a chronic illness. [Such an] odyssey offers us the possibility of recovering and cultivating our open, tender hearts. Without such labor we may remain hard and armored, 'fragmented,' 'distressed and sick of heart.' And it will show. It always shows. Perhaps because we are servants of the healing arts, this is our vocation and our blessing. Our degree of willingness to walk this way with another is a measure of our own brokenness and our own wholeness. They are inseparable. It is impossible to make contact with the life gushing up and out of these cracks if we are not opened."—Santorelli, 1999, pp. 97–98

Often, the very things that make hospice palliative care so rewarding make it difficult. Palliative care can be a source of great personal satisfaction and growth, yet it challenges professionals to face their own vulnerability and the fragility of life. For the most part, people bring to this work excellent professional or clinical skills, maturity, life experience, and the desire to make a difference. These are not enough to guarantee a sense of fulfillment or excellence in their work, however. Health care providers are at risk for high stress, illness, and burnout that leaves them with a "hardness of the heart or sadness of the soul" (Bowman, 1999, p. 7). They are asked again and again to form intimate relationships one day and to relinquish them the next. They accompany patients as they face death, are present during patients' pain and suffering, and witness grief and sorrow following the death of a loved one. This constant exposure to death and grief results in a loss of innocence that separates palliative care providers from their family and friends, who may only experience such events a few times in their lives. Discomfort and fear, accompanied by a lack of understanding, means others are often unable or unwilling to listen to such difficult experiences.

Because health care providers, just like all people, have different personal styles, roles, training, or support networks, the impact of caring for individuals who are dying and bereaved will vary among members of the team. In addition, the impact within each person will shift and change over time, depending on life stages, accompanying stresses, and general resilience. It is not static or predictable.

COMMON STRESSORS IN HOSPICE PALLIATIVE CARE

Health care providers are prone to both internal and external stress in the hospice and palliative care field.

Internal Stressors

Internal stress occurs when health care providers experience discrepancies between their visions of what such care will entail and the reality of the experience. These discrepancies can occur within different aspects of the individual or the care experience. The following are some areas in which disparities between the ideal and the real often occur.

Beliefs and Attitudes

Care providers may experience stress when they

- Have incongruent expectations about themselves and the care they are able to provide
- Struggle with personal boundaries and define success by what they can do for others
- See death as catastrophic, rather than as a normal part of life
- Find their job doesn't match their initial motivations in seeking employment

Skills and Knowledge

Care providers may also experience stress when they

- Feel that their training, skills, or support are inadequate to help them deal with difficult situations

Personality and Coping Style

Individuals may not be comfortable working in hospice and palliative care if they

- Are shy or timid or have low self-esteem in the face of a need for intense involvement
- Feel emotionally overwhelmed by multiple needs or demands
- Struggle with repeatedly forming and losing relationships
- Employ insufficient self-care strategies

Personal Life Situation

Individuals' personal life situations may be incongruent with hospice and palliative care if

- Personal life responsibilities compete with professional demands and become overwhelming
- Grief and loss in their personal life adversely affect life at work

External Stressors

External stress occurs when health care providers involved with death, dying, and bereavement struggle with or find conflict within the nature of the work or context in which it is provided. Just as with internal stressors, people working in this field may experience external stressors in several areas.

Patients' and Families' Responses
Individuals may experience stress if they have difficulty working with people who are

- Dying, grieving, suffering, and fearful
- Angry, afraid, demanding, and uncooperative
- Stressed and not coping/communicating very well
- Facing multiple challenges and issues

Training and Experience
Individuals may experience stress if they are inadequately prepared to

- Work intimately with emotional/spiritual issues
- Support those from other languages/cultures
- Deal with the cumulative impact of death and grief
- Provide relief for pain and other symptoms

Team Issues
Because hospice and palliative care is a team effort, individuals within the team may experience stress if they work within a team whose members

- Display a lack of trust, support, or respect
- Are unclear about roles (uniqueness and/or overlap)
- Have unrealistic expectations of one another
- Have conflicting beliefs/values about teamwork
- Work in isolation or with minimal communication

Work Environment

External stressors are often evident in an organizational environment that has

- Inadequate resources to meet the need
- Unrealistic expectations (workload, schedules)
- Conflicting beliefs about care, decision making
- Poor communication
- Perceived lack of appreciation

(Bowman, 1999; Riordan & Saltzer, 1992; Santorelli, 1999; Vachon, 1995, 1998)

COMMITMENT TO SUPPORT

Regardless of how health care providers cope with the stresses inherent in this work, they all need some kind of support. Although support is a responsibility shared among the individual health care providers, the team, and the organization, it is the organization's commitment to ongoing support that can really make the difference. It is critical that organizations take a broad view of what is supportive and recognize that no single approach will address everyone's needs.

Support is most effective when it includes various approaches and activities such as social events, supervision and feedback, educational workshops, and team involvement in problem solving and decision making. Support needs to address the broad range of internal and external stressors experienced by the team. It can be formal or informal, planned or spontaneous, or within disciplines or interdisciplinary in nature. Support should include nurturing for the head, the hands, and the heart. A skilled, cohesive, and supported team will provide better care, deal more effectively with change and stress, and cope better with the grief and sorrow that accumulate over time. In addition, individual members will stay healthier.

Although each person may be concerned about support, it is most often the psychosocial professionals (e.g., social workers, counselors, psychologists, chaplains) on the team who take an active role in ensuring it happens. Their training, experience, and inclination prepare them to identify and acknowledge emotion, address issues, and facilitate the team process. They view people not in isolation but within their environment or community, which helps them see the big picture or the context of a situation. Although this may be a suitable role for the psychosocial care providers, they need to be cautious about providing support for others at the expense of their own support needs. They, too, need support. When the care team is less structured or not available, support for the individual health care provider becomes even more significant. In these situations, self-care strategies are important in order for people to maintain or nurture themselves as they provide end-of-life care. They will need to be proactive in finding ways to remain balanced and healthy.

Guiding Principles in Developing a Support Program

1. Professionals, volunteers, and others who work with dying patients and their families, before death and during bereavement, require support to ensure that both their health and a high quality of care are maintained.
2. Primary responsibility for self-care lies with individual team members, with support from the organization.
3. Support programs must address the needs of the team, while being sensitive to the needs of each individual.
4. Support programs must be valued, encouraged, formalized, and funded by the organization.
5. Support must be embedded in an organizational culture that acknowledges the impact of working with death and bereavement and that encourages open communication, shared decision making, and risk taking.

6. An organization's commitment to support of health care providers should be equivalent to its commitment to patients and families.

7. Support programs must be comprehensive, addressing various sources of stress and offering a continuum of strategies moving from prevention through crisis intervention, treatment, and rehabilitation. (Bell, 1997; Riordan & Saltzer, 1992)

Aspects of Effective Support Programs

- Ongoing training, mentoring, skill development, and consultation (e.g., care of dying and bereaved people, team building, self-care strategies)
- Communication mechanisms (e.g., memos, information forums, newsletters, message boards)
- Celebrations, appreciations, transition rituals (e.g., to acknowledge accomplishments or retirements, to say "thank you")
- Opportunities for renewal (e.g., vacation and sick time, sabbaticals, retreats, on-site massage/reflexology)
- Team building skill development (e.g., renewing vision and values, conflict resolution, planning, personal connections)
- Opportunities for humor and fun
- Counseling and support groups for team members (e.g., addressing personal issues, career planning, loss and grief, trauma, job loss, personal bereavement needs)
- Opportunities for closure (e.g., gatherings to memorialize and honor patients, debrief difficult situations, acknowledge team losses)
- Activities that attend to the whole person and are physical, emotional, intellectual, spiritual, and/or social in nature

"I have noticed within myself that helplessness sometimes comes clothed in a guise of helping that easily carries me into doing,

planning, frantically scurrying about, imposing concepts on self and others. Born of fear and self-dissatisfaction, it is a trap and a subtle form of manipulation. Have you ever noticed this within yourself?" — Santorelli, 1999, p. 143

RESOURCES

Books

Firth-Cozens, J., & Payne, R. (Eds.). (1999). *Stress in health professionals.* New York: John Wiley and Sons.

Kabat-Zinn, J. (1994). *Wherever you go, there you are.* New York: Hyperion Press.

Kearney, M. (1996). *Mortally wounded.* New York: Scribner.

Moore, T. (1992). *Care of the soul.* New York: HarperCollins.

Muller, W. (1999). *How then shall we live?* Toronto: Bantam Books.

Remen, R. (1996). *Kitchen table wisdom.* New York: Riverhead Books.

Vachon, M. (2000). Burnout and symptoms of stress in staff working in palliative care. In H. Chochinov (Ed.), *Handbook of psychiatry in palliative medicine.* New York: Oxford University Press.

Articles

Maddix, T., & Pereira, J. (2001). Reflecting on the work of palliative care. *Journal of Palliative Medicine, 4*(3), 373–377.

Marquis, S. (1993). Death of the nursed: Burnout of the provider. *OMEGA, 27*(1), 17–33.

Murrant, G., Rykov, M., Amonite, D., & Loynd, M. (2000). Creativity and self-care for caregivers. *Journal of Palliative Care, 16*(2), 44–49.

REFERENCES

Bell, D. (1997). *Report of the Victoria Hospice staff and volunteer support project* (unpublished).

Bowman, T. (1999). Promoting resiliency in those who do bereavement work. *Lifeline, 27* (spring), 7–9.

Riordan, R., & Saltzer, S. (1992). Burnout prevention among health care providers working with the terminally ill: A literature review. *OMEGA, 25*(1), 17–24.

Santorelli, S. (1999). *Heal thy self: Lessons on mindfulness in medicine.* New York: Bell Tower Publishing.

Vachon, M. (1995). Staff stress in hospice/palliative care: A review. *Palliative Medicine, 9,* 91–122.

Vachon, M. (1998). The stress of professional caregivers. In D. Doyle, G. Hanks, & N. Macdonald (Eds.), *Oxford textbook of palliative medicine* (pp. 919–929). Oxford, England: Oxford University Press.

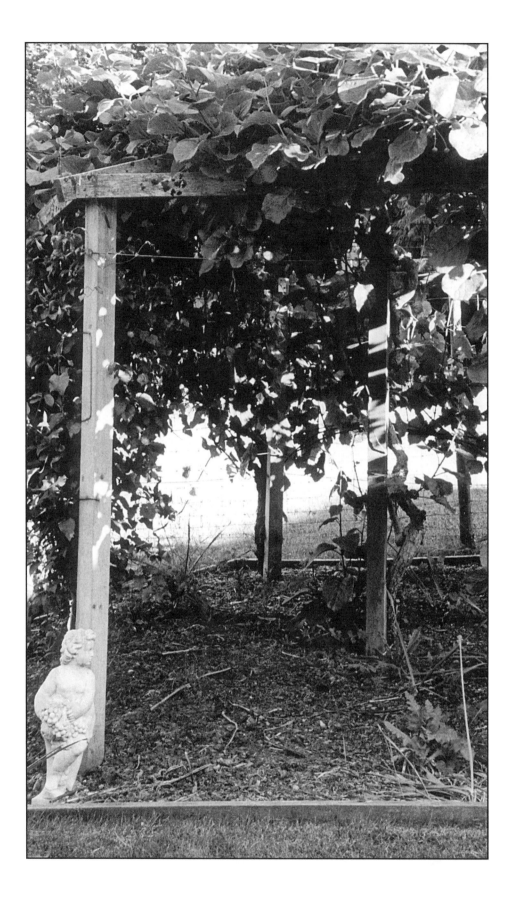

Establishing the Framework

INTEGRATION OF PSYCHOSOCIAL AND PALLIATIVE CARE

When health care providers are able to identify the psychosocial issues that may arise during various transitions, they have a normative context that can be used to appropriately assess needs and plan interventions. When patients and families understand what is happening, unexpected events often feel less frightening and random. When patients know what to expect, they can prepare somewhat for the changes ahead. Doyle-Brown suggested that forecasting and translating disease symptoms "allows the family to take a proactive stance—as problem solvers, not simply helpless reactors" (2000, p. 357). Forecasting and translating the phases of grief helps family members and others to be proactive in moving through the transitions of bereavement.

If it were widely understood in the health care field that certain transitions in the disease trajectory and particular phases of grief trigger psychosocial issues, then teamwork within the diverse group of professionals providing end-of-life care might be enhanced. Health care providers would be better able to anticipate concerns and articulate them with more clarity and confidence. Typically within hospice and palliative care, each discipline has a degree of understanding and comfort with other realms of expertise. Physicians and nurses explore existential questions and family dynamics, for example, whereas social workers and hospice chaplains become familiar with disease trajectories and basic principles of pain and symptom management. Yet, understandably, each discipline remains quite distinct in its approach, methods, responsibilities, and language. Linking disease progression and the resulting physical changes to psychosocial concerns in an understandable way should significantly improve overall patient and family care through enhanced communication and interdisciplinary relationships.

FRAMEWORK FOR PSYCHOSOCIAL CARE

The pace of the journey from diagnosis through death and bereavement varies greatly; every experience is unique. At the same time, it is important to have a general framework or map of the journey, which lays out some predictable transitions that occur as people face advancing disease. A framework that links these transitions to psychosocial issues can

- Support a model of holistic care that integrates both patients' and families' physical and psychosocial needs
- Improve communication among colleagues, volunteers, patients, and families about the psychosocial issues that arise as people move from diagnosis through death and bereavement
- Help patients and families prepare for the psychosocial impacts of the physical and cognitive declines associated with dying
- Improve accountability and influence resource allocation within health care
- Provide a framework for teaching psychosocial care to health care providers, hospice volunteers, and interested others

TEAM ROLES IN PSYCHOSOCIAL CARE

It is easy to make assumptions about the role of various disciplines within a hospice or health care team. It can be useful to understand how others see their responsibilities and contributions. As seen in Table 1.1, members of the Victoria Hospice team explain about their general role within the team and how they believe they contribute to the psychosocial care of patients and their families.

TRANSITIONS AND PSYCHOSOCIAL CARE

Most counselors in hospice and palliative care understand through intuition, experience, and observation that the grief process is ongoing. Parallels exist between

Table 1.1. Team roles in psychosocial care

Team member	Role on the team	Contribution to psychosocial care
Marjorie Woodroffe, Registered Nurse	The team is integral to palliative care. We all add our pieces to the total picture of the patient and family's diverse needs. The nurse is the negotiator, advocate, and liaison between the patient and family and the other team members.	Being with patients and families day and night means being there for emotional or spiritual support at that moment when there is a need to talk or to ask questions.
Rachelle Campbell, Licensed Practical Nurse	My role on the team is pretty important as we are there first in the day getting care going, with the help of the volunteers.	I talk to patients about how they're feeling or how things are going with them—friendly, everyday sort of things. It's like visiting—talking about everything and anything they want to talk about. I'm approachable; I guess that would be a good word.
Jill Sartorio, Registered Nurse	Patient advocacy is my role. The nurse is the bridge between the patient and the rest of the team.	I'm there as a listening post, a sympathetic ear, or a hand to hold; I offer what people need, when they need it. I help families understand the process and what the physical changes mean. I support them through the process of their family member dying.
Ruby Chapman, Occupational Therapist	I help patients to be mobile and comfortable. Occupational therapy (OT) is based on the mind, body, and spirit. Spirit is at the core of enabling.	It is important for the OT to respect and accommodate "where the patient is." Through building rapport and creating safety, people can talk about their concerns and feelings. Offering ongoing mobility offers hope that the patient's level of wellness may continue for a while.
Ruth Simkin, Medical Doctor	I am responsible for symptom management from the medical perspective. On behalf of the patient, I integrate what team members say with what I see, into one treatment plan.	It is my role to be honest, offer advice and encouragement, and help people face the reality of what's going on.
Dave Cheperdak, Executive Director	My role is twofold: one is "servant leader," in ensuring paid and unpaid staff members have the support and resources to do what they do best. The second is envisioning where we are going and why.	My personal objective is, at all times, to know at least one patient, so there is always a personal connection between administration and the people cared for. My social interactions with families add to the ambiance of support, comfort, and community.
Eileen Rutherford, Volunteer	I do emotional support volunteer work. I liaise with the counselor on the inpatient unit about who to see and how best to approach patients and families. I see people if they are new and have questions or if they are upset and need a little TLC.	I try to make a good connection to help them discuss worries or talk through feelings. My role is a catalyst—but it's a very individual thing. I have to be aware of their response to me and be guided by them in what I do.

the transitions that grieving people encounter before and after a death. Changes in the dying person trigger painful emotional, social, spiritual, and cognitive consequences. Similarly, the different phases of grief following a death stimulate responses and changes in these same areas. As diseases and grief progress, patients and/or families may experience some fairly predictable reactions and challenges.

When people feel unprepared for these reactions, their expectations of themselves and others may be unrealistic. For example, when patients do not understand what is happening in their bodies, they may unwittingly place themselves or their caregivers at risk. When bereaved people experience intense responses to loss, they may feel frightened or overwhelmed. Having a way to compare changes, reactions, and responses with expected transitions can help by normalizing the challenging journey patients and families take through diagnosis, illness, death, and bereavement.

TRANSITIONS FROM DIAGNOSIS TO DEATH: THE PALLIATIVE PERFORMANCE SCALE (PPSV2)

In 1995, a group of medical colleagues from Victoria Hospice Society developed the Palliative Performance Scale (PPS) (Anderson, Downing, & Hill, 1996), a modification of the Karnofsky Performance Scale (Karnofsky, Abelmann, & Craver, 1948). The PPS has been slightly revised to clarify usage in a second unpublished version (PPSv2). The PPS is an assessment tool used to monitor palliative patients' general functioning, mobility, and cognitive changes as disease progresses. The PPS number, expressed as a percentage (e.g., PPS 50%), is referred to as the patient's PPS score. This terminology is used frequently by nurses, physicians, and others in sharing information about a patient's functional status. It has also been shown to have benefits in prognostication and may be useful in resource allocation related to patients' physical needs. Although the scale has fairly well-defined categories, individual variations in disease progression will always require cautious interpretation. For a detailed explanation of how the PPS score is determined and the meaning of the categories, please refer to the instructions that follow the scale (Table 1.2, pp. 28–29).

Although many hospice and palliative care counselors recognize the clinical and educational value of normative scales and measurement tools for other disciplines, they sometimes struggle to see its practical uses in psychosocial care. It became apparent to our team, in using the PPS over several years, that a relationship exists between the physical and psychosocial realms encountered in practice. Because the PPSv2 and other similar tools are widely used in hospice and palliative care, it seemed timely to examine and develop a more formal connection between the scale and psychosocial transitions. In our practice, the PPSv2 serves as a guide or template that helps counselors and others understand the psychosocial journey taken by patients and families when faced with illness, death, and bereavement. The PPSv2 is shown in its entirety in Table 1.2. It is then divided into sections later in this chapter to illustrate each of the stages of functioning.

> "In offering a patient and his family a tiny roadmap of the last part of their lives together, and assuring safety along the way, the health care worker may allow them a peace and final serenity which has no price."
>
> —(Doyle-Brown 2000, p. 357)

TRANSITIONS VIA THE PALLIATIVE PERFORMANCE SCALE

The following sections outline a framework that provides a link between the patient's transitions in functional status (via PPSv2) and the issues and concerns experienced by patients and families.

Beginning the Journey: Early Diagnosis and Treatment

As shown in Table 1.3, during early diagnosis and treatment, an individual's functioning is still high.

Physical Indications

The diagnosis of a life-threatening illness may occur through a routine physical examination or as the result of an investigation to discover what is causing particular symptoms. It is very common for patients to feel deceived by their apparent good health if they feel well and have no observable signs of disease.

Psychosocial Impact

Regardless of how well or ill they feel, patients and families will struggle to comprehend the seriousness of the disease. Although they may be overwhelmed and unclear about what to feel, think, or do, patients still need to make critical decisions about treatment. Their lives often center on the disease and the effects of treatment during this transition.

The Path Not Chosen: Recurrence and Chronic Illness

As shown in Table 1.4, an individual's ability to maintain self-care remains even as ambulation is somewhat reduced.

Table 1.2.   Palliative Performance Scale (PPSv2)

PPS Level	Ambulation	Activity and evidence of disease	Self-care	Intake	Conscious level
100%	Full	Normal activity and work No evidence of disease	Full	Normal	Full
90%	Full	Normal activity and work Some evidence of disease	Full	Normal	Full
80%	Full	Normal activity *with* effort Some evidence of disease	Full	Normal or reduced	Full
70%	Reduced	Unable to do normal job/work Significant disease	Full	Normal or reduced	Full
60%	Reduced	Unable to do hobby/housework Significant disease	Occasional assistance necessary	Normal or reduced	Full or confusion
50%	Mainly sit/lie	Unable to do any work Extensive disease	Considerable assistance required	Normal or reduced	Full or confusion
40%	Mainly in bed	Unable to do most activity Extensive disease	Mainly needs assistance	Normal or reduced	Full or drowsy +/- confusion
30%	Totally bed bound	Unable to do any activity Extensive disease	Total care	Normal or reduced	Full or drowsy +/- confusion
20%	Totally bed bound	Unable to do any activity Extensive disease	Total care	Minimal to sips	Full or drowsy +/- confusion
10%	Totally bed bound	Unable to do any activity Extensive disease	Total care	Mouth care only	Drowsy or coma +/- confusion
0%	Death	–	–	–	–

Note: See explanation and definitions of each column on page 29.

Palliative Performance Scale (PPSv2)—Usage and Definitions

PPS scores are determined by reading each row horizontally to find a "best fit" for the patient. Begin at the second column from the left and read downward until the current ambulation level is reached, then read across to the next column and downward again until the activity/evidence of disease is located. These steps are repeated until all five columns are covered before assigning the actual PPS for that patient. In this way, leftward columns (columns to the left of any specific column) are stronger determinants of the final PPS score and generally take precedence over others. For example, a patient who has quadriplegia and requires total care would be PPS 30%. Although this patient may be using a wheelchair (and perhaps seems initially to be at 50%), the score is 30% because without caregivers lifting and transferring the individual, he or she would be otherwise totally bed bound.

Ambulation

The items *mainly sit/lie, mainly in bed*, and *totally bed bound* are clearly similar. The difference between sit/lie and bed is proportionate to the amount of time the patient is able to sit up versus the amount of time the patient needs to lie down. *Reduced ambulation* is located at the PPS 70% and PPS 60% level. Reduction of ambulation is tied to inability to carry out one's normal job, work occupation, or some hobbies or housework activities.

Activity and Evidence of Disease

Some, significant, and *extensive disease* refer to physical and investigative evidence that shows degrees of progression. The extent may also refer to progression of disease despite active treatments. The extent of disease is also judged in context with the ability to maintain one's work and hobbies or activities.

Self-Care

Occasional assistance means that most of the time the patient is able to transfer out of bed, walk, wash, toilet, and eat by his or her own means. *Considerable assistance* means that every day the patient needs help, usually from one person, to do some of the activities noted above. *Mainly assistance* is a further extension of considerable. This may fluctuate according to fatigue during the day. Total care means that the patient is completely unable to eat, toilet, or do any self-care without help.

Intake

Normal intake refers to the person's usual eating habits while healthy. Changes in intake are quite obvious. *Reduced* means any reduction from normal and is highly variable according to the individual's unique circumstances. *Minimal to sips* refers to very small amounts of food (usually pureed) or liquid intake, which are well below nutritional sustenance.

Conscious Level

Full consciousness implies full alertness and orientation with good cognitive abilities in various domains of thinking, memory, and so forth. *Confusion* denotes presence of either delirium or dementia and is a reduced level of consciousness. *Drowsiness* implies fatigue, drug side effects, delirium, or closeness to death and is sometimes included in the term *stupor*. *Coma* is the absence of response to verbal or physical stimuli; some reflexes may or may not remain.

Table 1.3. Palliative Performance Scale (PPSv2) 100%–90%

PPS Level	Ambulation	Activity and evidence of disease	Self-care	Intake	Conscious level
100%	Full	Normal activity and work No evidence of disease	Full	Normal	Full
90%	Full	Normal activity and work Some evidence of disease	Full	Normal	Full

Physical Indications

Progression of the disease, either from significant recurrence or lack of response to initial treatment, results in one or more symptoms such as nausea, pain, or weakness. This progression may occur with wide swings of remission and relapse, as in cancer or multiple sclerosis, or be more gradual and insidious, as in diseases such as emphysema or chronic heart failure. Some weight loss and fatigue are also common.

At the beginning of this transition, normal activities require extra effort. Over time, people in this stage need to curtail or reduce strenuous activities such as heavy chores around the house and yard. Eventually, they become unable to continue their regular job or employment, housework becomes more difficult, and hobbies and exercise need to be adapted.

Psychosocial Impact

As patients find they are less able to participate in work and/or physical activities, they struggle to adjust their lives and redefine themselves. The aftermath of recurrence leaves them feeling vulnerable and betrayed. Patients and families must choose how to face the disease (e.g., hopeful, resigned, fighting).

Table 1.4. Palliative Performance Scale (PPSv2) 80%–70%

PPS Level	Ambulation	Activity and evidence of disease	Self-care	Intake	Conscious level
80%	Full	Normal activity *with* effort Some evidence of disease	Full	Normal or reduced	Full
70%	Reduced	Unable to do normal job/work Significant disease	Full	Normal or reduced	Full

Table 1.5. Palliative Performance Scale (PPSv2) 60%–50%

PPS Level	Ambulation	Activity and evidence of disease	Self-care	Intake	Conscious level
60%	Reduced	Unable to do hobby/housework Significant disease	Occasional assistance necessary	Normal or reduced	Full or confusion
50%	Mainly sit/lie	Unable to do any work Extensive disease	Considerable assistance required	Normal or reduced	Full or confusion

Entering the Unknown:
The Shift Toward Hospice and Palliative Care

Table 1.5 shows that as the disease progresses, the individual's ambulation and activity level is greatly reduced, whereas food and fluid intake may remain largely unchanged.

Physical Indications

Through this period, the disease has become extensive. For patients with cancer, this often means widespread metastases; for those with chronic diseases associated with the heart or lung, there is a very limited response to active treatments and more frequent hospital admissions. As a result of the associated fatigue and progressing weakness, neither work nor hobbies are now possible. In fact, most patients require assistance with some activities of daily living. People may experience a decreased interest in food. By the end of this period, they will spend most of the time sitting or lying down. Unless a medical complication occurs, cognitive functions remain intact.

Psychosocial Impact

As people's daily lives are increasingly affected by the illness, patients and families must adjust their roles and responsibilities to accommodate these changes. As they contemplate the future, people struggle with the frequent fluctuations between hope and despair, and look for concrete information and reassurance about what is ahead.

The Long and Winding Road:
Illness Predominates

Table 1.6 shows the increasing fatigue and difficulty maintaining personal care that individuals experience during this transition.

Table 1.6.   Palliative Performance Scale (PPSv2) 40%–30%

PPS Level	Ambulation	Activity and evidence of disease	Self-care	Intake	Conscious level
40%	Mainly in bed	Unable to do most activity Extensive disease	Mainly needs assistance	Normal or reduced	Full or drowsy +/- confusion
30%	Totally bed bound	Unable to do any activity Extensive disease	Total care	Normal or reduced	Full or drowsy +/- confusion

Physical Indications

At the beginning of this transition, patients are weak and fatigued and spend most of their time in bed. They require help, on a regular basis, with much of their personal care. By PPS 30%, they are totally bed bound, requiring complete assistance to bathe, dress, shave, and eat or drink. With the disease now very advanced, overall weakness and fatigue are often unrelenting, and people require sleep for significant periods of the day as well as night. Drowsiness may be a combination of this fatigue and the adverse effects of medications. Intake of food and fluids varies but is usually limited.

Psychosocial Impact

As progression of the disease triggers unexpected or unwanted changes, patients and families face many difficult issues. They often wonder about the future, both in the short and long term. Patients may feel ambivalent about living and dying and may be concerned about their limited strength and energy and their increased dependence on family for care. Families also feel ambivalent about the future and find that giving care leaves them increasingly stressed and exhausted.

Watching and Waiting: As Death Approaches

As individuals approach death, their food and fluid intake is minimal and they require total care for all personal needs, as shown in Table 1.7.

Physical Indications

Along with physical changes in breathing, skin tone, and body temperature, patients' minds and cognitive abilities are noticeably affected as death approaches.

Table 1.7. Palliative Performance Scale (PPSv2) 20%–10%

PPS Level	Ambulation	Activity and evidence of disease	Self-care	Intake	Conscious level
20%	Totally bed bound	Unable to do any activity Extensive disease	Total care	Minimal to sips	Full or drowsy +/- confusion
10%	Totally bed bound	Unable to do any activity Extensive disease	Total care	Mouth care only	Drowsy or coma +/- confusion

Patients will become unresponsive at some point, sleeping continuously, or they will go into a coma. Some people seem to relax, but there are many who experience varying degrees of restlessness, agitation, or delirium. Swallowing soon becomes impossible. These profound physical changes require alternate care approaches such as different medication routes, catheters, and regular repositioning.

Psychosocial Impact

As patients become increasingly unresponsive and approach the time of death, families search for new ways to communicate and "be present" with them. They must now rely on others' interpretations and explanations regarding what is happening and make decisions for the patient. Families are anxious if patients become delirious, restless, or agitated. When patients stop eating and drinking, families often worry that they are starving or becoming dehydrated.

The Parting of the Ways: Time of Death

Table 1.8 shows an end to all functioning, from ambulation to conscious level, as the person dies.

Physical Indications

Depending on circumstances, the actual death may occur very quietly or quite dramatically. Some patients simply stop breathing, but for most there are periods of

Table 1.8. Palliative Performance Scale (PPSv2) 0%

PPS Level	Ambulation	Activity and evidence of disease	Self-care	Intake	Conscious level
0%	Death	–	–	–	–

apnea before death. If symptoms have been well controlled, death is often peaceful. Otherwise, patients may experience some degree of air hunger, pain, or restlessness, depending on the underlying disease process. After death, the patient's eyes may or may not be open, and often the fingers, hands, toes, and feet are cold and discolored.

Psychosocial Impact

When patients die, families often feel shocked, relieved, and/or surprised. Families and individuals within the family will each say good-bye in their own way.

TRANSITIONS IN BEREAVEMENT: PHASES MODEL OF GRIEF

A number of phase models (Martin & Elder, 1993; Rando, 1984) have been developed to describe phases of the grief process. Caution has been expressed as to whether phase models adequately demonstrate individual variation and difference. They are, however, helpful as a way to normalize and demystify the commonly intense experiences of bereaved people. This framework is an overview of the range of normal reactions to loss within which individual experiences can be considered.

The bereavement framework offered in the tables that follow are an adaptation of Rando's (1984) phases of grief and Worden's (1992) tasks. This framework is broad enough to be inclusive and structured enough to be informative and is a valuable tool that provides a welcome roadmap for the continuing journey of people experiencing bereavement. People who are bereaved often feel they are lost or going crazy, or fear that their grief will never end. This model portrays grief as a process with a beginning, middle, and end—a hopeful idea for bereaved people and practitioners alike. It helps people to understand and grow through grief in an actively engaged way rather than making grief something to suffer through, hide from, or deny.

Beyond the model of phases and grief tasks, the image of the labyrinth is also offered as a metaphor for this journey toward healing and wholeness. "The labyrinth is an archetypal image of wholeness that helps us rediscover the depths of ourselves" (Artress, 1995, p. 2). Unlike a maze, a labyrinth has no dead ends and no wrong turns, thus it symbolizes the grief journey on its movement toward central issues of meaning. The labyrinth has many turns and involves going back and forth over what seems like the same territory. Bereaved people journey to the center of grief, to the center of their selves, and then slowly reenter the world. Grief is like any significant journey; the traveler is changed by experiences along the way and the once-familiar world is different upon the traveler's return.

THREE PHASES OF GRIEF

Phase 1: Walking the Edges: When a Death Occurs

In the first phase of grief, bereaved people must face the reality of the death (see Table 1.9). They may experience a feeling of disbelief or a sense of unreality, be shocked at the news of the death, and feel bewildered or stunned. This may be a time when people need care and assistance. Bereaved people know intellectually that the death has occurred but can have moments of denial when they think or feel as if it has not really happened. They are walking the edges of the labyrinth. Denial acts as protection from the intense feelings and allows people to absorb

Table 1.9. Phase 1: When a death occurs

Description	Transition and image	Grief task(s)
Immediately following a death, there is a sense of shock, numbness, and disbelief that can last hours or weeks. Panic and strong physical and emotional reactions are common. This period allows people to take information in at a slower rate and to prepare for the adjustments that lie ahead.	The patient dies and, for the family, bereavement begins. Bereaved people face grief. Image: walking the edges	To move from denial to acceptance that the death really has occurred.

Social	Physical	Emotional	Cognitive	Spiritual
On "autopilot" Withdrawal or fear of being alone Unrealistic expectations of self and others Poor judgment about relationships	Shortness of breath, palpitations Digestive upsets Physical symptoms of shock Low energy, weakness, or restlessness	Crying, sobbing, and/or wailing Indifference, emptiness Helplessness, outrage	Confusion, forgetfulness, poor concentration Daydreaming and denial Constant thoughts about the person who died and/or the death itself	Blaming God or "life" Lack of meaning, direction, or hope Wishing to die and join the person who died

things at their own pace. Emotional numbness allows bereaved people to do the things that are necessary following a death. Others may interpret this numbness as strength and be surprised when feelings of distress are later expressed. At this time, the loss and subsequent grief are bereaved people's primary experience.

Phase 2: Entering the Depths: Adjusting to Loss

As shown in Table 1.10, the middle phase of grief in which people adjust to loss may last for an extended time, with episodes of intense grief interspersed with times when bereaved people feel more like their usual selves. Emotional responses include a range of feelings such as anger, despair, and loneliness. The intensity of these feelings can be unexpected and overwhelming. Bereaved individuals are traveling inward, entering the depths of their own pain and sorrow. Their values, beliefs, or faith may be challenged by the ways in which their worlds have changed. Bereaved people often review their relationship with the person who died. They consider how the relationship changed through time, with all the ups and downs,

Table 1.10.   Phase 2: Adjusting to loss

Description	Transition and image	Grief task(s)
As the numbness subsides, bereaved people begin to deal with the emotional pain of grieving. The intensity of this may surprise and frighten them, but it is natural and can be resolved. The time needed for this work is affected by the quality of support, other losses, and the bereaved person's approach to life.	Grief deepens and is the focus of attention and energy. Bereaved people live their grief. Image: entering the depths	To acknowledge, experience, and work through feelings related to the loss To adjust to life without the person who died

Social	Physical	Emotional	Cognitive	Spiritual
Continued withdrawal and isolation Wanting company but unable to ask Rushing into new relationships Self-consciousness	Tight chest, sharp pangs, shortness of breath Digestive upsets Aimless activity, gnawing emptiness Changes in appetite or sleep patterns	Intense and conflicting emotions Anger, sadness, guilt, hopelessness Generalized anxiety Magnified fears for self, others	Sense of going crazy Memory problems Understanding and concentration poor Vivid dreams or nightmares	Sensing the presence of the person who died; visitations Continued lack of meaning or purpose Attempts to contact the person who died

and may experience feelings of regret or guilt. Emotional pain can cause physical distress as the body reacts to these feelings. Bereaved people may respond quite differently to those around them. Family and friends often lack understanding and want people to feel better than they do. Grief is the central focus in bereaved people's lives at this time.

Phase 3: Reconnecting with the World: Mending the Heart

At some point in the grief journey, bereaved people become aware that the loss is becoming a part of their past experience (see Table 1.11). The good days outnumber the bad days more and more. They have more energy for family, friends, work, and other interests. They are able to remember things about the person who died with a sense of composure. Of course, grief is not over for the bereaved individual and there are times when the person who died is intensely missed. It is important for bereaved people to find natural, comfortable, and meaningful ways to remember, honor, and talk about the person who has died. At this time, bereaved people

Table 1.11. Phase 3: Mending the Heart

Description	Transition and image	Grief task(s)
As grief becomes more resolved, bereaved people have the energy and desire to reconnect with the world. Their loss begins to be seen in perspective as part of their past experience.	Grief lightens and bereaved people live with ongoing grief as a part of their life. Image: mending the heart	To re-invest energy in activities and relationships To create an appropriate relationship with the person who died

Social	Physical	Emotional	Cognitive	Spiritual
More interest in daily affairs of others Ability to reach out and meet others Energy for social relationships Desire for independence resurfaces	Physical symptoms subside Sleep pattern and appetite return to normal Gut-wrenching emptiness lightens	Emotions are less intense Feeling of coming out of the fog More peace and happiness Some guilt about how life goes on	Perspective about death increases Able to remember with less pain Memory and concentration improve Dreams and nightmares decrease	Connection with religious and/or spiritual beliefs Life has new meaning/ purpose Acceptance that death is a part of life

may acknowledge the personal growth that results from surviving, and continuing to survive, the loss. They reenter their world, changed and energized. They reevaluate their lives and make significant personal choices that increase their quality of life.

SUMMARY

In order to provide competent and consistent psychosocial palliative care, practitioners require a theoretical understanding of human development, principles that articulate their values as professionals and volunteers, and a framework that reflects patients' and families' journeys from diagnosis to bereavement. This combination will provide health care providers with the tools to normalize people's experiences, while celebrating and honoring their differences. Through the frameworks provided in this book, the various activities of hospice and palliative care will be clearly defined and internalized by the professionals. The PPS provides a way to conceptualize and respond to the needs and issues of patients and families as they approach death. The Phases Model of Grief similarly considers the transitions experienced by families once death has occurred.

REFERENCES

Anderson, F., Casorso, L., Downing, G.M., Hill, J., & Lerch, N. (1996). Palliative performance scale: A new tool. *Journal of Palliative Care, 12*(1), 5–11.

Artress, L. (1995). *Walking a sacred path: Rediscovering the labyrinth as a sacred tool.* New York: Riverhead Books.

Doyle-Brown, M. (2000). The transitional phase: The closing journey for patients and family caregivers. *American Journal of Hospice and Palliative Care, 17*(5), 354–357.

Karnofsky, D., Abelmann, W., & Craver, L. (1948). The use of nitrogen mustards in the palliative treatment of carcinoma. *Cancer, 1,* 634–656.

Martin, K., & Elder, S. (1993). Pathways through grief: A model of the process. In J. Morgan (Ed.), *Personal care in an impersonal world: A multidimensional look at bereavement (death, value and meaning).* Amityville, NY: Baywood Publishing.

Moules, N. (1998). Legitimizing grief: Challenging beliefs that constrain. *Journal of Family Nursing, 4*(2), 142–166.

Rando, T. (1984). *Grief, death and dying: Clinical interventions for caregivers.* Champaign, IL: Research Press.

Weisman, A.D. (1979). A model for psychosocial phasing in cancer. *General Hospital Psychiatry,* 187–195.

Worden, W. (1992). *Grief counseling and grief therapy: A handbook for the mental health professional* (2nd ed.). New York: Springer Publishing.

THE ROLE OF COUNSELORS IN HOSPICE AND PALLIATIVE CARE

What role do counselors play in hospice and palliative care? To formulate answers to this question, Victoria Hospice undertook a research project to identify the specific activities performed by counselors and social workers that are directly related to the care of patients and families in the hospice and palliative care setting (Thompson, Rose, Wainwright, Mattar, & Scanlan, 2001). Computer searches of several electronic databases, including PsycLIT, ERIC, Medline, Cinahl, Age-Line, and Social Work Abstracts, yielded key papers to inform the project. Some authors referred to social work roles (Amar, 1994; Hudgens, 1978; Hudson, 1989; Rusnack, Schaefer, & Moxley, 1988; Sakada-kis, Bonar, & MacLean, 1987; Stark & Johnson, 1983), whereas others described tasks (Black, Morrison, Snyder, & Tally, 1977; Kennedy, 1996; Monroe, 1994) or activities (Kulys & Davis, 1986/1987; MacDonald, 1991).

Overall, empirical investigations into the social worker's role in hospice and palliative care have followed one of two streams of inquiry: 1) identifying who on the palliative care team is perceived to be the primary provider of psychosocial care and/or 2) identifying the kinds of tasks performed by social workers that differ from those of the other hospice team members, such as nurses, clergy, and volunteers.

In 1996, Ryan found that service directors he surveyed perceived social work services in a dichotomous way; they perceived them as either for counseling issues only (usually for difficult issues that other staff feel unable to handle), or for practical issues only (financial and legal issues in particular) (p. 52).

Reese and Brown (1997) found that social workers were the principal providers of care in the psychosocial realm, particularly for those issues pertaining to death anxiety and social support, even though it was shown that other team members might also address these issues. Rusnack et al. (1988) found that social workers occupied the roles of advocate, counselor, educator, enabler, facilitator, mediator, participant, assistant, collaborator, consultant, maintainer, sustainer, innovator, liaison, negotiator, and organizer with patients, families, colleagues, and the service network.

Hudson (1989) focused exclusively on specific roles of social work, both direct and indirect. He examined these roles to determine their importance and how involved social workers were in performing each of them. He identified assessment, advocacy, communication/education, enablement, mediation, and social brokerage as direct services; he considered administration, coordination, fundraising, planning, professional development, program development, quality assurance, record keeping, research, and supervision to be indirect services. These roles were also identified in several studies from the medical and oncological social work literature (Egan & Kadushin, 1995; Hudgens, 1978; Kennedy, 1996).

There were two unexpected outcomes to our review of the literature: 1) the realization of the lack of understanding and agreement that exists about the unique functions of social workers in the health care setting and 2) how minimally their actual work has been formally documented (Keigher, 1997; Kulys & Davis, 1986; MacDonald, 1991; Oliviere, 2001; Ryan, 1996). We realized that no single piece of work fully reflected the practice of hospice and palliative care counselors. Very few resources spoke specifically about the psychosocial interventions of hospice and palliative care social workers and counselors. Even fewer resources addressed how social workers and counselors applied their skills and knowledge to the experiences of patients and families or if their interventions even made a difference. It became apparent that a common language concerning hospice and palliative care counselor's roles on the team would be beneficial.

THE VICTORIA HOSPICE "COUNSELING ACTIVITIES" RESEARCH PROJECT

Although we did not disagree with the literature findings, the articles only partially represented the diverse work of counselors and social workers in hospice and palliative care. To complete the picture, we surveyed our counseling team, asking each person to identify which work activities did and did not directly relate to patient and family care. Seven distinct themes emerged: 1) companioning; 2) psychosocial assessment, planning, and evaluation; 3) counseling interventions; 4) facilitation and advocacy; 5) patient and family education; 6) consultation and reporting; and 7) team support. These are described further in Table 1A.1. Each of these themes or categories was used to represent a discrete set of closely related activities.

The next step was to identify when, with whom, and how these themes appeared and how the counseling activities changed over time. Two separate checklists, the Psychosocial Activities Checklist (see p. 43) and the Bereavement Activities Checklist (see p. 44), were developed to capture how the themes related to what hospice and bereavement counselors were doing with patients and/or families.

Each counselor used the Psychosocial Activities Checklist to track the PPS, his or her time, and counseling activities related to the seven themes. Similarly, the counselors used the Bereavement Activities Checklist to track the number of months past death, counseling time, and activities. The results of this project are still being analyzed and prepared for publication.

Table 1A.1. Thematic analysis of counselor activities in a hospice/palliative care environment

Companioning	Psychosocial assessment, planning, evaluation	Counseling interventions	Facilitation and advocacy	Patient and family education	Consultation and reporting	Team support
"Be" with people	Prioritize counseling requests	Use active listening	Facilitate groups	Educate, clarify, and interpret regarding:	Write and verbalize reports to other professionals	Team building (emotional support, debriefing, and feedback)
Build rapport	Take histories	Explore issues and emotions	Facilitate family discussion and decision making	a. community resources	Consult with other professionals	Assist nursing colleagues with physical care and practical tasks
Comfort	Assess individual mental functioning, emotional status, loss history, social supports, coping styles, strengths and challenges, financial and legal concerns, spiritual needs	Reframe, empathize, challenge, question, summarize	Facilitate interdisciplinary meetings	b. agency services	Refer to internal/external services and programs	Support and encourage self-care practices within the team
Establish safety		Provide guidance and modeling		c. family systems		
Support what is sacred			Mediate conflict	d. patient personal care		
Share silence		Normalize grief process and individual differences	Advocate for patients and families	e. patient and family self care		
Connect physically (hugs, massage, therapeutic touch)		Invite spiritual exploration		f. estate and funeral planning		
Connect spiritually	Assess group and family dynamics	Facilitate disclosure		g. implications of disease progression		
	Assist clients in setting goals	Provide feedback		h. contact with MDs and RNs		
	Plan interventions	Problem solve				
	Carry out discharge planning	Offer coping strategies				
	Evaluate effectiveness of interventions	Provide opportunity to increase self-awareness				
		Assist with creation of rituals				

Psychosocial Activities Checklist

(A Victoria Hospice Society Research Project, 01/08/01)

Patient's first name: _____ Age: _____ Sex: _____ M _____ F

Diagnosis: _____

	Counselor ID# Visit 1				Counselor ID# Visit 2				Counselor ID# Visit 3				Counselor ID# Visit 4				Counselor ID# Visit 5				Counselor ID# Visit 6			
	Unit PRT Community / PPS				Unit PRT Community / PPS				Unit PRT Community / PPS				Unit PRT Community / PPS				Unit PRT Community / PPS				Unit PRT Community / PPS			
	Pt.	family	both		Pt.	family	both		Pt.	family	both		Pt.	family	both		Pt.	family	both		Pt.	family	both	
Companioning																								
Assessment, Planning, and Evaluation																								
Counseling Interventions																								
Facilitation and Advocacy																								
Education																								
Consultation and Reporting																								
Team Support																								

Bereavement (psychosocial) Activities Checklist
(A Victoria Hospice Society Research Project, 01/08/01)

Bereaved first name: _____   Bereaved age: _____   Sex: _____ M   _____ F

Date of death (d/m/y): _____   Relationship to deceased: _____

Cause of death: _____   _____ Program   _____ Community

	Counselor ID# Contact Date (d/m) Month Post-death Contact 1			Counselor ID# Contact Date (d/m) Month Post-death Contact 2			Counselor ID# Contact Date (d/m) Month Post-death Contact 3			Counselor ID# Contact Date (d/m) Month Post-death Contact 4			Counselor ID# Contact Date (d/m) Month Post-death Contact 5			Counselor ID# Contact Date (d/m) Month Post-death Contact 6		
	Phone	1:1	Group	Phone	1:1	Group	Phone	1:1	Group	Phone	1:1	Group	Phone	1:1	Group	Phone	1:1	Group
Companioning																		
Assessment, Planning, and Evaluation																		
Counseling Interventions																		
Facilitation and Advocacy																		
Education																		
Consultation and Reporting																		
Team Support																		

REFERENCES

Amar, D.F. (1994). The role of the hospice social worker in the nursing home setting. *The American Journal of Hospice & Palliative Care, 11*(3), 18–23.

Black, D.B., Morrison, J., Snyder, L.J., & Tally, P. (1977). Model for clinical social work practice in a health care setting. *Social Work in Health Care, 3*(2), 143–148.

Egan, M., & Kadushin, G. (1995). Competitive allies: Rural nurses' and social workers' perceptions of the social work role in the hospital setting. *Social Work in Health Care, 20*(3), 1–22.

Hudgens, A.J. (1978). The social worker's role in a behavioral management approach to chronic pain. *Social Work in Health Care, 3*(2), 149–157.

Hudson, J.E. (1989). An analysis of social work tasks in Canadian hospital-based palliative care programs. *Dissertation Abstracts International, 50*(9), 3059–A.

Keigher, S.M. (1997). What role for social work in the new health care practice paradigm? *Health and Social Work, 22*(2), 149–155.

Kennedy, V.N. (1996). Supportive care of the patient with pancreatic cancer: The role of the oncology social worker. *Oncology, 10*(2), 35–37.

Kulys, R., & Davis, M.A. (1986). An analysis of social services in hospices. *Social Work, 31*, 448–456.

Kulys, R., & Davis, M.A. (1987). Nurses and social workers: Rivals in the provision of social services? *Health and Social Work, 12*, 101–112.

MacDonald, D. (1991). Hospice social work: A search for identity. *Health and Social Work, 16*(4), 274–280.

Monroe, B. (1994). Role of the social worker in palliative care. *Annals of the Academy of Medicine, Singapore, 23*(2), 252–255.

Oliviere, D. (2001). The social worker in palliative care: The eccentric role. *Progress in Palliative Care, 9*(6), 237–241.

Reese, D.J., & Brown, D.R. (1997). Psychosocial and spiritual care in hospice: Differences between nursing, social work, and clergy. *The Hospice Journal, 12*(1), 29–41.

Rusnack, B., Schaefer, S.M., & Moxley, D. (1988). Safe passage: Social work roles and functions in hospice care. *Social Work in Health Care, 13*(3), 3–19.

Ryan, M. (1996). Walking in a minefield: Findings from a survey of social workers in Australian hospice and palliative care programs. *Australian Social Work, 49*(3), 47–54.

Sakadakis, V., Bonar, R., & MacLean, M. (1987). The role of the social worker in terminal care with institutionalized elderly people. *Journal of Palliative Care, 3*(2), 19–25.

Stark, D.E., & Johnson, E.M. (1983). Implications of hospice concepts for social work practice with oncology patients and their families in an acute care teaching hospital. *Social Work in Health Care, 9*(1), 63–70.

Thompson, M., Rose, C., Wainwright, W., Mattar, L., & Scanlan, M. (2001). Activities of counselors in a hospice and palliative care environment. *Journal of Palliative Care, 17*(4), 229–235.

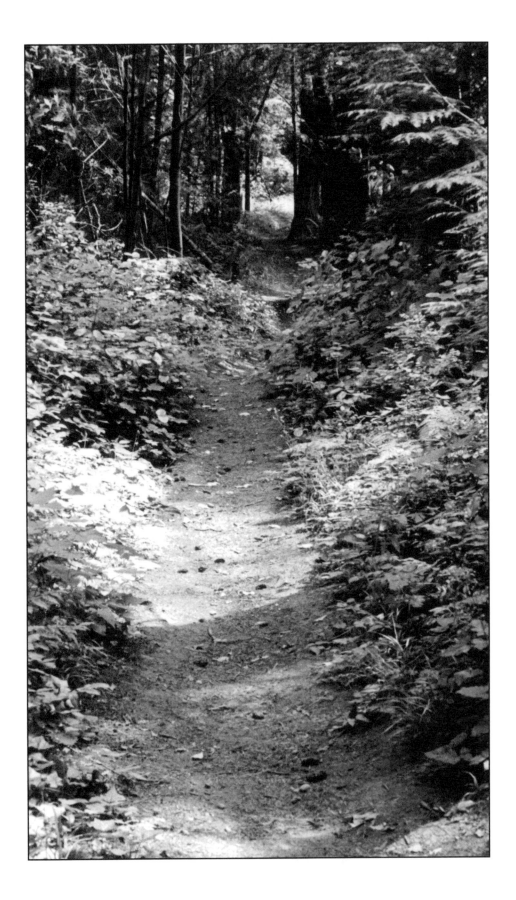

2

Beginning the Journey

EARLY DIAGNOSIS AND TREATMENT
(PPSv2 level: 100% to 90%)

Although some people learn of their diagnosis through a routine examination, most enter this early phase of life-threatening disease looking fine, but knowing something is not right. They seek a medical opinion or investigation to discover what is making them feel unwell. Preparing themselves for the worst, yet hoping and praying for something better, most people nonetheless want to know what is happening to them. Others want to avoid investigation and the potential for bad news and have to be pushed toward diagnosis by family members who want answers. As patients and families cope with the experience of diagnosis and treatment, there are five key areas (indicated by capital letters in the following paragraphs) in which issues most commonly arise. The first consideration, BECOMING A PATIENT, looks at the impact on people when they are first introduced to the unfamiliar world of health care that can often be complex and rigid.

The health care system has its own culture, language, and pace. Appointments, medical terminology, hospitals, and new faces can leave patients feeling lost and overwhelmed—like strangers in a strange land. Health care providers may be unaware of the struggles faced by people new to their system. Needing to trust these people with their lives, patients are sometimes hesitant to criticize or ask for help. With trepidation and awe, they begin their journey, looking for answers and determined to find a cure or miracle.

RECEIVING A DIAGNOSIS of any life-threatening disease is life changing. People face the fragility of life and realize how vulnerable both they and their loved ones are, perhaps for the first time (Weisman, 1979). An uncertain future initially triggers feelings of FEAR AND POWERLESSNESS. Some patients consider the possibility of death and imagine a journey marked by physical deterioration, dependency, pain, and loss. Others acknowledge this possibility, but become determined to fight and survive the crisis. Family members anticipate suffering and helplessness, wondering how they can make things better, yet knowing the future is out of their control.

> "Hope is a journey, not a destination; its value lies in the exploration. Hope is the way we live life and the journey of hope should last until we end."
>
> —David Kessler
> (Cotter, 1999, p. 321)

Once diagnosed, patients will have to MAKE CRITICAL DECISIONS. Although patients are still reeling in shock and disbelief, they face a barrage of information about their disease. Specialists make recommendations based on their knowledge of the disease and its current stages, the best available treatments, and the patients' and families' wishes. Family and friends make recommendations based on a desperate need to offer hope or find a cure, others' stories, or their own search for information. Some patients rely heavily on the advice of their physicians; trusting their skill and knowledge. Others will want to blend traditional and alternative approaches to treatment or reject what is offered altogether. Regardless of how people approach decisions, they often find there is little time to process the abundance of information and opinion. Although they may feel overwhelmed and on shaky ground, patients decide on a course of action that will shape their lives over the coming weeks, months, or years.

Once treatment begins, patients and families find that it can become the center of their world. Whether it involves surgery, chemotherapy, radiation, medications, or rehabilitation, the whole family is DEALING WITH THE IMPACT OF TREATMENT. Treatments determine when patients feel well or dreadfully ill, when they can work, and when they have energy for important activities. Families must grapple with changing routines and roles as they care for a person who may be frightened and miserable. They need to figure out how to support the patient, share extra responsibilities, and keep the family functioning together.

At this time, support groups can be invaluable for helping patients deal with issues that arise (see Table 2.1).

Table 2.1. Therapeutic goals and methods useful for groups addressing special issues of cancer patients

Stage	Issues	Goals	Methods
At diagnosis	Distress over diagnosis Confusion (disease, treatment, prognosis)	Stress management Emotional support	Information giving Interactive (new skills) Discussion (diagnosis)
During treatment	Discomfort (nausea, fatigue, weight change) Reality of illness sets in	Adjusting to life with cancer (changes, realities) Coping with treatments Emotional support	Interactive (new skills) Discussion (treatments)
End of treatment	Self-image, sense of control Questioning life activities Relationships Recurrence and death Attitudes/behaviors affecting health	Active coping, skill development Spiritual support (examining life values, beliefs) Considering the future Living a healthy lifestyle	Interactive (new skills, behavior therapy) Discussion (fears, control over disease)
Recurrence and dying	Emotional distress Death and dying Treatments Loss of control Family and friends Physical symptoms	Active coping Pain and stress management Emotional/social support Existential issues addressed Living fully in the moment	Interactive (new skills) Discussion (fears, losses, relationships)

Source: Spira, 1998.

JAN AND KATHY

Jan was a banker; her partner Kathy is a high school English teacher. At the age of 47, Jan was diagnosed with lung cancer. Although only one tumor was visible in her left lung, the diagnosis was very serious and the prognosis highly variable. Jan smoked as a young woman but had been physically active for many years; playing tennis and squash, jogging, and sailing. She had been a dynamic person, a force to be reckoned with; and her bank colleagues and business contacts respected her greatly for her dedication, drive, and extraordinary problem-solving abilities.

When Jan received her diagnosis, she became distressed and highly anxious. Upon entering the world of cancer care; she was quickly overwhelmed by the process of investigation, diagnosis, and decision making about treatment approaches. She was not able to sleep and became physically and emotionally exhausted. The more information she received about her disease, the treatment options, and unclear prognosis, the more agitated and fearful she felt. When her oncologist spoke with her about available treatments and their impact, Jan became immobilized and was unable to process the information or make any decisions. When she was overwhelmed, she missed important information and heard only negative or bad news. A successful problem-solver all of her life, she was unable to tackle or solve this problem. Fear gripped her spirit; she was in deep despair and felt no hope.

Jan decided to include Kathy and her brother James in every doctor's appointment and treatment decision. Now, on her behalf, they ask questions, explore options, and remember what is said. Jan still becomes fearful and terrified at the thought of suffering and dying, but, with less clutter in her mind, she is now able to make the decisions that are important to her. This has also allowed her to focus on taking care of herself during surgery and follow-up treatments.

Jan is still uncertain whether the side effects of surgery or other aggressive therapies would be worth it. She hates the idea of being a patient and wonders how Kathy will manage the dual role of caregiver and school teacher. Despite these concerns, she stills wants to live as long as possible, and Kathy and James want her to have the operation.

Where previously Jan felt she had to control her life's circumstances and solve any problems that came her way, she no longer feels that she has to find the solution to this dilemma of having a life-threatening illness. She has come to realize that she cannot cope with this situation by continually focusing on the enormity and reality of her disease. She now concentrates on living day to day and looks within this smaller world to find hope and strategies for coping.

KEY CONSIDERATIONS

Becoming a Patient

Jan had been a dynamic person and a force to be reckoned with; her bank colleagues and business contacts respected her greatly for her dedication, drive, and extraordinary problem-solving abilities. However, upon entering the world of cancer care, She was quickly overwhelmed by decision making about the process of investigation, diagnosis, and determining treatment approaches. Faced with physicians and others who assume her ability to "rise to the occasion," Jan could initially focus only on the bad news and her experience of this illness.

Once investigation and treatment begin, people may experience the role of patient for the first time. Not only do they struggle with the possibility of serious illness, but they must also learn to navigate a foreign territory.

In awe of the knowledge, skills, and authority of the medical professionals, patients and families can feel ignorant and powerless when faced with diagnosis and treatment. These feelings are further reinforced if patients are treated as a disease or set of symptoms rather than as people. Health care providers sometimes underestimate the strengths and abilities of families and may end up patronizing them. Feeling frightened, yet grateful for the attention, some patients are reluctant to challenge the status quo and to demand, or even to expect, that it be different (Lederberg, 1998). Others will take a very proactive stance in learning about their illness and directing their care.

This new world has a language of its own. Latin- and Greek-based words, statistics, and medical shorthand are quite foreign to patients and families. Many terms are difficult to understand, reinforcing the inequality of the patient–professional relationship. Add in patients' anxiety and fear, and it is not surprising that people do not know what questions to ask and often misunderstand what they hear. Some people quickly learn the terminology, but others remain on the outside, relying on someone else to interpret for them.

TRANSITIONS

Time
I have time
I have sadness
I have joy

Cancer
Is a gateway
To mortality
To the underworld

Goodbye
To my old life
A new one
Not yet found or created

Limbo
The place in-between
Painful, confused
Full of possibility

Myself
I walk a journey
Towards acceptance
Which holds the key to peace

I am not there yet

—(Fran Norris, 1997, p. 90)

Access to the health care system usually comes through a medical referral, with little practical and emotional preparation for what is ahead. Once in the system, referral to other services may be dependent on the specialist. For example, a referral for counseling may depend on the specialists' beliefs about the value of psychosocial interventions, their judgment about patients' needs for such support, or their own ability to work within an interdisciplinary team. Access is further influenced by the size of the community in which a patient lives, the type of disease encountered, and the resources available for information and support.

A number of preexisting factors such as financial stress, high levels of conflict, and difficulties in coping place patients at risk for social or emotional breakdown. Although some are able to advocate for themselves, many do not receive the psychosocial and practical support they need during diagnosis and treatment. This occurs for a number of reasons. Some people are too overwhelmed and unable to ask for help.

"Some think a request for support indicates an inability to cope, a loss of independence, or an acknowledgement of the presence of mental illness. They do not perceive their needs clearly, in part because there is little approval for admitting such needs in our society. [They are] unaware that counseling may help assuage the existential terror evoked by a diagnosis of cancer or alleviate grief over the loss of body function or appearance, or that it may restore a sense of control." (Christ, 1991, p. 303)

Interventions

These psychosocial interventions have been designed to specifically address the key consideration *becoming a patient*. Following are several assessment questions that will help open up a discussion, followed by more focused comments or tips that will facilitate further exploration of the issues that frequently arise at this time; each tip is followed by a sample dialogue.

Assessment Questions

- Tell me about any previous experiences you've had as a patient.
- Tell me what your experience has been since your diagnosis.
- What information have you received about how your specialist will work with you?
- What have you been told about the different kinds of support you can get?

Normalize feelings and validate experiences. Information based on others' experiences helps people put words to their experience and gives them a language to describe their thoughts, feelings, and needs.

> *"You say it has been quite frightening coming to the clinic and you don't seem to get the answers you want. Many people feel overwhelmed by all of the information, new words, and investigation schedules. There may be some questions that I can answer for you now. Then we could decide which questions you need to ask your physician, and you could write them down and take them to your next appointment. How would that work for you?"*

Provide information on how to navigate the system and link it to pre-existing systems. For example, clarify the role of the patient's specialist and family physician; explain procedures, expectations, and services available. When people understand how the system works, they feel more confident and are better able to advocate for themselves.

> *"Even though the specialist, Dr. Meredith, is seeing you right now to investigate your heart condition, it is important to remember that your fam-*

ily physician will still want to see you. She will want to know how your medications are working and, generally, how you are. What questions might you have for your next appointment with her?"

Provide opportunities for patients and families to explore the facts and meaning of the investigation. This helps people understand what is being said and allows them to clarify complicated words, statistics, non-verbal cues, or tone that may be confusing for them.

> *"Dr. Stevens explained what happens during a CT (computed tomography) scan and what he hopes to find out. Can you tell me what you understand about the procedure?"*

Receiving a Diagnosis: When the News Is Bad

When Jan received her diagnosis, she became distressed and highly anxious. She was not able to sleep and became physically and emotionally exhausted. The more information she received about her disease, the treatment options, and the unclear prognosis, the more agitated and fearful she felt. A successful problem-solver all of her life, she was unable to tackle or solve this problem.

Regardless of whether people expect the diagnosis, most tend to react with shock and disbelief. Some immediately anticipate death, some block out all or part of what is being said, and others quickly focus on cure and survival. People may have many questions about the investigation and the results, looking for mistakes or possible omissions. More likely, they will feel numb and may be unable to ask anything until the information has a chance to sink in. They may not have told family and friends about the investigation and worry about how to break the bad news to them.

People who have a preexisting high risk for developing a particular illness feel extremely anxious and vulnerable during any investigations that may lead to diagnosis of that illness (Kash & Learnen, 1998). Family history, environment, or lifestyle may mean they have fears of death based on past experience or personal misconceptions. They often express guilt because they could, potentially, pass this disease on to their children; or because they have survived while others have not. They may feel powerless to change their fate. Some people use denial as a coping strategy and, therefore, have avoided early testing or screening that may have prevented the disease from occurring.

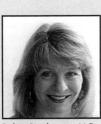

In My Own Voice
Breaking Bad News

Debra Braithwaite

Debra Braithwaite, M.D.,
is a physician with
Victoria Hospice Society.

Breaking bad news is a task not normally associated with palliative physicians because most patients come to palliative care following the diagnosis of a terminal illness. However, we are frequently involved in "rebreaking" bad news to patients as disease progresses and death approaches and know that the communication of difficult information is more an ongoing process than a single event. We are also frequent witnesses to the stories patients tell regarding their personal experiences in receiving bad news and know that they are affected long after the telling by the circumstances and manner in which it was delivered.

When I first started in palliative care, I noticed a wide range of patient reactions to being informed of a life-threatening illness. Many recalled the event in strongly negative terms, some had more neutral experiences, and a few were positive in their recollections. Although each was deeply affected by the information itself, some patients described additional distress due to the method in which it was communicated. In a few cases, it was remembered as the most painful experience of the entire illness.

What, I wondered, accounted for these differences? Why were some patients traumatized by the process of hearing bad news, while others emerged comforted and well supported? Was it because, as some patients suggested, the physician involved seemed cold in manner, unnecessarily blunt, and provided overwhelming amounts of medical information they didn't understand? Was the problem that the physician was rushed and evasive in manner, spent little time, and seemed reluctant to provide straight answers to patient or family questions? Perhaps the real difficulty lay with the patient? Had the individual unwittingly focused his or her own grief and dissatisfaction on the unfortunate "bearer of bad news"?

Clearly, patients and physicians have individual styles of communication and different perceptions of when frankness becomes brutality or gentleness wanders off into obfuscation. Although these differences are real, they are likely peripheral to the heart of patient–physician miscommunication. In fact, the most frequently noted determinant of patient distress or satisfaction concerned the attitude of the person delivering the bad news and how he or she approached the task. Did the person treat the patient with gentle dignity, communicate in a compassionate manner, and recognize the moment as the important event it is? Did they acknowledge that this conversation represented a "profound" or "sacred" moment in the patient's life and treat it with the respect it required?

Hearing that one is going to die is one of life's defining moments and serves to mark the transition from one stage of life to another. Time is measured against such moments. In human society, such events are typically associated with rituals that signal their importance to ourselves and others. Most "sacred moments," such as weddings, graduations, births, and funerals, are richly steeped in customs and traditions. Yet as a society we have few acknowledged rituals around the giving and receiving of catastrophic news, and, perhaps, we need them.

Physicians who are most successful in breaking bad news know the benefits of creating an atmosphere of respect, dignity, and reverence to support patients and families. Rituals that acknowledge the impact of life-altering news both decrease patient distress and lighten the burden of those delivering it.

The above principles apply any time bad news is broken or rebroken. Palliative patients, who deal initially with the fact of terminal diagnosis, may be further distressed by bad news along the way. Information that cancer has spread to another site is difficult as it foreshadows additional physical loss. Confirmation that treatment is no longer working may be devastating as evidence that disease is now progressing unopposed. Acknowledgment of general decline brings fears of physical dependence and indignity. Over the entire course of the illness, the reality of approaching death may be rebroken many times.

Although physicians are most commonly identified as the "bearers of bad news," almost everyone involved in the care of terminally ill patients and their families participates in the communication or confirmation of bad news at some time. News about recurrent disease may be broken by the oncologist, but it might be a counselor who confirms the significance of the patient's weight loss; a volunteer who lets the family know the person is now too weak to get out of bed unassisted, or a nurse who acknowledges, in the middle of the night, that little time remains.

In palliative care, we are intimately involved with breaking and rebreaking bad news on a continual basis. By understanding the benefits of good communication, we can dramatically improve patient well-being along with our own. The ability to break bad news skillfully— the gentle art of truth telling—is essential not just for physicians but for all members of the care team. Ongoing education in this area is required. If we break bad news poorly, our patients will suffer and we will likely avoid the conversations required to keep them well supported and informed. If we do it skillfully, we provide both counsel and comfort and gain the satisfaction that we have done a difficult thing well. *How to Break Bad News: A Guide for Health Care Professionals* (The Johns Hopkins University Press, 1992) by Buckman and Kason is a particularly good resource.

Once diagnosed with a life-threatening illness, patients struggle with difficult questions about what this disease means to them and their families. Illness and death are no longer impersonal and they wonder how they will manage. These patients will often ask, "How can I cope with this?" "What am I willing to do in order to live?" "What will this do to my family?" In the context of these questions, it is also important for patients to put the diagnosis into perspective. Since it is early in the disease, many patients will do well for long periods of time, even decades, or be cured. Most patients will find a balance between these two ends: living and dying.

Interventions

These psychosocial interventions have been designed to specifically address the key consideration *receiving a diagnosis*. There are several assessment questions that will help open up a discussion, followed by more focused comments or tips that will facilitate further exploration of the issues that frequently arise at this time; each tip is followed by a sample dialogue.

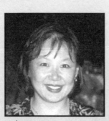

Helen Wong, B.S.W., is
a patient and family
counselor with the British
Columbia Cancer
Agency, Vancouver
Island Centre.

In My Own Voice
Death and Despair

Helen Wong

I came into the hospital with the words "malignant spinal tumor" on the admissions paper I held in my hand. The look in people's eyes told me how grim the situation appeared. The medical team sent me for bone scans, ultrasounds, blood work, and, finally, a biopsy. Although the biopsy came back negative for malignancy, they were not satisfied and still wanted to know what kind of malignancy I had.

I knew what a spinal tumor meant; after all, I had worked as a social worker in The Cancer Centre for the past 10 years. I knew the symptoms of the cord compression and the likelihood that a spinal tumor meant metastatic disease, rather than a primary cancer.

The news was very bad. My colleagues were stunned with the news. My family was not fully cognizant of the implications of the diagnosis. I had to share the possibilities with my husband and, eventually, with my 9-year-old daughter and 12-year-old son.

I found myself strangely calm going through the numerous tests. I had 40% cord compression. My legs were weak and unsteady. All those years of being supportive to patients in their emotional turmoil had taught me the value of living moment by moment and to appreciate what I had. I had hope.

I felt in my heart that everything was all right. Was this hope? My mind questioned why I felt so calm, unafraid, and peaceful. My mind methodically turned over possibilities. I decided that I would not return to work if I had metastatic malignancy. I envisioned renovating our home to accommodate a wheelchair if I were not able to walk again. I considered chemotherapy and radiation and how difficult it would be for me to come into the clinic where I work to be treated by colleagues.

I intuitively felt that this tumor had been in me for a long time. It was nothing new. I could live with it. Being a realist, I entertained the possibility that I might have a much shorter life because of it. I wept and grieved over all the unfinished business I had with my children.

The doctors focused on the bad news. Their task was to keep me in their reality. As my family doctor put it, "Helen, you know too much. We can't hide anything from you." Was it so bad that they would hide information from me to protect me?

I focused on being thankful for what I had. I felt strong mentally, physically, and spiritually. I gathered all the "hopelets" that came to me—the negative test results that found no malignancies; the opportunity to be mindful, to meditate, to pray; the loving, caring thoughts and prayers from family, friends, and colleagues. I was glad to be alive. I felt fortunate. I was in excellent hands and confident in the abilities of my care team, even though they despaired of my diagnosis. I did not let their despair affect my energy or touch my hope and inner peacefulness.

The tumor wrapped around my spine was removed along with pieces of my vertebrae. Two 6-inch titanium rods were screwed in place to support my spine. The pathology report was negative for malignant cells. My surgeon had been doubtful that the tumor was benign until the pathology report came back after surgery. Even then, my internist cautioned me that the tumor samples were undergoing further pathology review. I was warned that I was not "in the clear" yet and a malignancy might still be evident. I was not allowed to be hopeful.

I had good reason to be overwhelmed with despair and to feel hopeless. Most of the professionals around me were extremely negative and offered me no hope. Fortunately, my family doctor and one oncologist colleague were able to allow that I might *not* have cancer, as test results came back negative, one by one. I was eventually diagnosed with hemangioma, a benign tumor around my spine.

I had always encouraged patients to break their experiences down into small, manageable pieces. I would ask them to look not at the "big hope" (i.e., of being cured of disease) but instead to look at all the little "hopelets," at what exists and what one has. Now, I believe in this more than ever.

To flower, we need hope. Despair can wither our spirit and take up precious energy and time. Hoping can generate energy. It pulls us forward even when we are not always sure where we are going. It allows us to harvest the love and hope of others around us. It makes healing possible in the best sense—in our spirits, in our minds and, perhaps, in our bodies.

We must allow individuals in overwhelming circumstances to gather up their "hopelets," allowing each drop to collect into a pool of inner strength and peacefulness. Ronne Jevne says, "Hope is about possibility, not probability." In the realm of our spirituality and mindfulness, each step of the way that hope leads us, leads us through the path of finding ourselves.

Assessment Questions

• Has anyone else in your family had this illness? What was their experience like?

• What news were you expecting the doctor to give you today?

• When you've had very bad news in the past, how did you cope?

Clarify what patients understand about their diagnosis. It is important to use clear language and to correct any misconceptions or perceptions that will hinder understanding. Patients may have been given too little or too much information or simply been unable to hear what was said. Patients often remember nonverbal behaviors more than the words used.

> *"You mentioned that Dr. Crane looked very uncomfortable during your meeting but you're still not clear what she was telling you. In my experience, people usually come to the cancer clinic for three reasons. They are seeking a cure, they need treatments to control their disease, or they need treatments to treat the symptoms. Which group do you think you fit into right now? Can you tell me why that is?"*

Address practical concerns such as arranging transportation home, notifying family, or assigning a supportive volunteer. Patients may be disoriented and need someone to help them make decisions.

"Sandra, I understand you drove yourself to this appointment. I imagine it would be very hard to drive home again. Who could I call to pick you up?"

Offer quiet, calm time. Patients may need time to collect their thoughts and begin to deal with their feelings about the diagnosis.

"I wonder if you'd like to sit in my office for a minute and I could ask someone to bring you a cup of tea. Would you prefer that I stay with you until your sister arrives, or would you like to have some time alone?"

Explore patients' feelings about their diagnosis and hearing this bad news. This will provide an opportunity to acknowledge and normalize their reactions, and help you understand their concerns and coping strategies more clearly.

"I understand that Dr. Irwin just told you that there is a tumor on your lung. It must be hard for you to put things into words right now, but can you tell me how you are feeling?"

Encourage parents to give children in the family information about the diagnosis and/or treatment. Honest information, given in age-appropriate language, helps children understand what is happening in the family. It opens the door for ongoing conversations about what they are seeing and feeling.

"Although you may not be ready to tell your son everything about ALS, it will be helpful if he has some basic information about the cause of this disease and treatments you are going to have over the next months. Without accurate information, children often invent their own stories about the cause and outcome of an illness. What might you want to tell him now? Later?"

Fear and Powerlessness

When Jan received her diagnosis, she became distressed and highly anxious. The more information she received about the disease, the treatment options, and unclear prognosis, the more agitated and fearful she felt. Jan became immobilized and was unable to process the information or make any decisions. A successful problem solver all of her life, she was unable to tackle or solve this problem. Fear gripped her spirit; she was in deep despair and felt no hope.

Although people dread hearing bad news, they usually prefer to know what's wrong as soon as possible. Receiving the diagnosis marks a critical transition at which people begin to have a tangible sense of what lies ahead. The disease is now a certainty and becomes part of their lives. Once this news sinks in, treatment options and prognoses loom in the future. Something is answered, but many questions linger. Patients and families begin to see what is possible and what to expect, while realizing this illness may or may not have a predictable path. Many people sense they are generally quite powerless to alter the outcome.

Feeling frightened and perhaps facing their own mortality for the first time, people may have a heightened sense of vulnerability and impermanence. Trying to rationalize or make sense of their situation, people may ask, "What did I do to deserve or cause this?" Fran Norris captured this feeling in her poem, "Why?" (at right).

WHY?

Why me?
If I hear one more person
Who dies of cancer
Quickly, cruelly and in their
   40's

I want to be different—
Arrogant, offensive even to
   state it
There is nothing that makes
   my situation
Deserving of better
Or worse

But then I say goodnite
To my sweet boy
I look at the moon with my
   husband
I know all the things I have
   left to do
And I hope, not me, not yet

I know the answer
To the question
Of "Why me?"
The answer for all of us is
"Why not me?" I seek to
   make use of this ordeal

   —(Fran Norris, 1997, p. 8)

Once decisions have been made about treatment, patients and families look ahead with trepidation. Although, treatment is dreaded, it is, at least, action in an untenable situation and a hopeful path to cure or remission. It offers a way to pull back from the farthest point in their future—death—and focus on the here and now. The present, however, is also fraught with challenges, fears, and feelings of great helplessness. Patients may fear side effects of the treatments: changes in body, self-image, and wholeness that leave them embarrassed and ashamed, feeling ugly and unloved. Along with this is a fear of loneliness and isolation that will come with their possible withdrawal from work or from social or daily activities.

Serious illness threatens the whole family and every member in it (Baider, Cooper, & De-Nour, 1995; Northouse, 1995). It disrupts their sense of continuity, threatens their hopes and ability to plan for the future, and produces feelings of helplessness and guilt. Treatment brings forward family members' feelings of powerlessness as, once again, they are unable to protect the patient from the consequences of terrible illness. Family members may have internal conflict "between their own fears and their desire to reassure the patient" (Sales, 1991, p. 5) and often don't let the patient know how the disease is affecting their lives. They fear they cannot sustain their support, energy, and optimism. They anticipate life without their loved one. To protect themselves and one another, people may withdraw into avoidance or silence (Kristjanson & Ashcroft, 1994). Alone in their thoughts, distanced from those who could support them, patients and family members fear the pain and sorrow that lies just beneath the surface.

Fearing that this may be as good as it gets, patients struggle to pick up some of the pieces of their previous life. Even for those individuals intent on cure, the reality of the disease is never far from their minds, and fear and anxiety will never return to "normal" pre-illness levels again. Life is now experienced in a new, less permanent, and uneasy kind of way. Nothing is ever quite the same as it once was.

Interventions

These psychosocial interventions have been designed to specifically address the key consideration *fear and powerlessness*. There are several assessment questions that will help open up a discussion, followed by more focused comments or tips that will facilitate further exploration of the issues that frequently arise at this time; each tip is followed by a sample dialogue.

Assessment Questions

- Tell me what concerns you the most right now.
- Are you the kind of person who feels optimistic about how things will turn out, or do you generally feel pessimistic? How do you know that?
- How do your family members communicate about their concerns and worries?
- Tell me about your strengths. What gets you through tough times?

Address fears of the unknown and provide the information that is available. When people are able to separate out those things that can be known (now or in the process of time) from those for which there is no answer, it helps patients and families focus their attention on that which can be changed or known.

> *"You have asked a lot of questions about what will happen to you. I want you to know that many of those questions can be answered. Perhaps we can figure out what you want to know today and which things can wait until*

a little later. Then we could decide together who could best answer your questions. What is most important to you now?"

Provide practical information and assistance with financial concerns such as income, food, shelter, insurance, and drug costs. Patients and families are often legitimately concerned about the financial impact of caregiving. It is important that they receive information about income assistance and security programs, available benefits, and charitable organizations to which they can gain access.

> *"I understand that you are very concerned about how you can take time off from work to look after your mother during her treatments. Sonya, have you talked to your employer to see what support is available through your job? I could help you find out what financial assistance you can apply for and go through the paperwork with you."*

"The general public has limited knowledge regarding the various forms of systemic therapy. Their knowledge is often derived from personal experiences and from the media, whose content may be outdated and/or dramatized. These limited sources of information coupled with society's fear of cancer have led to many negative attitudes, irrational fears, and misperceptions about cancer therapy among the general public and health care professionals alike [and] have led to several commonly held, but erroneous, beliefs. Emotional distress for individuals anticipating, receiving, or completing a course of therapy is often universal."

—(Knobf, Pasacreta, Valentine, & McCorkle, 1998, p. 277)

Create opportunities for emotional and spiritual support. These opportunities will shift patients' focus solely from the physical to include broader aspects of healing. This offers patients ways to take control and regain some of their power.

> *"Although you are naturally expecting to benefit from this treatment, what other things can you do for yourself? What might you do to increase your interest and energy for pleasurable activities? Where else in your life do you find strength and support?"*

Use metaphors that reflect the transitions being faced by patients and families. Metaphors from the natural world (e.g., weather, oceans, life cycles) and traveling (e.g., journey, roads, trains, ships) resonate with many people, and allow them to parallel their experience with something familiar and predictable.

"Sometimes this journey can seem like traveling a twisting, bumpy road that goes up hills and down into valleys. This is normal, Jose. If you keep an eye directly in front of you and stay on the road, you can focus on healing and the next leg of your journey. There are people who can help you anticipate the next hill or dip in the road, people who will travel alongside of you and interpret the signs."

Identify, develop, and practice strategies for coping with people's feelings of fear and powerlessness. Activities that affirm strengths, reduce stressors, or develop new skills help people face their fears and move forward with their lives. If people feel unable to re-engage, they may withdraw or give up trying.

"Sometimes it may be helpful to look at a situation one page at a time. Instead of looking at 40 or 50 pages spread out in front of you, think of them bound into a book that you can open whenever you choose. You may look at one page or one chapter at a time. There may be chapters that are familiar and helpful, and you may look at them often. Other chapters you may look at later or never open."

Making Critical Decisions

Jan decided to include Kathy and her brother James in every doctor's appointment and treatment decision. When she was overwhelmed, she missed important information and heard only negative or bad news. Now, on her behalf, Kathy and James ask questions, explore options, and remember what is said. Jan still becomes fearful and terrified at the thought of suffering and dying, but, with less clutter in her mind, she is now able to make the decisions that are important to her. This has also allowed her to focus on taking care of herself during surgery and follow-up treatments.

Once people have received news of their diagnosis, their first questions often relate to next steps. "Is there any treatment for this disease?" "What can you do to help me?"

Patients need to process information about their disease and its treatment and make decisions about treatment (Christ, 1991). This is no easy task. People are often initially overwhelmed with the enormity of what may lie ahead. They often have difficulty listening to and understanding what is being said. Although they are in no condition to make measured decisions, make decisions they must.

People seek information from many sources such as specialists, friends, books, and the Internet. Depending on the accuracy of the information, people can become knowledgeable very quickly. They may challenge options offered to them because they are familiar with treatments and alternative therapies available in other places. If the information is unreliable and inaccurate, people may have unrealistic expectations about their care or make poor decisions. If treatments are unavailable or prohibitively expensive locally, patients may feel angry and let down by their health care system.

Often family members and friends want to understand what is happening and what can be done (Kristjanson, 1989). Patients can be inundated by opinion and information about diets, herbs, vitamins, surgery, medications, and alternative approaches to care. Although well intended, this kind of frenetic activity and the volume of information often creates confusion for patients and conflict within families.

When physicians outline possible treatment options, discussing the risks and benefits of each, they will generally recommend one particular approach. The plan will vary from one person to the next depending on the extent of the illness, the resources of the community, standard or clinical treatment protocols, and the judgment of their physician. This is a critical juncture in decision-making. Patients must decide whether they will accept a particular treatment plan (see Table 2.2).

ACTIVITIES TO COUNTER FEAR AND POWERLESSNESS

- Use affirmations such as scripture, sayings, poems, prayers, or statements that are meaningful to the person.
- Focus on healing activities that enhance well-being in the body (e.g., eating well, resting, paying attention to physical needs, using healing imagery).
- Encourage books that focus on positive or uplifting thoughts and activities that reinforce competence.
- Explore spirituality or religious beliefs through reading, reflection, or guidance from a religious leader or mentor.
- Use relaxation, guided imagery, nature, or music to calm or center the person.
- Encourage in normal or usual activities as possible.
- Enlist the support and strength of others through prayers and supportive thoughts to sustain the person's emotional and spiritual well-being.

—Helen Wong, British Columbia Cancer Agency, Vancouver Island Centre

If patients decide not to accept conventional treatment, they must make additional important decisions. Will they seek a second or third opinion? Will they explore alternative or complementary approaches? Will they look for a compromise? Will they reject everything that is being offered to them and choose no treatment at all?

Table 2.2.   Factors that influence patients' decision making through diagnosis and treatment

Factors	Example
Culture	Belief that only medical people or certain family members make decisions
Fatalism	If you speak of something, it will happen; death will happen regardless of decisions
Religion	Strict guidelines that direct choices such as no transfusions or medication
Coping skills	Problem-solving ability, dependency issues, adaptability, stress hardiness
Past experiences	Good or bad decisions, encounters with health care systems and professionals, illness
Personal characteristics	Age, frailty, gender, education
Current support and information	Family, health care providers, Internet, other patients

Patients refuse treatments for a number of reasons, such as a desire for quality time, a fear of side effects, or strongly held beliefs about life and death. Regardless, patients likely will be challenged to reconsider their positions. Family members and the health care team may be shocked and disappointed with a refusal to be treated. They may think that the patient is giving up or simply making a really bad decision. They may be concerned that those offering patients natural or nonconventional remedies are misleading them.

FOCUS ON: THE IMPACT OF EXPECTATIONS

A young woman was diagnosed with a treatable cervical cancer. Her physician offered her the usual course of treatment, but she refused. She said she did not want to "poison her body" in order to kill the cancer and did not consider the long-term possibility of cure worth the short-term cost. The medical team placed considerable pressure on her to agree to chemotherapy. They felt confused and angry about her continued refusal and found it hard to talk with her about her ongoing symptoms and medical problems. Family members eventually gave up trying to change her mind. They withdrew from her emotionally and could no longer talk about her disease or dying.

People have expectations—of themselves and others. During diagnosis and treatment, patients are surrounded by the expectations of health care providers, families, friends, and the broader community. When expectations match, there is a sense of harmony and common purpose. When something unexpected happens, however, this congruence is easily lost. Difficulties occur, and patient support is compromised (Baider, Cooper, & De-Nour, 1995).

The idea that patients will seek treatment within the framework of conventional medicine and, conversely, that this will be offered to them is generally assumed. Similarly, it is expected that patients will accept that treatment. This does not always happen, however. People may refuse treatment altogether or delay it until a future date. They may accept some treatments, but not others. They may wish to combine mainstream medicine with alternative or complementary approaches.

People make these decisions for a number of reasons. They might have been influenced by what they have heard and read, or by personal factors such as age, religious beliefs, or cultural values. They may be fearful of drugs and invasive treatments or believe that one therapy offers them a greater chance of cure than another. They may have been misled about the benefits of a particular treatment. They may believe that the side effects of treatment are not worth the benefits predicted.

Families usually expect patients to do everything they can to fight the disease, even when that may no longer be realistic. There can be conflicting ideas about what "fighting the disease" or not "giving up" means. When such conflicts occur, they create a tension in the relationship between patient and family. The result may be negative judgments, withdrawal, and feelings of betrayal for both sides.

When treatments end, family and friends often assume that patients will get back to normal routines and activities. They want to return to life as it was before the diagnosis. Perhaps driven by a need to stop worrying about the patient or to protect themselves from their own fears and vulnerability, these other people do not want to hear about life, for example, with cancer or multiple sclerosis. The permanent impact that life-threatening illness and treatment have on a patient's psyche is seldom acknowledged or expected. Certain short- and long-term effects leave people physically and emotionally changed. Patients may be unwell and chronically tired. Having faced fear, uncertainty, and death, people have a new perspective on life and what's important. They are forever changed and life will never be as it was before diagnosis.

Finally, it may be the disease that fails to match people's expectations. Treatments are offered and accepted, but the cure or remission that is predicted does not occur. Helplessness and confusion are felt by everyone involved, as they try to understand what went wrong, what they missed, or what else they could have done to prevent this.

Interventions

These psychosocial interventions have been designed to specifically address the key consideration *making critical decisions*. There are several assessment questions that will help open up a discussion, followed by more focused comments or tips that will facilitate further exploration of the issues that frequently arise at this time; each tip is followed by a sample dialogue.

Assessment Questions

- Have you had to make decisions under stressful circumstances in the past? Can you tell me how you did that?

- What kinds of things help you make good decisions? With whom can you talk things over?

- How are decisions made in your family? Who is involved in these kinds of decisions?

Help patients strategize about decision making. When they have information and understand the implications of their choices, they can make better decisions.

> *"You've been given a great deal of information about treatment options that are available to you. There are pros and cons to each approach. Nathan, are there other things you need to know or consider before you can make a decision? How will you go about making this decision?"*

Identify beliefs, wishes, and coping styles related to decision making. It is important that everyone knows how a person approaches decision making so that cultural, religious, or family beliefs and traditions can be supported and honored.

> *"It helps our team support you if we understand how you want to approach making decisions. How much information do you wish to receive about your treatments? Do you wish someone else were included in your decision-making? What else is important to you at this time?"*

Create a sense of time and space for decision making to help patients cope with the sense of urgency that often follows diagnosis. People need time to process what is happening to them.

> *"Susan and Ted, you have been given a lot information today, and I can imagine you might feel overwhelmed by it all. Would it be helpful for us to go over the main points again, so that you make sure you understand it all? Even though you may feel rushed, you don't have to make any deci-*

sions right now. Sometimes people need a little time to go away and think things through. It may be helpful to get a second opinion or make another appointment with Dr. Bruce to ask any questions you have."

Normalize different perspectives, concerns, and styles through information and open discussion. When families understand patients' needs and wishes, they are more able to follow and respect them.

> *"Everyone in your family is having a different reaction to Mary's diagnosis because you are different people with different ways of coping. Each of you is traveling along a road that began with your daughter's diagnosis of heart disease, and, while those roads may be parallel, they are separate and unique to each of you. Would it be helpful to ask Mary what is most important to her right now and talk about ways to support her?"*

Offer support for whatever decisions patients make. This includes those decisions that contradict medical advice. They may feel judged or pressured to reconsider. It is important that people know that they can change their minds about treatment in the future, although what will still be possible depends on the stage of the disease.

> *"I know this has been a difficult decision for you to make, and you may wonder if you did the right thing. What would be helpful at this time? What would be helpful in the future? How would it be for you down the road if you changed your mind but the treatment is no longer possible?"*

Dealing with the Impact of Treatments

Jan is still uncertain whether the side effects of surgery or other aggressive therapies would be worth it. She wonders how Kathy will manage the dual role of caregiver and schoolteacher. Despite these concerns she still wants to do everything she can to live, and Kathy and James want her to have the operation.

Whatever challenges treatment brings, this is still a time for reasonable optimism and hope. In fact, this is the best time for those diagnosed with a serious illness. Most patients still have good strength and energy. Their disease is at an early stage. Treatment may bring about significant improvement in both symptoms and control of disease and even the possibility of cure.

Both the disease and its treatment have major physical, emotional, social, and spiritual impacts, however. Everyone will feel vulnerable and forever changed. The short-term effects of undergoing treatment often leave people feeling debilitated, fatigued, and vulnerable. These effects will vary widely depending on the type of disease. For example, with congestive heart failure the use of diuretics and digoxin/ACE inhibitors usually result in immediate improvement with minimal side effects. With cancer, the patient may require surgery plus extensive chemotherapy. Regardless of disease, people feel anxious about treatment and its outcome, hoping that it all will be worthwhile.

Treatment may mean leaving home and taking time off from work. It can result in sleepless nights and missed family dinners. Families must find ways to adapt their preexisting lifestyle to what will work with this situation. This is a time of change for everyone: routines, responsibilities, and relationships must alter in order to accommodate treatment and illness (Kristjanson & Ashcroft, 1994). Many people willingly endure this upheaval because they are determined to fight the disease and overcome this invasion in their lives.

Studies show that patients facing surgery experience additional stress beyond that which normally accompanies a life-threatening diagnosis. They often feel extremely vulnerable, facing separation from home and family or even fearing death under anesthesia. Hospitalization can be difficult for families as they travel back and forth, wanting to be with the patient while maintaining routines at home. Furthermore, they are often expected to assist with the patient's meals, grooming, or baths and find themselves advocating on the patient's behalf for information and timely medications (Jacobsen, Roth, & Holland, 1998).

Patients and families will struggle with the various side effects of treatments. The following list suggests some ways health care providers can help people cope with and adjust to the huge impact treatment has on their lives. It includes practical ways to control physical side effects, supportive strategies to facilitate the rebuilding of self-esteem, and arrangements that can improve family life (Christ, 1991).

Develop ways to control side effects.

- Get information in advance and prepare for the side effects.
- Learn practical ways to cope (e.g., diet, wigs, ways to improve appearance, relaxation and visualization techniques, equipment to aid daily living).

Cope with ambivalence about treatment that is caused by its negative aspects, such as physical symptoms and lifestyle changes.

- Acknowledge and express ambivalence.

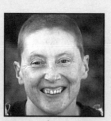

Mairi Scanlan, B.S.W., is a counselor with Victoria Hospice Society.

In My Own Voice
Bald Truths

Mairi Scanlan

It is a fact. If you choose to receive the vicious and vital combination of drugs to combat your breast cancer, you will lose your hair.

It is a fact. It will fall out in bits. When it is very, very short—less than a quarter inch long—those bits fall less noticeably. I was in a juice bar with Susan the day mine started coming out, having a smoothie and a burrito. I was thinking, "Chemo ain't so bad," liking the way my red hair was shaved so close to my head it was golden! "Hey," I said, tugging on the tiny strands, "It's coming out!" She made me stop yanking out little pinches full of hair, citing hygiene. They were amazing and tiny in the palm of my hand; the type and length that guys like to leave, upon shaving, in the sink.

It is a fact. I loved being bald. For the first 3 months, I was damn proud to wear my head outside. It is also a fact that my "community" respects and celebrates baldness. (Lesbians. We're lesbians.)

And it is another fact that—thanks Mom, Dad—I have a nicely shaped head. There were no heretofore hidden birthmarks, no flat bit, no phrenological phenomena. Just a nice round head. White, though. I mean really white. My head, when bald, is a glowing orb, the Irish phosphorescent skin gleaming in the sun. And in the rain. Possibly in the dark.

I offer the following: Shave your hair close before you lose it. Baldness can be camouflaged in many stunning ways, say turbans, and celebrated thus. Baldness can be accentuated in many other ways, like temporary tattoos, and celebrated thus. (In all cases, avoid the oversize baseball cap.) But when your hair goes, the loss is deep. It becomes painfully profound when you wake to a hank of hair on the pillow, or stand in the shower, crying softly, watching it wash into the drain.

It is a fact that what we choose to do with being bald is forever linked to what we believe about ourselves, about being a woman, about the place of hair in the display of our being. It is no shame, nor crime nor insult nor particular misery to be bald. It is often others who struggle with your baldness more. The husband who finds you briefly exotic, then lastingly strange. The partner who doesn't want to make a big deal of it, but says, with longing, "I miss your hair." The children who are frightened—in fact, they are the only people I consistently covered up for. Except baby Laurel who was as bald as me.

Feeling the sun on my head for the first time in the memory of my life was a magnificent experience; I was vibrating with pleasure. My head! In the sun! Without sunscreen! It is a fact. Skin that has never seen the light of day will burn faster than chicken under the grill.

I bought hats. People made me hats. There was a little striped acrylic number—my chemo hat. Or the itchy, yet stylin' green wool one. I still wear that hat. It is a fact. Your head will be cold.

As the drugs do their manifestly cruel and crucial job of destroying cells—indiscriminately—you will feel seriously unwell. There are drugs for this. Find out about them.

It is also a fact that hair, once fallen out, does not stay *uniformly* fallen out. IT GROWS BACK. Not a lot. Nothing you could comb or anything. Yet, softly, a fuzz appears across the dome of your thoughts, a scree of hair at the precipice of your ears, a cluster of distinguishable strands curl on the slope of your neck.

It is a fact. This looks terrible. My favorite hair, of all the hairs—and they are THAT individual—grew from just above my ear, straight out, an inch long. One day I was bald, the next, poof—a giant hair! There is an item on the market. Purchase it now. It is a swivel-head razor, designed to shave heads, and it comes in cool primary colors. It is a fact. Shaving your own head is both empowering and difficult; these states of being complement and reinforce each other. Have a friend or lover do it if you trust that person. Husbands, brothers, and boyfriends are a good bet because they have experience. Remember that all of them—women, men, lovers, friends, siblings and, cousins—are often bereft by your loss of hair, and may cry. Most of them will demonstrate this by flinging the razor into the sink and proclaiming shaving a "stupid %#&# idea!" Trust me, they're crying.

- Seek the support of others along with practical assistance (e.g., wigs, sex, mobility).

- Develop coping strategies (e.g., relaxation and meditation techniques, focusing on long-term benefits).

Rebuild self-esteem in the face of side effects such as fatigue, hair and weight loss, loss of mobility and/or body parts, and so forth.

- Address losses and begin to grieve them.

- Adjust life and appearance to compensate for these.

- Focus on the positive and humorous.

Accommodate the demands and effects of treatment into personal and family life and stay connected with normal life.

- Seek practical support with household tasks, family responsibilities (e.g., errands, child care, transportation).

- Plan "normal life" activities for well times (e.g., time with friends, work, gardening).

- Identify the anticipated improvements that may occur, hope for the best possible outcome.

- Identify personal strengths that may assist general well-being.

(From Christ, G. [1991]. A model for the development of psychosocial interventions. In *Recent Results in Cancer Research* [Vol. 2, p. 306]. Berlin: Springer Verlag; adapted by permission.)

Interventions

These psychosocial interventions have been designed to specifically address the key consideration *dealing with the impact of treatments*. There are several assessment questions that will help open up a discussion, followed by more focused comments or tips that will facilitate further exploration of the issues that frequently arise at this time; each tip is followed by a sample dialogue.

Assessment Questions

- What are you hopeful about? What helps you to be hopeful?

- What side effects are you expecting with this treatment? What are your concerns about this kind of treatment?

- What are you finding most difficult about your chemotherapy treatments?

- What will help you manage right now?

- Tell me how you will juggle your job, young children, and having your spouse in the hospital, all at the same time?

Offer opportunities to speak with others who have undergone similar diagnoses and treatments. Peer support is a powerful tool that gives patients credible information about what to expect and what helps.

"Often, it is very helpful to talk to other people who have the same illness. They can tell you about their experiences and offer tips about how to deal with things like hair and weight loss, nausea, and other side effects of treatment. Jessica, would you like someone to call you with more information?"

Teach skills such as relaxation and visualization to enhance patients' ability to cope with the side effects of treatments. These techniques are useful in managing stress prior to and during appointments, as well as reducing the impact of physical symptoms.

"Our experience has shown us that certain kinds of breathing exercises can help you stay calm during stressful situations. Would it be helpful if I show you some simple exercises that you can practice at home? Then you will be able to relax yourself when you go for your first treatment."

Identify concerns patients and families have about care and treatment, and support discussion of these. Acknowledging issues in a non-defensive way can help people identify their underlying concerns. It is then possible to reframe or strategize how to address these issues in ways that fit for them.

"I understand that it is very difficult for you when your treatments are scheduled five days a week and you want to travel home before dark on Friday afternoons so you can prepare for your Sabbath. How could we accommodate you in planning your schedule?"

Help the patient and family to understand one another's experience of treatment, and to communicate with one another. It is helpful to clarify the similarities and differences, looking for ways that everyone can feel supported.

"You mentioned it is very hard for you to work shifts and take care of the children. I know you are concerned that your wife isn't able to look after

them and she thinks it will be some time before she can manage. What are your concerns about this? What would help you share your frustration with your wife? What would help you look for solutions?"

Create opportunities for patients to discuss how their treatments are going. They may wish to modify or stop treatments, but may not realize they have a choice. Even if they decide to continue, this discussion will help them be clear about what they really want to do.

"It sounds like you have a number of concerns about your treatments and you say you might want to stop them. What do you think would happen if you stopped this medication? What other options do you think you have? What might help you discuss this with your specialist?"

Clarify patients' hopes, identify their inner strengths. Build on these in order to support positive energy, a sense of well-being, and a spirit of optimism.

"Tell me more about your hopes at this time. What will help you to achieve them? Are there other things that may bring added strength and energy to you? Is there any way that I can help you in this journey?"

OUR EXPERIENCE

SUPPORT GROUPS FOR PATIENTS

Groups "designed for people with cancer may very well be the most powerful psychosocial intervention available for the vast majority of patients [and] can garner the emotional support of persons with similar experiences and use the experiences of others to buffer the fear of future unknowns" (Spira, 1998, p. 701).

Depending on the stage of the illness and the therapeutic intention of the intervention, the most effective groups use one or a combination of the following approaches:

Providing information

• Lecture format with discussions about prevention, diseases, and treatments

Cognitive-behavioral therapy

• Training in coping skills
• Combination of information (stress or communication strategies) and practice (trying the skills being taught)

Social/emotional supportive therapy

• Exploring issues related to the disease
• Open-ended opportunities to acknowledge and express concerns and emotions

As health care professionals, we have considerable opportunity and experience working with people as they start the journey that begins with the diagnosis of a life-threatening illness. Diagnosis and treatment mark the first time we meet patients and their families. During this transition our goal is to help patients and families deal with this life-altering diagnosis, understand an unfamiliar environment, and make the best decisions possible. We want to optimize what we have to offer as well as the strengths patients and families bring.

We find that families can be more optimistic than patients, and tend to concentrate on cure or remission and the success of treatment. Although patients focus initially on the worst possible outcome, most of them quickly shift their focus from the harsh possibility of death to an instinctive drive to overcome the disease. These patients will often do better emotionally and physically than those who continue to feel overwhelmed and helpless with the enormity of what they are facing. People with a positive attitude and the belief that they can get better will have lower levels of distress. This, in turn, increases physical, emotional, and spiritual well-being (Spira, 1998). We want to acknowledge both optimism and pessimism as normal to help patients and families understand and support one another through the confusion and intensity of this transition.

We see patients who are overwhelmed and need people and places that are safe and reliable. They are frightened, yet ready for a fight. We look for ways to build on their life successes and strengths and help them move through the challenges that face them. We want to know who they are and what is important to them. Do they have particular beliefs or traditions that might affect their care? How do they normally deal with crises and illness? As health care providers, we know it is important to develop relationships that are respectful, calm, and hopeful. These relationships offer people a place to speak the unspeakable, to ask the unaskable, to share tender hopes, and to express deep sorrow and fear.

We help people sift through information about their disease, prognosis, and treatment options. We encourage them to explore options and alternatives and to make the best decisions possible. We talk about how to manage the physical and emotional upheaval that occurs at this time and how to navigate our system. We may need to address the limitations or realities of what medicine, or our particular organization, can do.

TEAM ISSUES

Health care providers can forget that patients and families know themselves best. Expectations about patients—or their diseases, or stress, or heavy workloads—can cause providers to lose sight of the person. As a result, it is easy to impose professional experience, views, and therapies on patients rather than explore their experience and insights and uncover what they need at this time. If health care providers do not examine their assumptions, they may provide unwanted care to families and then become irritated and confused by these families' perceived non-compliance.

Attitude, fear, or lack of skills may lead some professionals to operate in a one-way fashion—information is given in a particular way, assumptions are made, conclusions are drawn, questions are discouraged, and further opinions are not sought. This approach leaves little room for additional support and may prevent patients from gaining access to other disciplines (e.g., occupational therapy, physical therapy) and the services that they offer.

Breaking bad news is difficult at the best of times. When it is broken "badly," it affects not only the patient, but also the entire team. Some physicians, trying to be gentle, speak in such a vague manner that patients hear hope when none exists. At the other end of the spectrum, there are those whose bluntness causes additional stress, erodes whatever hope may be present, and damages the relationship with the physician and possibly the team. These situations can cause rifts within the team that, if left unresolved, will undermine trust and collaboration. Both approaches leave someone else to "pick up the pieces" and to guide patients and families to hear the message more accurately and have opportunities to deal with the news and strategize what happens next.

ABOUT CHILDREN

Children and teens are rarely present when someone in their family receives a diagnosis of life-threatening illness. Nor are they usually present during treatments, doctor's appointments, or meetings with other health care providers. What they are told about the illness will depend on what their informants know, how much information these people believe children should be given, and how comfortable they are giving this information. What children assume, or think they know, will be further influenced by how the information is given and how they interpret what is said.

Many adults hesitate over giving information to children and teens because they do not want them to worry, they believe children won't understand, or they are not comfortable talking about such a difficult subject. Adults may feel so shocked and overwhelmed by the news that they aren't able to talk about it. They may feel distracted by the emerging decisions and tasks that come with the diagnosis of a serious illness. They may believe that everyone must remain positive and hopeful of a miracle.

Whatever children are told, they will be hugely affected by the diagnosis and what lies ahead. They will see the side effects of treatments and the changes in family roles and activities. They will hear conversations about the illness. They will be aware of the stress, grief, fear, and powerlessness of the adults in their lives. They will notice how others behave differently toward the patient and to themselves.

It is important that children feel included and informed about what is happening in their family. Sometimes, parents do not realize how much information their children have gathered, or how accurate it is. Children will rely on their imagination or past experiences; including television programs, movies, or friend's stories, to fill in missing details. Support and appropriate information are crucial to how children will deal with diagnosis, recurrence, and chronic illness.

Key Points

Children and teen's reactions to diagnosis and recurrence will reflect the reactions of the adults around them. They will also be influenced by the information they are given and their level of understanding about the significance of the diagnosis or recurrence.

Children and teens will likely be more affected by what is happening in their daily lives than by what is anticipated or feared in the future. Changing routines and responsibilities, family stress, and the side effects of treatments experienced by the patient may disrupt their personal world in ways that create a sense of loss and chaos that needs to be addressed.

Children and teens are better able to understand and integrate the meaning of life-threatening illness when they are included in illness-related discussions and activities, encouraged to ask questions, and given information in age-appropriate language and manageable amounts.

Interventions

These psychosocial interventions have been specifically designed to address the needs of children. There are focused comments or tips that will facilitate further exploration of the issues that frequently arise at this time; each tip is followed by a sample dialogue.

Find out what children believe about the cause, treatments, and expected progression of the illness. Identify and help parents address any misconceptions or gaps in their understanding.

"Max, I know that your mom has a serious illness called multiple sclerosis. What do you know about this disease? What else would you like your mom and dad to tell you about it?"

Ask children and teens how this illness is affecting their lives and whether they have any solutions in mind. This helps families talk about the issues and, perhaps, adjust their routines or expectations to accommodate children's needs.

"What is the hardest thing about your sister being sick? How do you feel about that? How do you think your mom might help you and still give Kayelene the care she needs?"

Encourage families to include children and teens, where appropriate, in illness-related planning, discussions, and activities. Things that are known and familiar tend to be less confusing and frightening. Children need to have a balance between being involved with the ill person's life and maintaining their usual activities and normal childhood experiences.

"Alfonse, you are wondering what they're going to do to your aunt. I have a book that explains cancer treatments that you and your grandma could read together. Then you could ask us any questions you still have. I know you usually play with your friend at this time. Would you like to talk now or go outside now and talk later?"

SUMMARY

Diagnosis marks the beginning (see Table 2.3) of people's journey through illness, treatments, dying, death, and bereavement. Regardless of the outcome, these people's lives will never be the same again. Patients and families are catapulted into the health care system, perhaps for the first time. Once diagnosed with a life-threatening illness, they become involved in the world of treatment and disease. Soon, they are making decisions about the direction of their care and, in the midst of all of this, they are faced with the truth that they can and likely will die from this disease. With this reality, patients and families struggle to find a way to cope and function for the rest of their lives.

This journey can be a frightening, arduous, and overwhelming one. Yet, at the same time, people's lives can be enriched, creative, and meaningful. The road

Table 2.3.   Palliative Performance Scale (PPSv2) 100%–90%

PPS Level	Ambulation	Activity and evidence of disease	Self-care	Intake	Conscious level
100%	Full	Normal activity and work No evidence of disease	Full	Normal	Full
90%	Full	Normal activity and work Some evidence of disease	Full	Normal	Full

traveled is not uniform or straight. It has many rough spots and hazards that can surprise and jostle people as they try to navigate their way.

REFLECTIVE ACTIVITY

This simple reflection exercise can be used to help patients relax or as part of a visualization tailored to particular needs such as fear of treatment, feeling overwhelmed, or needing safety. The exercise is based on principles of guided imagery and relaxation and uses a scripted dialogue between a guide and listener that focuses on relaxation. It is recommended that each person involved alternate roles of guide and listener, either by using this script or expanding it to include a guided visualization for one of the above needs. For example, the guide could lead the listener to envision a place, known or imagined, where he or she can find strength and safety. Later, the roles would be reversed, then the pair could discuss the experience from the perspective of both guide and the listener. You may want to alter this script to include words that fit for you or a particular listener. It is important to maintain respect, choice, and safety throughout all guided exercises.

Many excellent books, recorded tapes, CDs, and web sites are available that offer information, guidance, and scripts for additional guided imagery, visualization, or relaxation exercises (see resources at the end of this chapter).

To begin, with your partner find a quiet spot to practice the following relaxation script. Soothing background music may help the listener feel at ease. Take your time going through the script and improvise as appropriate. Make sure your listener is comfortable, preferably in a reclining position. Have him or her loosen any constricting clothing, uncross legs and arms, and close his or her eyes if this feels comfortable. Once your listener is situated, allow your own body to sink deeply and comfortably in the chair/bed/floor that supports you. Notice how that feels. When you are comfortable, begin this script:

Focusing on the sound of my voice, allow all sounds in the background to fade away. Let the sounds of the room become dim and recede; they are not important.

Notice the coolness of the air in your nostrils. With each breath you take, you notice this coolness coming in, comforting and cool.

Feel the space between your brows soften with your breath. Your face relaxes, and any tightness or tension melts away with each easy breath, which takes no effort whatsoever.

Notice your breath, as its ease and comfort makes its way downward.

Like a cleansing wave of relaxation, it makes its way downward, flowing down your neck, and shoulders—let your shoulders soften and fall.

Your belly rises gently with your breath. No effort is required, your breath moves easily in and out.

Your mind is at ease; your mind is calm.

As you exhale, allow your breath to carry away any concerns, tensions, and blockages, releasing any tightness, thoughts, worries, memories. Let them go.

Allow yourself to rest in this safe, comfortable place, breathing in gently, deeply. Let your breath out with a sigh; you are safe, peaceful, at ease.

(At this point, the guide may insert a visualization or simply allow the listener to rest in silence or hear soothing music.)

Take in a deep breath and notice your body, the air around you, the sounds in the room; let your mind come back to this room, here, now, move your fingers and toes, your hands and feet. Stretch, move, open your eyes, feeling revitalized and refreshed.

RESOURCES

Web Sites

Canadian Association of Psychosocial Oncology
  www.cancercentre.com/CAPO
The Caregiver Network
  www.caregiver.on.ca
Journal of Psychosocial Oncology
  www.med.jhu.edu/cancerctr/ptfamsvc/jpo.htm
The National Institute of Arthritis and Musculoskeletal and Skin Diseases
  www.nih.gov/niams/healthinfo/lupusguide/chp6.htm
Relaxation/Guided Visualization Sites
  www.allthatwomenwant.com
  www.mcps.k12.md.us/departments/eap/visualization
  www.pages.zoom.co.uk/awake/Sense/Sagacity/relaxationexercises
  www.the-stress-site.com/Relaxation
  www.wholeperson.com/wpa/tr/30s/30s2toc

Books

Cunningham, A. (1992). *The healing journey: Overcoming the crises of cancer.* Toronto: Key Porter.

Holland, J. (Ed.). (1998). *Psychosocial oncology.* New York: Oxford University Press.

Holland, J., & Lewis, S. (2001). *The human side of cancer: Living with hope, coping with uncertainty.* New York: HarperCollins.

Kabat-Zinn, J. (1990). *Full catastrophe living: Using the wisdom of your body and mind to face stress, pain, and illness.* New York: Delacorte.

Kabat-Zinn, J. (1994). *Wherever you go, there you are: Mindfulness meditation in everyday life.* New York: Hyperion.

Miller, K. (2001). *The cancer poetry project: Poems by cancer patients and those who love them.* Minneapolis, MN: Fairview Press.

Mitchell, S. (1991). *The enlightened mind.* New York: HarperCollins.

Ontario Cancer Institute. (1997). *Skills for healing workbook.* Toronto: Princess Margaret Hospital.

Rosenberg, L. (1998). *Breath by breath: The liberating practice of insight meditation.* Boston: Shambhala.

Santorelli, S. (1999). *Heal thy self: Lessons on mindfulness in medicine.* New York: Bell Tower.

Thich, N.H. (1994). *The blooming of a lotus: Guided meditation exercises for healing and transformation.* Boston: Beacon Press.

Waxler-Morrison, N., Anderson, J., & Richardson, E. (1990). *Cross-cultural caring.* Vancouver: University of British Columbia Press.

Articles

Altilio, T. (2001). Learning from Liza. *Journal of Pain and Symptom Management, 21*(3), 251–253.

REFERENCES

Baider, L., Cooper, C., & De-Nour, A. (1995). *Cancer and the family.* New York: John Wiley & Sons.

Christ, G. (1991). A model for the development of psychosocial interventions. In *Recent Results in Cancer Research* (Vol. 2, p. 306). Berlin: Springer-Verlag.

Cotter, A. (1999). *From this moment on: A guide for those recently diagnosed with cancer.* New York: Random House.

Jacobsen, P., Roth, A., & Holland, J. (1998). Surgery. In J.C. Holland (Ed.), *Psycho-Oncology* (pp. 257–268). New York: Oxford Press.

Kash, K., & Lerman, C. (1998). Psychological, social and ethical issues in gene testing. In J.C. Holland (Ed.), *Psycho-Oncology* (pp. 196–207). New York: Oxford University Press.

Knobf, M., Pasacreta, J., Valentine, A., & McCorkle, R. (1998). Chemotherapy, hormonal therapy and immunotherapy. In J.C. Holland (Ed.), *Psycho-Oncology* (pp. 277–288). New York: Oxford Press.

Kristjanson, L. (1989). Quality of terminal care: Salient indicators identified by families. *Journal of Palliative Care, 5,* 21–30.

Kristjanson, L., & Ashcroft, T. (1994). The family's cancer journey: A literature review. *Cancer Nursing, 17*(1), 1–17.

Lederberg, M. (1998). The family of the cancer patient. In J.C. Holland (Ed.), *Psycho-Oncology* (pp. 981–993). New York: Oxford Press.

Norris, F. (1997). *A voice to be heard ... about breast cancer.* Victoria, British Columbia, Canada: Trafford Publishing.

Northouse, L. (1995). The impact of cancer in women on the family. *Cancer Practitioner, 3*(3), 134–142.

Sales, E. (1991). Psychosocial impact of the phase of cancer on the family: An updated review. *Journal of Psychosocial Oncology, 9*(4), 1–19.

Spira, J. (1998). Group therapies. In J.C. Holland (Ed.), *Psycho-Oncology* (pp. 701–716). New York: Oxford Press.

Weisman, A. (1979). A model for psychosocial phasing in cancer. *General Hospital Psychiatry, 1,* 187–195.

PSYCHOSOCIAL ASSESSMENT

"Having assessed the damage, social workers need to ensure that the diagnosis does not become a cornerstone of identity. Whatever else symptoms are, they may also be a sign of the soul's struggle to be alive, responsible, and involved. Care of the soul is a continuous process that concerns itself not so much with 'fixing' a central flaw as with attending to the small details of everyday life."—Moore, 1992, pp. 3–4

In psychosocial assessments, it is the person, not his or her illness, who comes first. Patients are much more than their diagnosis or prognosis. An individual has an identity within his or her family, culture, and community that supersedes one's identity as an ill or dying person. Patients and their families come to this point in their lives with preexisting expectations, needs, and beliefs. They bring with them an incredible store of knowledge, strengths, and abilities.

If care of people who are dying and bereaved is to be holistic, then assessment, planning, and interventions must include spiritual, psychological, social, emotional, physical, and practical components (Byock, 1997). The environment must support spiritual questioning and reflection, acknowledge family strengths or struggles, value cultural differences, and address caregiving needs.

A psychosocial perspective recognizes that there is a wide spectrum of normal healthy reactions to illness, death, and bereavement. Patients and families are respected as equals and their differences are acknowledged, honored, and appreciated. People are supported according to their abilities and strengths. Psychosocial assessment is guided by genuine compassion for others and faith in both the resilience of the human spirit and the potential for personal growth.

> *"For helpers, the goal may be not the heroic cure but rather the constancy of caring and connection and collaborative work toward improving the quality of day-to-day living."* —Saleebey, 1996, p. 303

Assessment and care based on human strengths honor two things: "the power of the self to heal and right itself with the help of the environment, and the need for an alliance with the hope that life might really be otherwise" (Saleebey, 1996, p. 303). The emphasis of interactions is on what is possible and desirable, rather than on what is wrong, missing, or abnormal. This approach does not assume health care providers know what people understand or need. Helpers can avoid putting labels or diagnoses on people's circumstances and, instead, recognize them as the experts on themselves. This perspective keeps the possibility of choice, control, and growth open. "The power to name oneself and one's situation and condition is the beginning of real empowerment" (p. 303).

WHY IS IT IMPORTANT TO DO PSYCHOSOCIAL ASSESSMENTS?

"Tools are for the sake of the workers, not necessarily the clients" (Price, 2001, p. 246). If the tool or framework is relevant, however, to the needs and interests of those clients (or patients and families), then it may be of considerable benefit. The remainder of this section highlights a number of the benefits in using a framework or guide to assess psychosocial needs and concerns. It examines these benefits from the perspective of patients and families, as well as the health care providers.

Psychosocial assessments provide health care workers with

- A core of standardized reference information regarding patients and families that is retrievable, comprehensive, and relevant

- A sense of the individual's values, experiences, emotions, thoughts, actions, and personality (Price, 2001)

- A picture of how patients and families see themselves, in the broader context of their particular communities

- An understanding of the strengths and struggles of patients and families from their perspective

- An opportunity to identify disadvantages, complications, or risks for patients and families

- A basis for determining patients' and families' current needs and issues

- A backdrop against which to understand new issues, concerns, or needs as they arise

- Support for clinical decisions regarding interventions (e.g., care planning, grief counseling, education)

- Clarity in determining priorities and how to meet needs with available resources

- Formal ways to measure impacts of therapies or supportive interventions from a quality improvement or research perspective

Psychosocial assessments give patients and families

- Opportunities to tell their stories

- Time to name their circumstances, struggles, and experiences themselves

- A place within the caregiving team and a voice in decision making

- Clarity about their strengths and abilities

- Opportunities to identify and build on their own resources: talents, knowledge, motivation, and community support

- Ways to communicate openly and face current issues of living and dying

WHAT SHOULD PSYCHOSOCIAL ASSESSMENTS INCLUDE?

Health care providers want to know about people's strengths and qualities; things that may complicate their ability to cope; people's approach to illness, death, or bereavement; and what help they require at this time. In order to understand people's resilience and their ability to adjust to difficult situations, assessments should consider past competence, adversities already faced, personal assets, perceptions of support, and individual definitions of stressful situations (Masten, 1994).

To help health care providers as they gather information and acquaint themselves with patients and families, the following assessment questions are organized into four categories: general questions, questions that are focused on strengths and on risks, and questions that address practical needs.

General Assessment Questions

- Who are the individuals in this family? How is this disease/death affecting their daily living and relationships?

- How do family members communicate with each other? With others?

- What do they believe about their illness/their bereavement? About death?

- What is most important to them now and as they look ahead?

- What do they most fear about dying, death, and bereavement?

Strengths-Focused Questions

- How do people describe themselves, their strengths, and capabilities?

- What is working well?

- What coping strategies have helped them manage loss or stress in the past?

- What meaning do they make of this experience? What beliefs and values sustain them? Where do their souls find nutrition and sustenance?

- How is the family managing together? What is working well? What is difficult?

- How are they managing ongoing health and safety issues?

- What do they find to be supportive at this time?

Risks-Focused Questions

- How do people assess their risk? What is worrying or distressing them?

- Do they have unresolved past losses, multiple losses, or concurrent life issues?

- Are there taboos, pressures, or cultural issues at play? Is empowerment an issue?

- Within the family, are there complex relationships, conflicts, or difficult circumstances (e.g., living situation, child with special needs)?

- Is there a history of addiction, abuse, or mental health problems?

- Do people feel connected to others spiritually, socially, or emotionally? Do their lives have meaning? Do they have hope?

Practical Needs Questions

- What practical assistance do people need now or in the future?

- What help do people need with care planning, finances, estate business, funeral arrangements, decision making, or living arrangements?

- Do people need assistance to find support and comfort for themselves?

- Are people already connected with other helping professionals (e.g., mental health counselor, spiritual mentor, social worker, physician)?

- What other community resources (e.g., professionals, support networks, activities) would be helpful?

Psychosocial assessment is an opportunity for patients, families, and health care providers to discover and name the strengths and resources to be found within individuals, groups, and communities. The risks people identify, now and in the future, complete the picture of how they are doing as they face life-threatening illness, death, and bereavement. The gathering of this information is an ongoing process that will help people work together to identify, address, and manage the needs of dying patients and their families.

REFERENCES

Byock, I. (1997). *Dying well: The prospect of growth at the end of life.* New York: Riverhead Books.

Masten, A. (1994). Resilience in individual development: Successful adaptation despite risk and adversity. In M. Wang & E. Gordon (Eds.), *Educational resilience in inner city America: Challenges and prospects* (pp. 3–25). Mahwah, NJ: Lawrence Erlbaum Associates.

Moore, T. (1992). *Care of the soul.* New York: HarperCollins.

Price, S. (2001). Has something changed? Social work, pastoral care, spiritual counseling and palliative care. *Progress in Palliative Care, 9*(6), 244–246.

Saleebey, D. (1996). The strengths perspective in social work practice: Extensions and cautions. *Social Work, 41*(3), 296–305.

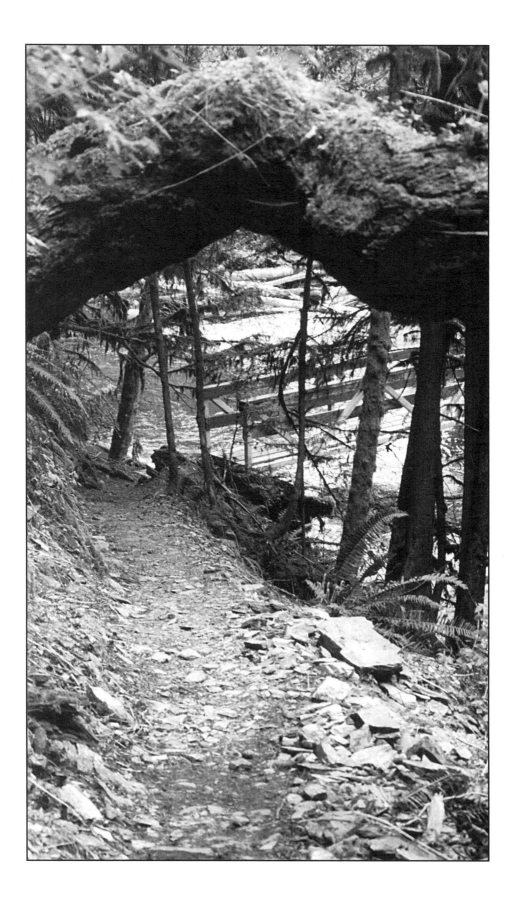

The Path Not Chosen

RECURRENCE AND CHRONIC ILLNESS
(PPSv2 level: 80% to 70%)

*O*nce diagnosed with a life-threatening illness, people live with the possibilities of recurrence and disease progression. Reactions may vary, but it is, universally, a time marked by trauma, fear, and grief. People are faced with a NEW AWARENESS of the disease and its significance in their lives. Some patients report that a return or progression of their disease is more difficult than the initial diagnosis. Although a few are relieved that the waiting is over, many patients are still determined to survive and look for new ways to overcome this illness.

News of recurrence or progression is stressful for everyone in the family. Concerns for the patient's well-being are mixed with resentment at the re-intrusion of illness into their lives. Once again, the family must deal with uncertainty and changing expectations, along with the issues that arise out of the stress and fears for the future. FAMILY DISSONANCE is not uncommon as people struggle to redefine their relationships with one another and adjust to this new situation.

Patients, in a state of limbo in which they are neither healthy nor dying, may feel or be disconnected from others. They feel let down and betrayed by their bodies, treatments, health care providers, and the health care system. People experience many physical, emotional, and social losses that confirm that they no longer fit within the mainstream. This ISOLATION prompts some people to seek supportive environments and ways to anchor themselves in this new reality; others need to break from this and seek an alternate reality where their world gets better, not worse.

Time takes on new meaning as the perspectives of patients and families are changed by each recurrence. Life expectancy may be foreshortened, and the prospect of dying appears on the horizon. Faced with UNCERTAIN TIME, some will seize the moment and live life to the fullest, while some will withdraw and become afraid to look ahead. Others reject this uncertainty and remain single-minded in attempting to reach their goal of surviving or finding a miracle. Hope and denial are important coping strategies as priorities and perspectives change. For some people, hope is an easy, natural response that adapts to the situation at hand. Others must work hard to remain anchored in hope. There are many FACES OF HOPE as people seek ways to create meaning in their lives and define what endures in the face of recurrence and progression.

FRANK AND LENA

Frank is a 51-year-old man who was diagnosed with early chronic obstructive pulmonary disease (COPD) 12 years ago. For many years, he has had ongoing problems with emphysema and chronic bronchitis. He was recently treated for pneumonia, and during his last doctor's appointment was told he now has advanced COPD. His wife, Lena, was shocked to hear that his condition had become so much worse, but Frank knew his breathing was becoming more labored and had wondered what was happening. Lena is finding it very hard to be supportive of Frank. She and her children tried to get Frank to stop smoking for many years. He always said that he had smoked from the age of 10 and can't—or won't—quit now. Lena gets very angry when he talks this way. She desperately wants Frank to get better and is often tearful and afraid when he can't get his breath.

Frank and Lena were born in the Philippines and immigrated to the United States in their thirties. They have five children; three young adults in their twenties and two teenagers still living at home. Frank's mother, Maria, has lived with the family for many years and cares for the children when the parents work. She speaks little English, but is able to understand much of what is said to her.

Frank has worked with a road crew for many years, starting as a laborer and working his way up to job foreman. Although Frank has considerable sick leave available, he has continued to work through much of his illness. His supervisor recently asked him whether he is able to continue with his present position and wondered if he should move to a part-time or less strenuous job. Frank is proud of how well he has done with this company and feels considerable grief about the idea of leaving his foreman's position. He wonders how long he will even be able to manage lighter work.

> "Can there be a worse sickness than that we are never well or can be so?"
>
> —John Donne

Frank's condition has gradually limited his activities and ability to get out. He and Lena have become increasingly isolated. Initially, their extended family and friends were very supportive, but, over the years, many have slowly withdrawn contact. When Frank was well, he regularly played golf with several men from the neighborhood. Over the last few months, he has managed only to play nine holes a few times. He found it hard to keep up with the others. Although Frank misses the camaraderie, he feels apologetic for his shortness of breath and slow pace when he does play.

Lena works long hours at a large care facility as a nurse's aide and finds herself too tired to do more than look after Frank, the house, and the children. She worries how they will manage to survive on her salary and, in very bleak moments, wonders what they'll do if she has to take time off of work to care for Frank. The older children all come for dinner on a regular basis and, while Frank enjoys this time, he is often quite fatigued and goes to bed early. His sons help with extra chores around the house and garden, but they are both busy with their own lives.

One son has been searching the Internet for information on his father's condition and wants his dad to look into a couple of the sites and try some of the new therapies he has read about. Lena has Frank taking large doses of vitamins to keep up his strength and energy. Frank takes these to please her but doesn't believe they help. He hopes that he will be well enough to go home to the Philippines in the next year. They have not been back for many years, and his mother wants to visit her family. She hopes she might get him to go to a faith healer while they are there.

KEY CONSIDERATIONS

A New Awareness

Frank is a 51-year-old man who was diagnosed with early COPD 12 years ago. Over the years, he has had ongoing problems with emphysema and chronic bronchitis. He was recently treated for pneumonia, and during his last doctor's appointment was told he now has advanced COPD. His wife, Lena, was shocked to hear that his condition had become so much worse, but Frank knew his breathing was becoming more labored and had wondered what was happening.

During the course of a life-threatening illness, it is not uncommon for people to have one or more remissions followed by a recurrence of the disease (Sales, 1991). Those with chronic illness may eventually experience many such recurrences of illness, always living with the fear of recurrence in what is known as the Damocles syndrome (Koocher & O'Malley, 1981). In varying degrees, people live with the threat of recurrence day in and day out, wondering if every ache, every pain, signals the return of the disease. In a chronic, progressive illness, this insecurity is ongoing. With successful treatment in early-stage cancer, patients continue to struggle with this threat for varying periods of time. After being given one or more "clean bills of health," most people progressively set these worries aside, however. Later, when cancer recurs, they are immediately catapulted back into this world of uncertainty.

Whether or not a recurrence is more difficult for patients and families than the original diagnosis, it is clear that recurrence is a traumatic event (Mahon & Casperson, 1997; Northouse, Dorris & Charron-Moore, 1995). It is now impossible to ignore "that the scales have been tipped in favor of the disease rather than the individual, that the balance is disturbed" (Burnet & Robinson, 2000, p. 30). One individual described his experience this way:

> I knew all along that it could come back, but let me tell you, nothing could ever prepare you for it. Even when I knew it was happening, I got real lightheaded when the doctor told me. It is so horrible when you hear it. It's one thing to think about it and another to have someone say it to you. (Mahon & Casperson, 1997, p. 182)

People's personalities, coping styles, expectations, and past experiences influence the impact of recurrence. Patients who believe themselves cured, or, conversely, who expect recurrence, report higher anxiety, depression, social withdrawal, and intrusive dreams than those who simply fear recurrence or who have previously faced recurrence (Cella, Mahon, & Donovan, 1990). People's previous experiences with treatment and the health care system also influence their reactions, as do their observations of other people's recurrences. They may believe their experience will be the same as that of others, even if they have been given a different diagnosis.

Many patients say adjusting to recurrence is harder than adjusting to diagnosis because recurrence is more damaging to their sense of hope. It becomes harder to believe that you can fight "this thing" or live to old age when recurrence tells you the disease is still growing or progressing. At this time, people talk about their feelings of shock, depression, and anxiety. They are shaken by the reality that, in spite of best efforts, this disease is progressing.

> It's not just the dying thing. It's just that you realize that there are things you have no control over…[that] will probably never go away. I might get another remission but it will always be there. It makes you feel very vulnerable…[it] could come back at any time without any warning. I know that now and I'll never forget it. I didn't feel as vulnerable the first time. (Mahon & Casperson, 1997, p. 184)

For some, progression occurs gradually. For others, changes happen suddenly. Once again, they must face their fears about death and disability, and there is a profound sense of injustice at this renewed assault (Northouse et al., 1995). Why has their disease recurred when others have not experienced recurrence? How has the system failed to cure them when others are doing well?

Some patients and families may express relief when recurrence occurs. The waiting is over, Damocles' sword has fallen and the worst has happened (See sidebar at right). This transition sees patients and families coming to a deeper awareness of the significance of the disease (Mahon & Casperson, 1997). In spite of treatments, prayers, or lifestyle changes, the illness has not gone away. The patient is very sick and everyone struggles to learn how to live with it rather than warring against it.

> What is certain is that when diagnosed with recurrent disease, the patient embarks on a journey. This journey is very different for different individuals, depending on their own truths and life perspectives. [Professionals] need to work with the patient and family agenda, make no presumptions, and create focused time to be supportive, facilitate adjustment and promote well-being. (Burnet & Robinson, 2000)

THE SWORD OF DAMOCLES

A Greek legend tells of Damocles, a courtier to the tyrant Dionysius, who was extravagant in praising his sovereign. One evening, Dionysius invited Damocles to a sumptuous feast. During the entertainment, Damocles looked up and saw that Dionysius had seated him directly beneath a sword that was suspended from the ceiling by a thread. For Damocles, this sword was a symbol of the precariousness of life and how one's fortune could change from being in favor at court to falling out of favor, causing the sword to fall down on one's head. For people who have had cancer, that sword represents the frailty and precarious nature of life itself. The threat of recurring disease and death always looms over them.

Interventions

These psychosocial interventions have been designed to specifically address the key consideration *a new awareness*. There are several assessment questions that will

help open up a discussion, followed by more focused comments or tips that will facilitate further exploration of the issues that frequently arise at this time; each tip is followed by a sample dialogue.

Assessment Questions

- What problems, if any, is the recurrence (or progression) causing for you?
- How much impact is this (symptom, recurrence) having on your life right now?
- What were your initial reactions to this recurrence?
- What things helped you deal with your initial diagnosis (or last recurrence) that might be helpful now?

Explore the physical, social, and emotional impact recurrence has had on patients. Understanding the impact can help clarify what is distressing and suggest what may be helpful.

> *"Alicia, these relapses of MS are really beginning to affect your mobility and you are now unable to walk without a cane. How are you feeling about this new development?"*

Determine how prepared people were for this recurrence. Their expectations, previous experiences, and beliefs about recurrence can influence how well they are able to adjust.

> *"Often people talk to me about being worried that their cancer will come back. They sometimes say that while they hope it won't recur, they're always waiting for the other shoe to drop. How has it been for you?"*

Ensure that patients and families get the information they need about the disease, treatments, and procedures. They may have forgotten previous information and instructions. They could have new questions or be remembering an earlier experience that was frightening or difficult.

> *"Juanita, I know that you received chemotherapy treatments when you were first diagnosed with breast cancer. It's sometimes helpful to review the process with your nurse or physician before starting treatment again, however. What concerns or questions might you have for them?"*

Explore the fears patients and families have about the progression of this illness. A realistic perspective helps people cope with their responses and make good decisions for themselves.

"While we're all together, it might be helpful to talk about what you expect will happen to your dad next. What particular worries or thoughts do you have about what's ahead?"

Support people's reactions. Encourage them to talk about their recurrence or progression and help them to find the strengths or skills to get through this time in their lives.

"John, I hear you talking about new ways to fight your disease. Tell me more about this. I am also wondering what would help you to accomplish this."

Family Dissonance

Lena is finding it very hard to be supportive of Frank. She and her children tried to get Frank to stop smoking for many years. He always said that he has smoked from the age of 10 and can't—or won't—quit now. Lena gets very angry when he talks this way. She desperately wants Frank to get better and is often tearful and afraid when he can't get his breath. Lena works long hours at a large care facility as a nurse's aide and finds herself too tired to do more than look after Frank, the house, and children. She worries how they will manage to survive on her salary and, in very bleak moments, wonders what they'll do if she has to take time off work to care for Frank.

Adjustment to recurrence and chronic illness is an ongoing process that affects the entire family. It will be influenced by how patients and families deal with ambiguous feelings, share common beliefs and values, and communicate and maintain relationships within the family. Many people are able to draw on past experiences. Having received "bad news" previously, they may have already cemented some new strategies into their repertoire of coping skills. These families will likely be able to mobilize well and help one another deal with the stress of chronic and progressive illness (Weisman & Worden, 1986). Others find each step of the way a struggle, with many obstacles and few strategies for overcoming them. Dissonance occurs when families are unable to resolve the various issues, such as giving up versus fighting, that arise as they move through these challeng-ing times.

The transition from PPS 80% to 70% raises issues that come with the reali-ties of progressive illness, such as changing responsibilities, increased limitations, and fears about the future. Families have already had a taste of caregiving and re-ceiving care and understand some of what lies ahead. Dudgeon et al. (1995) re-ported that the two main concerns for patients at this time are the well-being of their families and the worry of becoming a burden. Looking to the future, some realize that as they become increasingly ill and limited in their physical or men-tal abilities, their care will take its toll on family members. Increased expenses, re-duced income, social limitations, and physical demands will likely contribute to family hardship in the months or years ahead (Carosella, 1988).

Family needs are often concealed in the shadows, while the spotlight of con-cern and support is focused on the patient. Some people may be less supportive of patients at this time; they may resent the impact of the illness on their own lives, anticipate further physical and emotional sacrifices, or worry if they will be able to cope with these demands. They may come to resent the changes in lifestyle forced upon them because of the patient's changed occupation, reduced finances, and altered roles and activities. Some may direct anger toward patients whose lifestyles are perceived to have caused their disease (e.g., a smoker who has con-tracted throat cancer). At times, family dynamics are so complicated by illness, caregiving, guilt, and resentment that people may not want to engage in problem solving; they may even see death as the solution. Family members may feel trapped, at the mercy of the disease (Carosella, 1993; Cella et al., 1990).

Dissonance occurs on a number of different levels within families. Communi-cation may be hindered by conflicting beliefs or ideas about such matters as treat-ments, hope, and finances. It can also be affected by each person's wish to protect others from their grief, fears, or negative feelings. When people find it difficult to talk about resentment, anger, or uncertainty about their future (Chekryn, 1984), they may avoid talking about their feelings for fear of increasing stress in the fam-ily. Conversations related to the illness may be limited to daily activities, symptoms, medications, or appointments rather than recurrence, disease progression, and dying. Family members dealing with contagious or hereditary illnesses may find them-selves in an unenviable place, perhaps watching their own future unfold before them.

Family members want to know, and need to feel, they have done everything possible to fight this disease. They are often still looking for information about cures or new treatments. They try to be useful and involved, to maintain hope in the face of advancing disease. This can create dissonance when the patient and/or health care providers are following a different course. For example, if patients choose not to fight for a cure any longer or if health care providers recommend treatments to minimize symptoms or give comfort only, families may accuse them of giving up. The further apart people find themselves in attitudes and goals, the more difficult

"Courage is being scared to death and saddling up anyway."

—John Wayne

it can be for patients and their families to adjust to recurrence and chronic illness (Northouse et al., 1995).

Interventions

These psychosocial interventions have been designed to specifically address the key consideration *family dissonance*. There are several assessment questions that will help open up a discussion, followed by more focused comments or tips that will facilitate further exploration of the issues that frequently arise at this time; each tip is followed by a sample dialogue.

Assessment Questions

- Tell me how you are coping as a family with the recurrence (or progression) of your son's illness.

- How has starting this new treatment changed things in your family?

- How is your family talking about the differences that have arisen since the recurrence?

Explore what is most difficult for individual family members and how they deal with these stresses. What is most stressful for one person in the family may not be difficult for another. Understanding and talking about these differences helps family members to support one another better.

> *"Sally mentioned how it worries her that you get really anxious when she is feeling short of breath. Robert, what do you think about this? What kinds of things are most stressful for you?"*

Help family members talk about changing roles, expectations, and responsibilities. It is often easier to discuss difficult choices and make plans ahead of time rather than in the midst of a crisis.

> *"We've been talking about some of ways that chemotherapy can really change your life and how hard it may be to keep normal activities going. From your previous experience, what will be most challenging for you as a family? How could you begin preparing for this?"*

Learn about any new concerns or issues within the family. Stress and differences will often arise as an illness progresses or recurs, and families may need help identifying and dealing with them.

> *"I remember that your children were very supportive when you first underwent open-heart surgery 2 years ago. Pierre, you mentioned that your physician is now recommending more extensive bypass surgery. Your son is against this and worries that it would be too hard on you, especially because you are already short of breath. How is this sitting with you and the rest of your family?"*

Isolation

> Frank's condition has gradually limited his activities and ability to get out. He and Lena have become increasingly isolated. Initially, their extended family and friends were very supportive, but, over the years, many have slowly withdrawn contact. When Frank was well, he regularly played golf with several men from the neighborhood. Over the past few months he has only managed to play nine holes a few times. He found it hard to keep up with the others. Although Frank misses the camaraderie, he feels apologetic for his shortness of breath and slow pace when he does play.

Many patients with chronic or recurrent illnesses find themselves in a paradoxical situation that Landsman described as the world of the "marginal man." They are "suspended in a state of limbo between the world of the sick and the well, belonging to neither yet a part of both" (1975, p. 268). People struggle to find within themselves a way to live normally in a life that is not normal; to fight hard, yet be realistic; to balance their fear of death with the likelihood of a compromised life.

For patients with progressive illnesses, a forced reduction of activities and social life increases isolation and may create stress on personal relationships. The lack of opportunity to share regular activities begins to create gaps or barriers in relationships. This is illustrated in the story of Frank, who is now unable to play golf with his friends as much as he used to. An individual's need to talk to others who understand can become paramount (Dudgeon et al., 1995). A study of recurrence of cancer cited patients' feeling isolated, having "no one to talk to" and "no one who understood" (Dudgeon et al., 1995, p. 7). Patients dealing with immune-compromised diseases such as AIDS and hepatitis B find that the myths and misconceptions about the infectiousness of their particular illnesses may serve to isolate them further. People encounter losses on many levels and in many aspects of their lives at this time.

People may describe themselves as "in the community of people with the dreaded disease" or as "different and less than others" (Christ, 1991, p. 310). If the focus of their care is now changed, pa-

> "Somebody asked me if I was less scared of death and I said no, I just like life a whole lot more."
>
> —(Hilton, 1988, p. 229)

tients can feel abandoned or let down by changes in attitude, treatment, or commitment that they experience. Some people, ashamed or embarrassed by the effects of the illness on their bodies, may also withdraw from the larger community. Others will reach out in new directions for support, such as seeking counseling or joining groups or disease-specific networks. Those who continue with an aggressive "cure and survival" attitude may be isolated unless they are able to find support that matches their hopes and approaches. Within these supportive environments, people are often able to integrate their experience of recurrent and progressive illness in a positive way, learning from one another, building on strengths, and learning new coping strategies.

During this transition, families also struggle to maintain the semblance of a normal life under what Rolland called the "abnormal presence of a chronic illness and heightened uncertainty" (1984, p. 255). Rolland suggested that they need to find a way to "maintain maximal autonomy for all family members in the face of a pull toward mutual dependency and caretaking" (p. 255).

Interventions

These psychosocial interventions have been designed to specifically address the key consideration *isolation*. There are several assessment questions that will help open up a discussion, followed by more focused comments or tips that will facilitate further exploration of the issues that frequently arise at this time; each tip is followed by a sample dialogue.

Assessment Questions

- What supports do you have in your life right now?
- What changes have occurred in your daily activities because of this recurrence?
- Do you experience times when you feel lonely or alone? When does this happen?

Help patients and families identify activities and people in their lives that feel supportive. It is important not to make assumptions about what is supportive, as people's circumstances, perceptions, and needs can change.

> *"Lara, you used to tell me about your busy social life, going out with people from work and spending a lot of time with your friends or extended*

FREQUENTLY REPORTED CAUSES FOR PATIENT AND FAMILY ISOLATION

- Decrease in social life (due to reduced energy or interest, treatments, care-giving), less contact with others (due to stopped or reduced work, reduced participation in activities previously enjoyed)

- Restricted lifestyle and roles; "life can become regimented, complicated, and compromised" (Kasch, 1984, p. 14)

- Alterations in normal day-to-day activities

- Possible relocation for treatment

- Belief or reality that "no one understands"

- Social taboos, misconceptions, fears

- Conspiracy of silence (when illness has stigma attached), poor communication

- Social issues—housing, insurance, finances, living outside traditional/conventional culture (e.g., people who are gay, drug user populations)

- Issues within families—dissonance, fears, grief, family expectations about patients' capabilities/patient expectations of family, attitudes regarding illness, family being less supportive

Dudgeon et al., 1995; Kasch, 1984; Stajduhar, 1998

---

family. It sounds like you've not been wanting to socialize for some time and you rarely mention your family to me. How connected and supported are you feeling at the moment?"

Explore the paradoxes that people may be struggling with at this time. It can be difficult to live as a chronically ill person in a healthy world and patients may need support and new skills to find a balance that works for them.

"Now that you are receiving regular dialysis treatments, the doctor is suggesting that you can go back to work and start doing the things you used to do. I wonder about the expectation that you'll do all that and still come in for dialysis. What are you thinking and feeling about that?"

Clarify the causes of patients' and families' isolation. Knowing when they feel abandoned or alone will enable parents and family members to consider ways to address this situation.

"Cameron, you said that you felt abandoned by your specialist when she told you that there are few treatment options available to you because of the progression of your cancer. How are you feeling about what was said? Does your wife feel the same as your doctor about this? Are you able to talk about this with her?"

Offer opportunities for patients and families to talk about the many losses that come with progressive disease and recurrence. Giving voice to thoughts and feelings is cathartic and helps assuage people's sense of being alone with their grief.

"Over the past few months, you've had to give up a number of activities and routines that have been part of your life for years. You've mentioned that you are no longer able to play tennis or take your grandchildren on long hikes. You talked about your volunteer work at The Salvation Army, as well as the heavy yard work you often did for your neighbors. How does it feel for you as I list these things that you are no longer able to do?"

Help patients and families identify and mobilize their resources. Family, social, and professional supports are important at a time when people feel isolated and disconnected.

"You have both mentioned feeling somewhat alone at this time. There is a local ALS support group for patients and their families that meets once a month. Would you be interested to find out more? Would you like an introduction to one of the members?"

Uncertain Time

Although Frank has considerable sick leave available, he has continued to work through much of his illness. His supervisor recently asked him whether he is able to continue with his present position and wondered if he should move to a part-time or less strenuous job. Frank is proud of how well he has done with this company and feels considerable grief about the idea of leaving his foreman's position. He wonders how long he will even be able to manage lighter work. Lena works long hours at a large care facility as a nurse's aide and finds herself too tired to do more than look after Frank, the house, and the children. She worries how they will manage to survive on her salary and, in very bleak moments, wonders what they'll do if she has to take time off work to care for Frank.

After a first recurrence, people start thinking about the future of their family in a new way, about the possibility of disability, symptoms (pain), future recurrences, or dying (Burnet & Robinson, 2000; Chekryn, 1984). Their perspectives and responses to life change as they think about what is important to accomplish while they are still relatively healthy. Time is a precious commodity in life. As long as one can view an infinite amount of time ahead, one can literally take one's time. If, however, time suddenly seems limited, an increasing sense of urgency arises and an internal struggle takes place. A natural vacillation occurs for many during this transition period: "I intend to live longer and survive this disease" versus "I may not have a lot of time and I want to make the most of it." These oscillations are not easy yet will likely continue to some degree beyond this transition and even persist until close to death.

People often talk during this transition about living life to its fullest. How they define that for themselves and how they expect to accomplish that will vary greatly. Old age, retirement, grandchildren, and career can no longer be taken for granted. Some people challenge themselves to focus on living and making time count. They push themselves to the edges of their physical, emotional, or spiritual comfort zones. They may decide to cram in everything possible, taking risks and chances as never before. Others may empty their days of activities and focus on creating peace and order in their lives. They may take a dream vacation, delve into the concept of life after death, or heal a long-standing rift. For many, priorities shift away from seeking career advancement and toward building family relationships and fulfilling life-long ambitions and dreams (Mahon & Casperson, 1997).

The uncertainty that comes with recurrence brings with it a new perspective and renewed sense of vulnerability. Patients feel uncertain as they are not able to foretell the future and don't feel secure or safe from danger. They often doubt themselves and the advice or information they receive, which leads to uncertainty in making choices or decisions (Hilton, 1988). New symptoms, check-ups, the end of treatments, or family dissonance can increase uncertainty. Managing this uncertainty is an essential task in adapting to recurrence and chronic illness. People seek ways to feel supported and understood, to be positive or hopeful, and to know what can be depended on. Those people who value life, with strong beliefs and goals, tend to have a more positive outlook and actively seek ways to adjust. Those who are more anxious or passive will struggle to find direction or a sense of security. They may put their heads down and refuse to look into the future, afraid to face what they anticipate is ahead (White & Grenyer, 1999).

Uncertainty also comes when recurrence and chronic illness coincide with the movement into a new phase of family development. Each phase presents new challenges and requires families to take on new roles and responsibilities. As shown in Table 3.1, difficulties occur as patients and families try to complete these developmental tasks while at the same time coping with the stresses and changes that accompany recurring illness.

> "The clock provides only a mechanical measure of how long we live. Far more real than the ticking of time is the way we open up the minutes and invest them with meaning. Death is not the ultimate tragedy in life."
>
> —(Bob McDonald, 2002)

Interventions

These psychosocial interventions have been designed to specifically address the key consideration *uncertain time*. There are several assessment questions that will help open up a discussion, followed by more focused comments or tips that will facilitate further exploration of the issues that frequently arise at this time; each tip is followed by a sample dialogue.

Table 3.1. The impact of disease recurrence on development tasks of adults

Developmental tasks	Problems due to recurrence
Young adult (intimacy versus isolation)	
Learn to live with mate	Stress with new roles, parenting stress
Start a family	Sexuality, body image, fertility issues
Manage a home, finances	Added expenses, reduced income
Start a career	Delayed advancement, job loss/disruption
Find a congenial social group	Difficulties connecting with healthy peers
Middle adult (generativity versus stagnation)	
Become financially socially responsible	Difficulty fulfilling extra responsibilities
Relate to partner as a person	Fear of abandonment, separation
Accept normal changes of aging	Complicated by treatment, impairments
Assist children in becoming adults	Fear of premature abandonment
Develop adult leisure activities	Fatigue and malaise
Older adult (integrity versus despair)	
Adjust to decreasing health and energy	Complicated by treatment, dependence
Adjust to retirement, decreased income	Increased expenses, and forced retirement
Adjust to death of partner	Fear of abandoning partner, loss of grandparenting role
Adjust to new family roles	Early dependence on children or partner

From Mahon, S. (1991). Managing the psychosocial consequences of cancer recurrence: Implications for nurses. *Oncology Nurses Forum, 18*(3), p. 582; adapted by permission.

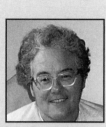

Betty Vining is a patient with recurrent cancer.

In My Own Voice
Special Celebrations

Betty Vining

The pain in my hip was so bad I couldn't walk; I could hardly stand. I told my doctor, "If I was the family pet, I'd be put down because it would be the humane thing to do." But I didn't believe the cancer could be back. After surgery and chemo, it was gone. Wasn't it? And the diagnosis came back "cancer," to be dealt with by a single, high-dose radiation treatment.

While I went through the tests and waited for the radiation, I had my fiftieth birthday. I wanted a picnic at the lake. I wanted to celebrate because I was so glad to still be alive at 50, having had a serious accident and breast cancer since turning 48. With help from family and friends, I made a suitable picnic feast and went in my wheelchair to the lake. It was a wonderful party—great food, a beautiful location, and 10 very special people. My nephew wheeled me into the lake, and I went swimming with the kids—who are my three main reasons for living after the accident. Afterward, the littlest one climbed onto my lap in the chair for a get-warm snuggle. No one has had a better fiftieth birthday party. I appreciated everything, each little detail, even more because the party almost got cancelled due to the cancer. I will soon be 51, and I want to have a picnic at the lake to celebrate.

Having the radiation turned out to be no big deal, not nearly as hard as the waiting. Two days later the pain was gone. After a few months, I walked the same as before the cancer metastasized. Some days are hard. Every little pain brings the question to mind. Is it back? And yet I still have things to do, reasons to live, people to love. I don't know for how long, but then I never really did. I know, statistically, things don't look wonderful, but I'm still alive and I feel great. Except, I feel sorry for the friends who talked about how awful they felt to turn 50. I'm really looking forward to 60.

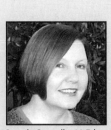

In My Own Voice
The Tick of a Clock

Brenda Pengelly

Brenda Pengelly, M.Ed.,
is Education Coordinator
of the Learning Centre
for Palliative Care at
Victoria Hospice.

Seven years after my mom had been treated for breast cancer, she was diagnosed with bone metastases. That Christmas she asked for a fancy new clock to display on the mantle. Mom was receiving radiation and chemo, but she still continued her other activities. She kept hopeful, at least in our presence. During a visit she showed me another new clock she had purchased for her kitchen wall. It was large, and she liked it because it was easy to see the time.

During the following months, time ticked by. These months were woven with a mixture of precious times. There were times of remembering and sorrowing, followed by times of despair when Mom, worried and weary, wanted to die. She didn't want to be a burden.

By the second year her world had shrunk to her bed, placed beside the window of the family room. There she could watch life, increasingly as an observer who marked the passing days and weeks. On her bedside table were the things she most needed and wanted, including a recently requested purchase—a pink alarm clock ticking loudly.

Assessment Questions

- What kinds of things are worrying you right now?
- How have you dealt with uncertainty in the past?
- As you think about the future, what's most important to you?

Clarify what is important to patients and families at this time. They may feel overwhelmed by what is before them and not know how to refocus their lives.

"Maria, before this recurrence I know you were very involved with the Sunday school in your church and found it very meaningful work. How is your illness affecting your ability to do this? What options do you have for staying involved in the future?"

Help patients understand the physical, emotional, and spiritual fatigue that comes with recurrence or chronic illness. When people know how much energy is expended on serious illness and daily activities, they are better able to prioritize and plan how best to use the energy they have.

"Jacob, you are surprised at how easily you become tired and how your energy varies from day to day. It is also hard for Mona when she can't plan activities in advance because you don't know how you'll feel. I'd like to tell you about a helpful tool called an energy circle. Think back to how much energy you had before this latest recurrence; a full circle would represent your energy then. (Have the patient draw a full circle.) Now, draw a wedge within that circle to show how much of your previous energy you have right now. You could do this exercise to assess how you are doing each day. You may find it helps you talk about what amount of energy is available for various activities during the day and how that feels. Would this be a helpful tool for you?"

Provide opportunities to review successes and positive qualities to guide and help people maintain their sense of self. The ability to reframe or view oneself from a different perspective can illuminate skills, qualities, and wisdom that can provide confidence.

"You say that you feel overwhelmed by more treatments, Terry. You've been a really successful long-distance runner. Tell me, what qualities made you so successful? Which of these are still valuable and useful in your life today?"

Provide opportunities for people to discuss any regrets or worries they may have, such as not being able to continue their normal work, see their grandchildren grow up, realize a dream or ambition, or heal a relationship. This may give them an opportunity to deal with their disappointment and decide what still can or must be done.

"Now that your ALS is progressing quite quickly, I know you are concerned that you might not see your grandson grow up. Often, when people learn that their life may be shorter than expected, they begin to review what they've accomplished and what they still hope to achieve. What might you do to leave a legacy for your grandson as he grows up?"

"Terminally ill patients cannot put life on hold while disability and treatment are endured."

—(Byock, 1996, p. 125)

The Faces of Hope

One son has been searching the Internet for information on his father's condition and wants his dad to look into a couple of the sites and try some of the new therapies he has read about. Lena has Frank taking large doses of vitamins to keep up his strength and energy. Frank takes these to please her but doesn't believe they help. He hopes that he will be well enough to go home to the Philippines in the next year. They have not been back for many years, and his mother wants to visit her family. She hopes she might get him to go to a faith healer while they are there.

Many opinions exist about the sources, targets, and value of hope. Hope has been described from theological, philosophical, biological, and psychological perspectives. For those involved in palliative care, concerns exist about the ethics involved in sustaining unrealistic hope. In spite of this, hope is seen as critical to the psychosocial well-being of patients and families as they struggle to find ways to cope with recurrence or chronic, progressive illness.

Hope is a complex process that occurs in the context of time. Not always logical or tangible, it is about creating the possibility of something better in the future. Hope is experienced in the context of people's past lives; influenced by their roles, culture, relationships, and expectations. It occurs in the present, as people grapple with the uncertainties before them. It considers a range of possible outcomes that are desirable. Hope is about possibility—not probability. It uses the strengths and wisdom of the past to build a bridge to the future (Jevne & Nekoliachuk, 1999).

For people experiencing recurrence and chronic illness, everyday living includes both hope and despair; they are not mutually exclusive. Hope is not a steady course that people set out on and follow to the end. Hope lies on a continuum that covers a range of possibilities going from despair (no hope) to denial

HOPE

Following is a list of some well-known quotations about hope. Reading or listening to the opinions of well-respected individuals can help patients and families generate their own, internal sense of what form hope takes in their lives.

The human body experiences a powerful gravitational pull in the direction of hope. That is why the patient's hopes are the physician's secret weapon. They are the hidden ingredients in any prescription. (Norman Cousins)

Everything that is done in the world is done by hope. (Martin Luther King, Jr.)

Hope is what you do until you know what you need to do. (mother of a child with leukemia)

Hope is a sense of the possible. (Edmund Lynch)

Hoping occurs most noticeably when one feels captive. (Paul Pruyser)

Hope is to see in the eyes of another that you are understood. (Henri Nouwen)

When you get to the end of your rope, tie a knot and hang on. (Anonymous)

Hope is the thing with feathers
That perches in the soul—
And sings the tune without words
And never stops—at all. (Emily Dickinson)

(false hope). People find themselves at different spots along that hoping continuum, depending on their changing situation and who they are.

> Denial is a defense mechanism that consists of avoiding the facts, whereas hope accepts painful facts but places them in a wider perspective that includes other, more acceptable aspects of those facts. [Hope is] based on reality, taking into account the obvious meaning of a tragic event as well as additional meanings that a person finds more acceptable. (Callan, 1989, p. 36)

During this time, some people feel powerless and hopeless about their situation. Their ability to hold on to hope may be threatened by many things including ongoing recurrences, the bad reputation of the illness, concerns about their families, uncertainty about the future, or the attitudes and behaviors of others (Lindvall, 1995). Patients need to find reasons to go on, ways to come back from this place of despair. They do this through hope. Patients who are unable to refocus away from despair and helplessness, often experience more distress and diminished physical well-being (Spencer, Carver, & Price, 1998).

It should be recognized that, at PPS 80% or 70%, good response to treatment is still a reasonable expectation for many, depending on the type of the disease, its prior response to earlier treatment, and individual variation. Hopes for extended survival may still be realistic. People seek and maintain hope in other ways as well. Sources of hope are tied to what gives their life meaning and a sense of worth. They may include spiritual or religious beliefs, family, friends, health care providers, nature, or self-exploration. For some, personal flexibility allows them to adapt constantly to the situation at hand and maintain hope. Others must be single-minded about hope because they find it too difficult to hold on to hope and prepare for ongoing illness or death at the same time.

HOPE IS

- A possibility (a way out)
- Transcendent (a reason for being/personal purpose, as part of a larger whole)
- Goal-directed (an expectation of reaching a goal)
- A state of mind (a brighter tomorrow)
- Multi-dimensional (a confident yet unclear expectation)
- An orientation of the heart (a conviction that things ultimately make sense)

—(Jevne, 1999, p. 11)

People may hope for different things. These may be related to the disease, certain dreams or ambitions, personal relationships, or spiritual connections. As people make the transition from focusing on the physical healing of their bodies to the possibility of healing their minds and spirits, they are letting go of what they cannot control and nurturing that which they are able to control. In the process of hoping and confirming what has meaning in their lives, people can find positive aspects in their journey through recurrence and chronic illness.

The beliefs, attitudes, and approaches of health care providers have a tremendous impact on hope. Opinion, tone, or behavior can give a person hope or take it away. On the one hand, health care providers sometimes worry about giving false hope and try to lower patients' and families' expectations about their future to avoid disappointment. As a result, patients may experience resentment or unnecessary despair and hopelessness. Patients and families may also fear being too hopeful—they may be afraid to get used to it, fearing it's too far to fall, or too painful when they again feel despair. On the other hand, some health care providers may want patients to be optimistic and hopeful and try to ease the bad news. They substitute false hope for realistic hope, suggesting to patients that they may do better than expected. Unfortunately, this approach can support ongoing denial and distract patients from preparing for the future or dealing with the emotional and spiritual issues of recurrence (Buchholz, 1990). As patients and families interpret information based on their need to have hope, it is critical that health care providers are clear about what they are saying and understand the influence they can have on people's hope.

The Hierarchy of Hope

Patients' experiences of life-threatening illness are by no means "linear." To help health care providers conceptualize patients' ever-changing hopes, it may be helpful to frame their experience in a hierarchical way. Based on Maslow's (1943) Hierarchy of Needs, the Hierarchy of Hope (see Figure 3.1) illustrates the shifts in people's hopes and needs as they progress from diagnosis to palliation and death.

Helen Wong, a Patient and Family Counselor at the BC Cancer Agency, Vancouver Island Centre, developed this model, which implies that there is always hope and that this hope shifts from being focused on the physical realm to comfort and quality of life to spiritual connectedness. It helps health care providers conceptualize these transitions of hope. They may then be able to support patients and families to clarify and uphold hope in the context of the medical situation.

When people receive a life-threatening diagnosis, they first focus on hope for a cure. Sometimes, this hope stays with patients and families through the remainder of their lives, until close to the time of death. For others, as the illness progresses or recurs, their early hopes for cure or management of symptoms shift to other levels and they begin to focus on day-to-day comforts and quality of life. As patients move upward in the Hierarchy of Hope and let go of some of their previous hopes, little by little, they are able to embrace the hopes that reflect their emotional needs and, ultimately, their spiritual needs.

Each level of the hierarchy is filled with many specific hopes and "hopelets" (Bombeck, 1989) that will be particular to each person. Patients are sustained by their ability to collect these small, tangible "hopelets" and string them together in a way that gives them increased hope and strength.

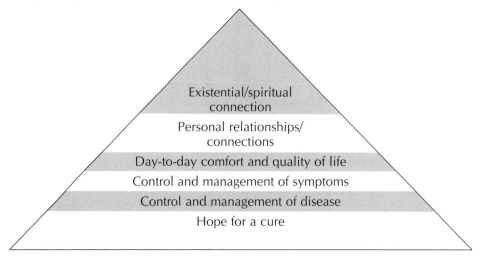

Figure 3.1. Based on Maslow's Hierarchy of Needs, the Hierarchy of Hope illustrates shifts in hopes and needs as people approach death.

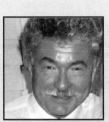

Michael Boyle, M.S.W., is a social worker and professional practice leader of patient and family counseling at the British Columbia Cancer Agency, Vancouver Island Centre.

In My Own Voice
The Medical Curse

Michael Boyle

One of the most subtle and tragic shifts that can occur in a patient's life is sometimes referred to as the "medical curse" (Dossey, 1995; Remen, 1998). In essence, the curse tells a patient that there is no hope. A patient comes to believe that the statistical chances for his or her survival are slim, whether or not they are. A professional (usually a medical oncologist, radiation oncologist, or some other specialist) can transmit the curse verbally and/or nonverbally. The curse is given with the best of intentions and, often, unconsciously. It happens when the patient's world of hope and the medical/scientific world of statistical probability collide. Like two weather fronts meeting, the collision creates a huge emotional downdraft for most patients, especially in the beginning phases of illness, when outcomes are uncertain.

The medical curse is based on fear. The health professional fears instilling a false sense of hope in the patient. Therefore, he or she feels responsible to give "the facts" to the patient in a clear way. These facts, which are statistical probabilities, may instill fear in the patient.

A caring physician I work with always tells his patients that their probability "from a statistical point of view" is simply that, a probability, and he cannot predict. This physician does not feel obliged to dwell on statistical prognostication. He encourages each person to see him- or herself as exceptionally able to overcome "the odds" in his or her own unique way. He chooses to help the patient find hope through a realistic and joint appraisal of what is possible. This may include complementary approaches. Other professionals are then called upon to assist the patient with making choices. This opening up of options gives relief to the patient and helps him or her avoid feeling abandoned when medical options are limited. By calling in others to assist at what could be a moment of utter hopelessness, the health care provider transforms the experience from "There is nothing more that we can do" into "There may be something (or someone) else that can help." This serves to honor and acknowledge the other aspects of a person's life that have meaning and significance to him or her. It is specifically in these social, emotional, and spiritual areas where the work of healing can now be done.

This highlights the importance of a team approach. When medical hope for cure fails, patients can look to other team members for help and support. Hope for other possibilities in life can grow. Patients are then able to regain their sense of personal equilibrium and control.

The antidote to the medical curse comes from the heart, not the head. The heart is always searching for hope.

WAYS TO ENGENDER HOPE

- Professionals must never underestimate the influence they have on the hopes of patients. This requires that they carefully consider the language they use, the kind of relationships they form, and their view of the situation at hand.

- Remember that while health care providers may be experts in medicine, nursing, or counseling, patients are experts on themselves. Approach them from your humanity rather than your role.

- Share information openly and leave room for alternative solutions or approaches.

- Hear their story; recognize symbolic hopes as well as those that are concrete.

- Be helpful; respond with action wherever possible.

- Focus on potential rather than on limitations or problems; recognize patients' and families' abilities.

- Remember patients' rights and your limitations; don't insist on always being right.

- Use hopeful humor; patients and families often need a reason to smile during this time.

- Suggest hope through your actions and language; expect a better day tomorrow.

From Jevne, R., & Nekolaichuk, C. (1999). A hope research manual: Points of departure, rays of hope. Approaching the 21st century conference, Edmonton, Alberta; reprinted by permission.

Interventions

These psychosocial interventions have been specifically designed to address the key consideration *the faces of hope*. There are several assessment questions that will help open up a discussion, followed by more focused comments or tips that will facilitate further exploration of the issues that frequently arise at this time; each tip is followed by a sample dialogue.

Assessment Questions

- What do you most hope for? How can that happen? What would it look like?
- How important is hope to you as you face this illness? How has your hope changed over time?
- What are your sources of hope? How do you maintain hope?

Normalize and support feelings of hope and despair. It is reassuring for people to know that hope and despair are expected and that these feelings are not mutually exclusive.

> *"We've been talking about how overwhelmed and out of control things feel for you right now. You have also talked about how you treasure every day that you feel well and look forward to more of these days. How is it for you to have feelings of hopelessness and hope at the same time?"*

Help patients and families understand that hope can change with time and circumstances. They may be able to redirect their hope to things that are within their reach.

> *"Fernie, I understand that you are very disappointed about not feeling well enough to go on the trip to Hawaii at this time. You're wondering if you will ever be able to make that kind of trip. Have you considered a trip closer to home that may not be so demanding on you?"*

Identify small hopes and possibilities that can be collected for a "rainy day." "Hopelets" feel so much more possible or achievable and can sustain patients through times of despair.

"We've been talking a lot about hope and you said your greatest hope was to be cured. Now that you've been told this isn't possible, you feel hopeless. I wonder if there are some other, day-to-day hopes that you have for yourself? What might you hope for over the next few months?"

Normalize whatever unhopeful feelings patients and families experience, such as despair or shame. People often don't talk about despair even though they are feeling that way, and it can be a relief to know they need not be hopeful all the time. Avoiding feelings can take as much energy as dealing with them.

"It sounds like you're having trouble being optimistic right now. It's pretty much impossible to feel hopeful all the time, isn't it? I'd like to hear some more about how you're feeling since today's treatment was cancelled because of your low blood count."

OUR EXPERIENCE

As we work with people during this time of recurrence and chronic progressive illness, our goal is to help them draw upon already learned strategies to cope with this crisis. By acknowledging their fears and hopes, we want to help them find meaning and a new perspective for their experience.

Recurrence brings patients and families back to us, seeking further treatment or support for what is happening. Once again, they are in crisis and we help them tap into the skills and strategies they learned through the time of diagnosis and early treatment. We help them understand new information about treatment or care options and make decisions regarding them. We know that recurrence brings increased awareness of the seriousness of their illness and the vulnerability of their life. Acknowledging this new level of understanding helps address the feelings of fragility and loneliness that patients have at this time.

Patients and families often report a deep despair during this time. They have done everything possible to fight the disease. They expected to do well and didn't. Feeling helpless and confused, they wonder how this could happen to them. We companion them in their grief and sorrow, looking for opportunities to comfort, reframe their helplessness, and encourage hope. We speak carefully and clearly with people who are interpreting what we say and how we say it based on their need to have hope. We do this by using their words, starting where they are in their perceptions, and checking out what they hear us saying. We do this by giving truthful information that is guided by what they want or need to hear, rather than our professional need for truth. We leave room for hope as, indeed, there is always something to be hoped for. Patients and families often tell us that they feel abandoned by their health care providers when any treatment offered is not curative, but palliative, in focus. While acknowledging these feelings, we want to clarify any misconceptions about the information that has been given and help people to adjust to this shift in focus of care. This should not be seen as abandonment of care. We make certain that they are directed or referred for appropriate psychosocial support, such as a palliative care program, peer support, web-based chat rooms, and other professional or lay counseling.

> "There is a weird power in a spoken word....And a word carries far—very far—deals destruction through time as the bullets go flying through space."
>
> —(Joseph Conrad, 1990, p. 106)

In all that we do, we look for ways to build on the strengths we find and to engender hope. Our experience tells us that those who remain optimistic and hopeful, and who look for what is positive and possible, will live more engaged and fulfilling lives.

TEAM ISSUES

When success and failure are defined differently within the team, it is difficult to support one another. If a patient rejects traditional medical treatment and pursues costly alternative treatment, only to find that the disease has progressed, some team members may feel that the patient had a right to seek alternative treatment no matter the outcome. Others may view it as a tragedy, however, since the patient would likely have responded well to medical intervention. Without discussing and understanding each other's views, including what the patient felt about the situation, it becomes easy to judge one another and the decisions made.

Team members have different beliefs and opinions about what people should hope for, how much hope is realistic, and when it is unhelpful. Some team members worry about instilling false hope or supporting "unrealistic" hopes. Others are comfortable with not knowing, and believe people can find their own truths. When individual team members make these kinds of judgments, they are more likely to be based on personal beliefs than on what actually helps patients and families get through the day. Without discussion, these differences can create stress and discord within the team and cause confusion for patients and families if they receive varying messages about hope and denial.

When decisions are made about ongoing treatment and care after recurrence and disease progression, they are typically the responsibility of the physician and patient. Good decision making is based on being well informed about many aspects of treatment, including the social, financial, and emotional implications. When left to one professional, the burden of covering all aspects is most difficult. Where a larger team is available, the ability of several team members to share their knowledge and views is generally most helpful. This requires good communication, planning, and sharing of roles—and this, too, can create challenges. Beyond this, when team input is ignored or discredited, dissonance or conflict can result.

SUMMARY

Recurrence is a fact of life with many life-threatening and chronic illnesses. It can signal the failure of treatment to cure or effect a remission in some diseases and reflect the progressive nature of others. Feeling vulnerable and helpless to stop what is happening, people struggle to maintain normalcy and a connection with the world. Time takes on new significance, as life becomes more uncertain. Hopes shift as people seek to gain some control in this predicament and make sense of what is happening to them.

Family members find their needs become secondary as they support patients and take on added responsibilities and roles. They may act as cheerleaders or coaches, caregivers, and steady companions. Traveling a parallel but separate path, families may struggle with the reactions and choices of patients. This can create dissonance and further stress within the family.

Some patients and families may live with the realities and limitations of this transition for a long time (see Table 3.2). The disease might sweep others along, with uncertainty ahead and reality pressing from behind. Regardless, people cannot turn back and must continue traveling "the path not chosen."

Table 3.2.　Palliative Performance Scale (PPSv2) 80%–70%

PPS Level	Ambulation	Activity and evidence of disease	Self-care	Intake	Conscious level
80%	Full	Normal activity *with* effort Some evidence of disease	Full	Normal or reduced	Full
70%	Reduced	Unable to do normal job work Significant disease	Full	Normal or reduced	Full

REFLECTIVE ACTIVITY

The following exercise is intended to demonstrate the influence that health care providers have on how patients and families adjust to this transition.

Role-Play Instructions

Take a moment to consider what you believe about relationships between professionals and patients, about hope and truth telling. With a partner, choose one of the following statements of belief and role-play an interview between a health care provider and a patient whose illness has recently recurred or progressed. The patient is trying to deal with bad news and find hope in his or her situation.

Person 1: You are a health care provider who holds a particular belief, outlined in the following table. Choose one statement from column A. Talk to the patient about what you expect will happen for him or her over the next months or years as his or her particular disease progresses.

Table 3.3. Contrasting beliefs of health care providers

	Statement of belief A	Statement of belief B
Hope and denial	Denial is bad. Patients who express hope disproportionate to survival statistics are being unrealistic and need to be corrected.	Denial is often functional. It gives people a way to control the amount of reality to be dealt with at any one time and may permit a level of coping that full acknowledgment of a situation may not. Hope and denial are not mutually exclusive.
Relationships	When talking with people about serious situations, I must remain emotionally detached and professional.	A balance between professionalism (demonstrating knowledge, skill, and objectivity) and being personal (connecting in a caring, human way) is ideal.
Truth telling	Patients must be told the truth.	Truth, as it relates to medical conditions, is usually a matter of statistics and patients may accept whatever is said, without question. Information given to patients is very powerful and must be communicated in a sensitive and careful manner.
Power	Professionals know best.	Although professionals may know more about the disease, patients have lived with it longer than the medics have treated it. Patients and families are the experts on themselves and need to feel in control whenever possible.

From Jevne, R. (1999). *Approaching the 21st Century conference*. Edmonton, Alberta, Canada; reprinted by permission.

Person 2: You are a patient who has recently experienced a recurrence or dramatic progression in an illness. In spite of the statistics or what is known, you are extremely hopeful about your future and express this in the interview.

Both: Take a moment to decide upon the situation to be role played, such as the "demographics" of your characters, the illness, your preexisting relationship, what is hoped for, and so forth. As you role-play the interview, notice your thoughts, feelings, and reactions. When finished, debrief the scene and discuss anything that arose during the interview. Next, replay your scenario using the parallel belief statement given in Column B. Again, debrief the experience and note any differences.

RESOURCES

Web Sites

American Lung Association
   www.lungusa.org
Canadian HIV/AIDS Clearinghouse
   www.clearinghouse.cpha
Chronic Obstructive Pulmonary Disease Professional Organization
   www.copdprofessional.org
Chronic Lung Disease Resource
   www.cheshire-med.com/programs/pulrehab/rehinfo.html
Chronic Hepatitis C: Current Disease Management
   www.niddk.nih.gov
Growth House, Inc.
   www.growthhouse.org/hospice.html
Hope Foundation of Alberta
   www.hopefoundation.org
Journal of the American Medical Association HIV/AIDS Information Center
   www.ama-assn.org
Renal Disease Information
   www.kidneypatientguide.org.uk
Living with ALS
   www.als.org

Books

Albom, M. (1997). *Tuesdays with Morrie.* Lake Forest Park, WA: Bantam Ballantine.
Cousins, N. (1989). *Headstart: The biology of hope.* New York: Dutton.
Jevne, R., & Nekoliachuk, C. (1999). *A hope research manual: Points of departure, rays of hope.* Approaching the 21st Century conference: Edmonton, Alberta, Canada.
Lynch, J. (1974). *Images of hope: Imagination as the healer of the hopeless.* Notre Dame, IN: University of Notre Dame Press.

Mitsumoto, H., & Forbes, H.N. (1994). *Amyotrophic lateral sclerosis: A comprehensive guide to management.* New York: Demos Publications.

Pollin, I., & Golant, S. (1994). *Taking charge: Overcoming the challenges of long term illness.* New York: Times Books.

Schwartz, M. (1996). *Letting go: Morrie's reflections of living while dying.* New York: Dell.

Wilber, K. (1993). *Grace and grit: Spirituality and healing in the life and death of Treya Killiam Wilber.* Boston: Shambhala Press.

Articles

Centers, L. (2001). Beyond denial and despair: ALS and our heroic potential for hope. *Journal of Palliative Care, 17*(4), 259–264.

Herth, K. (2000). Enhancing hope in people with a first recurrence of cancer. *Journal of Advanced Nursing, 32*(6), 1431–1441.

Teno, J., Weitzen, S., Fennell, B., & Mor, V. (2001). Dying trajectory in the last year of life: Does cancer trajectory fit other diseases? *Journal of Palliative Medicine, 4,*(4), 457–464.

REFERENCES

Bombeck, E. (1989). *I want to have hair, I want to grow up, I want to go to Boise.* New York: Harper and Row.

Buchholz, W. (1990). A piece of my mind. *Journal of the American Medical Association, 263*(17), 2357–2358.

Burnet, K., & Robinson, L., (2000). Psychosocial impact of recurrent cancer. *European Journal of Oncology Nursing, 4*(1), 29–38.

Byock, I. (1996). Beyond symptom management. *European Journal of Palliative Care, 3*(3), 125–130.

Callan, D. (1989). Hope as a clinical issue in oncology social work. *Journal of Psychosocial Oncology, 7*(3), 31–46.

Carosella, J. (1988, February). The phenomenon of the long-term dialysis patient: Coping and surviving. *Contemporary Dialysis & Nephrology,* 25–27.

Carosella, J. (1993). Reexperiencing loss: Diagnosis of end-stage renal disease in diabetic patients. *Dialysis & Transplantation, 22*(12), 722–733.

Cella, D., Mahon, S., & Donovan, M. (1990). Cancer recurrence as a traumatic event. *Behavioral Medicine, 16*(1), 15–22.

Chekryn, J. (1984). Cancer recurrence: Personal meaning, communication and marital adjustment. *Cancer Nursing, 7,* 491–498.

Christ, G. (1991). A model for the development of psychosocial interventions. *Recent Results in Cancer Research, 121,* 301–312.

Conrad, J. (1900). *Lord Jim.* Edinburgh & London: William Blackwood & Sons.

Dossey, F. (1993). *Healing words.* San Francisco: HarperCollins.

Dudgeon, D., Raubertas, R., Doerner, K., O'Connor, T., Tobin, M., & Rosenthal, S. (1995). When does palliative care begin? A needs assessment of cancer patients with recurrent disease. *Journal of Palliative Care, 11*(1), 5–9.

Erikson, E. (1963). *Childhood and society.* New York: W.W. Norton.

Hilton, A. (1988). The phenomenon of uncertainty in women with breast cancer. *Issues in Mental Health Nursing, 9,* 217–238.

Jevne, R., & Nekoliachuk, C. (1999). *A hope research manual: Points of departure, rays of hope.* Approaching the 21st Century conference, Edmonton, Alberta, Canada.

Kasch, C. (1984, June 14–19). Communication, adaptation, and the restoration of psychosocial competence: Helping patients cope with chronic renal failure. *ANNA Journal.*

Koocher, G., & O'Malley, J. (1981). *The Damocles syndrome: Psychosocial consequences of surviving childhood cancer.* New York: McGraw-Hill.

Landsman, M. (1975). The patient with chronic renal failure: A marginal man. *Annals of Internal Medicine, 82*(2), 268–270.

Lindvall, L. (1995). Hope in everyday living of cancer patients. *Hoitotiede, 7*(5), 223–232.

Mahon, S. (1991). Managing the psychosocial consequences of cancer recurrence: Implications for nurses. *Oncology Nurses Forum, 18*(3), 577–583.

Mahon, S., Casperson, D. (1997). Exploring the psychosocial meaning of recurrent cancer: A descriptive study. *Cancer Nursing, 20*(3), 178–186.

Maslow, A. (1943). A theory of human motivation. *Psychological Review, 50,* 370–396.

Northouse, S., Dorris, G., & Charron-Moore, C. (1995). Factors affecting couples' adjustment to recurrent breast cancer. *Social Science Medicine, 411,* 69–76.

Remen, R.N. (1996). *Kitchen table wisdom.* New York: Riverhead Books.

Rolland, J. (1984). Toward a psychosocial typology of chronic and life-threatening illness. *Family Systems Medicine, 2*(3), 245–262.

Sales, E. (1991). Psychosocial impact of the phase of cancer on the family: An updated review. *Journal of Psychosocial Oncology, 9*(4), 1–18.

Spencer, S., Carver, C., & Price, A. (1998). In J.C. Holland (Ed.), *Psycho-Oncology* (pp. 211–222). New York: Oxford University Press.

Stajduhar, K. (1998). Palliative care at home: Reflections on HIV/AIDS family caregiving experiences. *Journal of Palliative Care, 14*(2), 14–22.

Weisman, A., & Worden, J. (1986). The emotional impact of recurrent cancer. *Journal of Psychosocial Oncology, 3*(4), 4–16.

White, Y., & Grenyer, B. (1999). The biopsychosocial impact of end-stage renal disease: The experience of dialysis patients and their partners. *Journal of Advanced Nursing, 30*(6), 1312–1320.

FAMILY TYPES AND STAGES

Life and death happen in the context of a family. In palliative and bereavement care, the patient and family are considered the unit of care. To be able to offer care that is relevant, health care providers need to have a way to understand families and the psychosocial concerns and realities that they face. The following information suggests a context for that understanding.

According to the Canadian Hospice Palliative Care Association National Principles and Norms of Practice (2002), the family is defined as those closest to the patient in knowledge, care, and affection. Family may include

- The biological family

- The family of acquisition (related by marriage/contract)

- The family of choice and friends (including pets)

Often, professionals in health, palliative, or bereavement care assume that all patients come from a traditional family, which can be misleading because families come in a variety of types. Family type will influence how a family responds to people, events, and various health and human systems and may influence how the system responds to them. The characteristics of families, based on their type and stage in the family life cycle, are described next.

FAMILY TYPES

Table 3A.1 lists several variations on family, including nontraditional types. For example, it lists a *single person* as a family type to acknowledge the place of single people in the family life cycle. For *couples*, sexual orientation and marital status are acknowledged as important factors because they affect practical, social, and emotional issues. If *families with children* are blended or multi-generational, relationships may be more numerous and/or more complicated, which is why these factors are considered. It is important to acknowledge that the various categories or types of families are not mutually exclusive and that any number of combinations is possible. For example, a single parent or married couple may be gay or heterosexual, or a common-law couple may or may not have school-age children.

FAMILY STAGES

Defining families by type alone gives an incomplete picture of how they will be affected by the experience of illness, death, and bereavement. Professionals must also consider where families are within the family life cycle. Theoretically, families move from one stage to another in the family life cycle. In reality, things are not necessarily so straightforward. For example, a "couple again" family may suddenly find themselves at an earlier stage if another child is born.

Table 3A.1. Family types

Single person	Couple	With children
Heterosexual	Married	Single parent
Gay or lesbian	Common-law	Married
	Gay or lesbian	Common-law
		Gay or lesbian
		Blended
		Multi-generational

Family systems theorists have identified special fundamental tasks for families at various points along the developmental continuum (Hall & Kirschling, 1990; Knapp & Delcampo, 1995). Response to present events and circumstances, such as illness, death, and bereavement, are shaped in part by a family's current life cycle stage. From a life cycle perspective, these circumstances may be more difficult for families who are already experiencing normal stage-related losses (Jenkins, 1989), such as the loss felt by parents when young adults move away from home. Difficulties can also arise in families in which a member is estranged or has a disability or ongoing dependency. Some families have complex developmental issues before they come to palliative or bereavement care. Identifying these families and the issues surrounding them allows for early intervention.

VARIOUS FAMILY STAGES AND THE IMPACT ON CAREGIVING

This family life cycle information considers the various family stages and provides a brief comment about the developmental tasks and goals within each. Common psychosocial concerns and realities for families as they face life-threatening illness, death, and bereavement are highlighted, along with interventions that will guide professionals in assessing and planning care that is appropriate for each family stage.

Family Stage: Single Person

Single people may be at any stage of individual or family development. They may have ties to their family of origin or to a family of choice. As a family type, their task is to establish and maintain identity and independence. Most single people pursue personal, career, or educational interests. Many are building relationships with friends and/or partners. Some single people, either by choice or circumstance, will not have formed important work or social connections and their interests may be solitary.

Family Psychosocial Concerns and Realities

- Identifying possible caregivers
- Feelings of isolation, unfairness, incompletion; concern about lack of descendants
- Financial worries such as disability/health insurance, drug or treatment costs, and loss of income

Psychosocial Interventions

- Help patients maintain independence
- Identify and advocate for appropriate resources
- Explore and address feelings of incompletion and unfairness

Family Stage: New Couple

At any age, whether engaged, newly married, common-law, or gay/lesbian, couples are developing and defining their relationships. As they envision the future together, some of them may be considering parenthood. Their tasks include fitting into the kin network of existing families. As extended families come together, various roles and responsibilities shift from the family of origin to the new partner.

Family Psychosocial Concerns and Realities

- Negotiating who has primary decision-making and caregiver rights and responsibilities
- Feelings of burden, failure, and disappointment
- Financial worries such as disability/health insurance, drug or treatment costs, and loss of income

Psychosocial Interventions

- Support the new couple and maintain privacy and closeness
- Assess individual and family strengths, needs, and dynamics
- Facilitate communication about needs, wishes, and responsibilities

Family Stage: Established Couple

Long-term childless couples are often focused on their lives together now and in the future. Career, professional, or financial advancement may be of particular importance to them. They develop and pursue mutual and independent interests. Although some established couples might be quite exclusive, others enjoy interfacing with their social network.

Family Psychosocial Concerns and Realities

- Realities of burden and protection
- Concerns about loss of predictability and dreams or plans for the future
- Concerns regarding abandonment and survival
- Realities of possible career burnout

Psychosocial Interventions

- Facilitate planning for care, respite, and death
- Assess bereavement risk
- Facilitate communication about maintaining intimacy

Family Stage: Child Bearing

At this stage, the parents are trying to establish a satisfying home. They are adapting to the needs and interests of the children and coping with energy depletion and lack of privacy. They may also be coping with the pain of miscarriage and neonatal death. At any of the family stages with children, the family may be single parent or co-parent.

Family Psychosocial Concerns and Realities

- Concerns about healthy partner's dual role as parent and caregiver
- Realities of dying person's loss of parenting role
- Concerns about how to help the children

Psychosocial Interventions

- Develop an adaptive plan for family needs and priorities
- Educate and support key adults to address children's grief
- Encourage legacy work for and with the children
- Advocate for personal time in the adult relationship

Family Stage: School-Age Children

Families with children in school are establishing and maintaining the basic routines of family life. Time and energy go toward setting up children's activities and attending school and extracurricular functions. If the family has a child or children with special needs, this often requires the involvement of other systems. Blended families, at this or at any of the other stages, will have additional issues to consider.

Family Psychosocial Concerns and Realities

- Concerns about serious disruption of familiar routines
- Realities of coordinating child care, patient care, and career responsibilities
- Concerns about surviving as a family and maintaining cohesion

Psychosocial Interventions

- Work directly with the children
- Educate teachers, school counselors, and classmates about children's grief
- Facilitate family discussions and model helpful communication and information

Family Stage: Teenage Children

A significant developmental task for families with teenage children is to foster the teenagers' increasing independence. When teens are engaged in at-risk behaviors, the natural stress of this time is magnified. As the adults are able, they begin to establish postparenting interests.

Family Psychosocial Concerns and Realities

- Concerns about how the dying parent competes with the normal egocentric/peer focus of adolescence
- Expectations of maturity and caregiving in teens
- Accelerated loss of parental control
- Normal conflicts challenge hopes for harmony

Psychosocial Interventions

- Be direct, patient, and accessible with teens
- Assess expectations of teens
- Encourage parents and teens to find a balance between letting go and maintaining structure

Family Stage: Launching Center (Empty Nest)

The task for families at this stage is to release and support young adults to live independently, while maintaining a secure and safe home base. This transition may be over a prolonged period as young adults move in and out of the family home. Some families do not launch their young adults, and these adult children may or may not continue to live comfortably at home for many years.

Family Psychosocial Concerns and Realities

- Concerns of burden and protection
- Realities of the condition of the marriage
- Concerns about loss of "couple again" dreams

Psychosocial Interventions

- Address loss of dreams for couple and/or adult children

- Assess expectations of adult children
- Explore conflicting priorities for adult children who are also caregivers

Family Stage: "Couple Again" Family

As the couple find themselves alone again, the marriage relationship may be rekindled. They may plan for, or adjust to, retirement. This can be a time when they find themselves in the "sandwich generation" with young grandchildren, adult children, and elderly parents. At this stage, the family may live in a multigenerational home.

Family Psychosocial Concerns and Realities

- Concerns about the loss of retirement dreams
- Concerns about the loss of the grandparenting role
- Realities of multigenerational factors

Psychosocial Interventions

- Encourage legacy work for and with grandchildren
- Facilitate life review and completion work
- Assess the burden of caregiving on partner and adult children

Family Stage: Aging Family

As family members grow older, they are adapting to the effects of aging. They may have multiple needs and losses. Changes in health and ability bring them into contact with various systems. The loss of a life partner carries the family life cycle full circle, back to the single person again.

Family Psychosocial Concerns and Realities

- Realities of caregiver frailty
- Realities of dispersed or depleted family
- Concerns about attitudes and beliefs that affect care

Psychosocial Interventions

* Assess loss history and legitimize grief
* Encourage life reflection and life review
* Address isolation and loneliness

REFERENCES

Hall, J.E., & Kirschling, J.M. (1990). A conceptual framework for caring for families of hospice patients. *Hospice Journal, 6*(2), 1–28.

Jenkins, H. (1989). The family and loss: A systems framework. *Palliative Medicine, 3,* 97–104.

Knapp, E., & Delcampo, R. (1995). Developing family care plans: A systems perspective for helping hospice families. *The American Journal of Hospice & Palliative Care, 12*(6), 39–47.

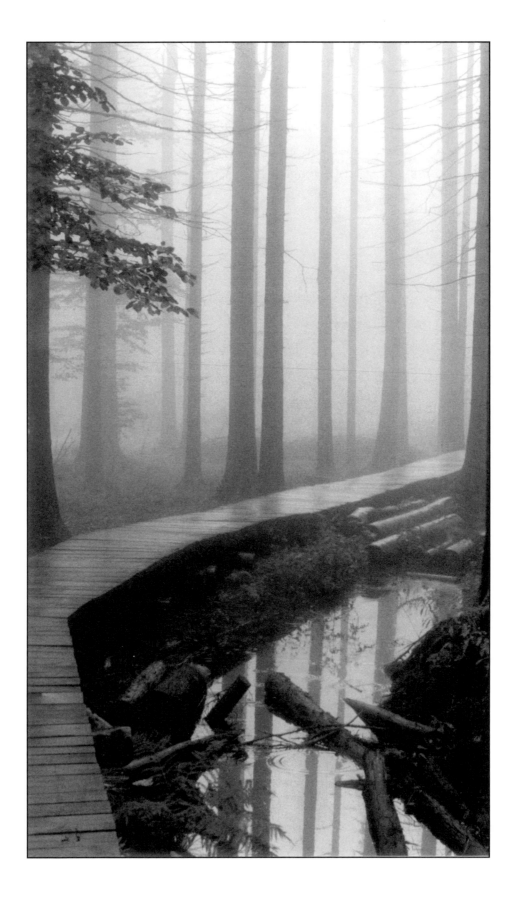

4

Entering the Unknown

THE SHIFT TOWARD HOSPICE AND PALLIATIVE CARE
(PPSv2 level: 60% to 50%)

The shift from treatment toward palliative care is difficult for everyone involved. This CHANGE IN FOCUS occurs when the disease is advanced and cure
is not possible. Even when health care providers work together to facilitate a
smooth transition for the patient and family, this is a painful shift for many. As
the shift occurs, most people see hospice as a bleak, final destination intended for
the last few days of life. Few patients and families are oriented toward dying. For
the most part they have retained the hope that the patient is getting better, and
they believe the individual deserves to have a better outcome after what he or she
has gone through in treatment. Health care providers' discomfort with "failure,"
coupled with the stress experienced by patients and families, causes some people
to move from treatment to palliation with minimal information, understanding,
or support.

During this time people carefully review their journey through early diagnosis and treatment, verifying that all potentially helpful treatments were considered and all avenues were explored. Some people will pursue aggressive treatment
options and hope for a cure until death. Others are quite accepting of their terminal status and do not wish for any further treatment.

At this time, the patient begins to experience the advanced nature of the disease and to anticipate decline and death. Undeniable physical change initiates deep emotional and spiritual shifts, and the patient begins to grieve the loss of both past and future life. The patient's decision to share his or her grief with friends and family is dependent on a variety of factors, such as personality, history, safety, and opportunity. Although PATIENT GRIEF may not be expressed in emotion or words, it may be observable in behavior. Often, patients wish to protect their family members from the sadness and hopelessness they feel and, therefore, internalize their grief. Grieving patients may focus on getting their affairs in order or completing unfinished projects. They may also want to take a dream trip or to revisit important past relationships or places.

Reeling after receiving the news of a now-advanced and extensive disease, many patients and families resolve to remain optimistic and positive. At the same time, they may feel abandoned by their bodies, each other, the treatments, or the health care system. They are concurrently preparing themselves for dying while rejecting the certainty of death. This is a time of finding a constructive balance between hope and denial. Patients face multiple unknowns and have many questions about their future and the future of their families. This may be a time of great ambivalence, when EMOTIONS are intense, unpredictable, and suppressed. People fear the depth of their own and each other's emotions and try to maintain the positive, hopeful attitudes they used to survive earlier encounters with the illness. Patients worry how their family members will survive the emotional and spiritual anguish of death and bereavement. People have fears about what death will be like. These common thoughts, feelings, and concerns can be paralyzing.

Patients and families have a lot on their minds, but have difficulty with open COMMUNICATION. Talking directly about realities may feel insensitive, and words cannot capture the enormity of what people are thinking and feeling. Family members are trying to prepare themselves and plan for the future, but do not feel comfortable talking to the patient about what lies ahead. Similarly, patients may not want to upset family members with their sadness or regret. Wanting to protect each other from the harsh reality, they keep most conversations simple, concrete, and positive.

It is not unusual for the patient and family to be grieving different losses in different ways, and at different times. This disparity often creates conflict and confusion that can result in FAMILY ISSUES. Changes in family roles and responsibilities are hard for patients and families to accept. When people must alter familiar patterns and routines, they may struggle to have confidence in themselves and each other. This can lead to a loss of identity; leaving people feeling bereft, unneeded, and anxious.

JOHN AND LOUISE

John was first diagnosed with lung cancer 1 year ago and underwent radiation treatment. Last week, he and his wife Louise learned that the disease has now spread, with metastatic tumors in his lungs, bones, and liver. Although the oncologist is offering treatment for emerging symptoms of pain, shortness of breath, and nausea, he was also clear that the cancer is now advanced with little chance for overall improvement. When John asked about his prognosis, he was told it was not good. He and Louise were shocked to find out that his cancer had progressed. Although he was experiencing some symptoms, John thought it was just indigestion from his renewed appetite for Louise's Cajun-style cooking. Now he is having episodes of pain and nausea several times a day, occasionally he vomits, and only able to walk short distances. John is obsessed with getting his affairs in order but does not discuss his wishes, feelings, or plans with Louise. He has recently had nightmares about drowning but says they are too upsetting to discuss. John asked Louise not to discuss his prognosis with their friends and family. Louise, however, wants and needs to talk to someone.

> "If people cannot speak of their affliction they will be destroyed by it, or swallowed up by apathy. It is not important where they find the language or what form it takes. But people's lives actually depend on being able to put their situation into words, or rather, learning to express themselves, which includes the nonverbal possibilities of expression. Without the capacity to communicate with others, there can be no change. To become speechless, to be totally without any relationship, that is death."
>
> —(Soelle, 1976, p. 76)

John and Louise have been married for 10 years. He is 62 and she is 49. This is a second marriage for both of them. John and his first wife divorced 13 years ago; Louise's first husband died from stomach cancer 15 years ago. Louise has a 20-year-old daughter, Tanya, who lives at home with John and Louise and is attending college full time. John has a 32-year-old son, Jeff, and a 26-year-old daughter, Sarah. Sarah, her husband, and their three young children visit John yearly, and she telephones frequently. Jeff and John have not spoken for 6 years. Jeff has a 2-year-old son whom he sees sporadically, but whom John has never met. Against the family's advice, John has been trying to contact Jeff.

Due to his lack of stamina, John recently retired and had to sell his self-owned house-painting business. Prior to and during the early treatments, he was an active and healthy man who diffused his stress through physical activity. He had coached junior boys' lacrosse for many years and golfed twice a week with long-time friends. Lately, he has been unable to participate in lacrosse or golf but says he will get back to it soon. Louise works full time as a receptionist at a busy dental office. John puts a lot of faith and money into the vitamin and ozone therapy regimes that he's using, but Louise doesn't feel they can afford to continue with them much longer. As she looks ahead, Louise also worries about having to take off work to look after John. She hopes the cancer center oncologist is able to continue as his doctor.

KEY CONSIDERATIONS

Change in Focus

John was first diagnosed with lung cancer 1 year ago and underwent radiation treatment. Last week, he and Louise learned that the disease has now spread, with metastatic tumors in his lungs, bones, and liver. Although the oncologist is offering treatment to the bones and lungs for emerging symptoms of pain, shortness of breath, and nausea, he was also clear that the cancer is now advanced with little chance for overall improvement. When John asked about his prognosis, he was told that it is not good. Louise hopes the cancer center oncologist is able to continue on as John's doctor.

Moving from aggressive to palliative care is overwhelming for patients and families. In an article on the impact of terminal illness in the family, Smith (1990) explained that when people receive the message that no more can be done and the family doctor or medical team suggest hospice care, "It is the latest in a long line of shocks and crises experienced during the course of the illness" (p. 129). The family may be feeling abandoned and rejected by a system they came to trust, and may lack the confidence or energy to familiarize themselves with a new one. To many people, palliative and hospice care is an unknown, dark entity. To others, a hospice is a place where people go to die. Often, when the guidance and familiarity of specialists and facility support that they have known stops, patients and families feel lost and overwhelmed. Despite this, people become experts at maintaining hope in the midst of the uncertainty, fatigue, and great obstacles that they face.

To hear from trusted doctors and health care providers that cure is not possible is a tremendous blow to the heart and soul. A patient may be hearing this news following a recurrence that comes in spite of treatment, or he or she may be hearing the diagnosis for the first time after seeking medical care for symptoms that

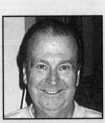

In My Own Voice
Dan Maloney versus ALS

Dan Maloney

Dan Maloney was
diagnosed with ALS
4 years ago.

I first noticed a problem with the strength in my legs. At my aunt's funeral, I found it difficult to get up from kneeling. I had to hold on to the pew and pull with all of my strength. I was tripping more frequently, but I did nothing about it.

Five months later, I told my doctor, who referred me to a local neurologist, but we didn't appear to be getting to the root of the problem. Another neurologist in Vancouver, however, was able to diagnose the symptoms as ALS, or Lou Gehrig's disease, within 45 minutes. I knew exactly what that meant as I recently had lost a neighbor to ALS. Here I am, 57 years old, and I know it is a fatal disease. The reality of the verdict hit me when I explained to my sister who was with me what this terrible disease is all about. We returned home and again I broke down. My wife had moved out. There I was alone with a broken marriage and a terminal disease that I had to face.

I took a couple of days off work to come to terms with my future. I started notifying my family. I was honest with them, and from them I gained my strength.

With one phone call to the local ALS Society, life got better. They made the assistance, support, and equipment I needed to assist with daily living available to me. I correspond with dozens of PALS (People with ALS) and belong to a local support group.

About this time I decided I was going to live with ALS rather than die with ALS. I had to be as strong for my family as they are for me. I could dwell on "Why me, Lord?" or count my many blessings. I have three wonderful daughters, two sisters, a brother, three sons-in-law, and eight grandchildren to be grateful for. I have many friends who truly care for me.

A year after my diagnosis, I knew I had to end my 38-year career. I was risking harm to myself. With tears in my eyes, I discussed my departure with my managers and thanked them for their support while I was adjusting to an unknown future. I faced my loyal coworker to tell him he didn't need to cover for me anymore.

With my marriage over and my career behind me, my daughters came forward to offer me a home with them. I had always promised myself I would never move in with any of them. I learned "You never say never." They convinced me that they'd worry less if I wasn't on my own. So here I am living with my daughter and her family. I'm very up front with my family about how ALS is affecting me and don't hide the truth from them. We deal with my setbacks on a daily basis.

The equipment and renovations I need will likely cost me more than $35,000. Renovations in my bathroom, for instance, to make it wheelchair accessible cost more than $10,000. The shower can accommodate an assistant, when the need arises, which I suspect isn't far off.

Today, I'm doing okay. Sure, my legs don't work, I'm confined to a wheelchair, my shoulders and arms are very weak, I no longer drive, but at this point I can still do most things for myself. Every day is good. I know God will give me and my family the courage and strength to face the future challenges, whatever they will be. There is no cure, but there is hope!

could no longer be ignored. One patient struggles with the failure of treatment, while another tries to deal with the impact of bad news coupled with a poor prognosis. However carefully this news is given, it feels cold, hopeless, and confusing; it is very difficult news to hear. It is common for people to repeatedly question or review the validity of the information, believing that some critical factor has been overlooked or new treatment untried. Writing about helping families through a life-threatening illness, Latimer explained that families "need to go over the same information about the illness, treatment, and future prognosis a number of times because their stress and anxiety prevent them from assimilating information" (2000, p. 82). This inability to accept the harsh realities of serious illness is one of the ways that people cope. It is not uncommon for people to use denial at various times throughout this transition and beyond.

The patient-centered approach of palliative care firmly places choice and responsibility in the hands of patients and families. Although patients have been at the center of decisions about treatment, this time marks a transition during which care shifts from making decisions about managing the disease and its treatment—a medically driven focus—to managing the rest of one's life—a quality-of-life focus. Although it may feel as though no critical decisions are left to make, there are still many decisions and opportunities that can make the patient's remaining time meaningful. Few people are relieved to learn, however, that palliative care aims to make dying as comfortable as possible. Hannicq stated that families "see palliative care as the slow but certain death of a loved one" (1995, p. 22). Although the gravity of the patient's condition is unavoidable, talking openly about death may yet be taboo. In their hearts and minds, people are often still fighting for the cure. Consequently, palliative care, and its expertise in death and dying, may be quite unappealing to patients and families.

Interventions

These psychosocial interventions have been designed to specifically address the key consideration *change in focus*. There are several assessment questions that will help open up a discussion, followed by more focused comments or tips that will facilitate further exploration of the issues that frequently arise at this time; each tip is followed by a sample dialogue.

Assessment Questions

- Tell me about your experience in acute care, the cancer clinic, and so forth.

- What were the most positive things about that time? The most negative things?

- What did you learn about yourself and what you need or value?

- What do you know about what's happening with your disease and treatment now? What are you still wondering about?

- What or who are your primary supports?

Normalize feelings and validate experiences. Overwhelmed by their present circumstances, people may have trouble finding words to express what they think and feel. When we put words to people's experiences, it gives them a language to build on and use when communicating their needs.

"I can understand that you are feeling abandoned and uncertain right now. You were really comfortable with the staff at the treatment center, and this feels like a huge step into the unknown."

Highlight strengths and coping strategies. Faced with a terminal diagnosis, people can become paralyzed by the enormity of the emotional and spiritual journey ahead. When we help people to identify their internal resources, it restores equilibrium and a sense of competence. Recognizing how they survived other difficult times helps people apply previous successes to their present situation.

"It sounds like it was very hard for you to stop working. I can also see how your managerial skills have helped you to access information and advocate for yourself during this illness."

Identify and introduce supports. Be sure to identify and explore existing supports. Many people have no prior experience with someone who is seriously ill. Listen carefully for their most important concerns and create a helpful link between the patient/family and the health care team. It is important to be specific about exactly how the services that you suggest will address their particular concerns.

"I'm noticing how your faith has been a major source of hope and peace in your life. Are there people from your faith community who have been particularly helpful to you and your family during your illness? I also heard that you and your wife have been unable to go to church because you cannot drive. Would you like me to ask one of our volunteers to drive you both to church on Sunday?"

Help patients and families identify and build meaningful opportunities that are still possible. It is important that they take advantage of their current independence and energy to participate in enjoyable or valuable activities, knowing that the future will soon bring increased debility and decline.

"Judith, you mentioned that you have always wanted to revisit your early roots. Have you and Caleb considered making a trip to your home town? What would you need to do to prepare for such a journey?"

Patient Grief

> Now John is having episodes of pain and nausea several times a day oc-
> casionally vomits, and is able to walk only short distances. Since receiving
> this news, he is obsessed with getting his affairs in order but does not dis-
> cuss his wishes, feelings, or plans with Louise. He has recently had night-
> mares about drowning but says they are too upsetting to discuss.

Although grieving occurs throughout the disease process, it is particularly
strong for patients at this time. In "The Crisis of Dying," Abiven explained that
a "crisis is triggered when the patient realizes that the serious disease has entered
its final phase" (1995, p. 29). In other words, patients now realize that they may
die sooner than they had expected. By this time, most patients are no longer working, their social lives are shrinking, and they are experiencing new or increased
physical limitations. Even quiet hobbies and household tasks may be too strenuous now. Maintaining normal activities and responsibilities is becoming impossible. Appetite may be reduced. At this time, patients anticipate and make many
unwelcome adjustments to their lifestyle and relationships. It may be very difficult for patients to accept assistance, even with their decreasing energy and increased vulnerability. Each of these changes signifies what is no longer possible
and alerts patients to further decline. The reality of their situation is deeply felt if
not always expressed. One study reported, "Some patients were unable to talk
about their feelings of depression or sadness" (Greisinger, Lorimor, Aday, Winn, &
Baile, 1997, p. 148).

The examination of present circumstances often leads people to review their
lives and reflect on transformational relationships and events. This process may
uncover sources of joy or sorrow that patients wish to revisit or resolve, and often
brings a source of much needed meaning and renewed purpose to the altered lives
of people (Kissane & Clarke, 2001). Completing projects, fulfilling dreams, and
spending quality time with family and friends may be especially important to patients now. Vachon (1998) contended that humor and reminiscence shared with
family and friends help to give patients a sense of purpose. This tends to be a time
of deep reflection and intense emotion for patients who are accounting for the lives
they've led and the deaths that await them.

The concept of who we are and how we feel about ourselves is closely tied to
the activities of our daily lives. If unable to interact in familiar ways, patients and
families must learn new ways of being together. The physical changes that happen
to patients, such as weight loss, fatigue, and weakness, contribute to their per-

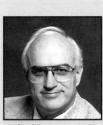

In My Own Voice
Total Pain

Michael Downing

Michael Downing, M.D.,
is the medical director at
Victoria Hospice, the
original physician with
the program.

If pain was a simple physical on/off switch (the Cartesian model) and we could provide the off switch, the fears of the dying might be eased. However, such an on/off mechanism for pain does not exist. Rather, with unrelieved pain, a complex and insidious process begins to develop at several levels for the individual. It has been called "total pain" because the multifaceted nature of pain includes not only physical stimuli but also one's reaction to or experience of pain. The perception, the context, and the meaning attributed to pain are aspects of *intellectual pain.* But, as people have feelings and reactions, *emotional pain* adds to the mix with varied tones of anxiety, frustration, guilt, hope, and ambivalence. Most people do not live in isolation, and so *physical pain* spills over to others around them, creating *interpersonal pain* among family or health care providers. Feelings of being a burden, "short fuses," or *unresolved pains* from the past can arise. *Financial pain* strikes with income loss, care expenses, and so forth. The next level is *spiritual pain,* as unrelenting pain leads to questions like "Why me, God? Why now? Where is the pain leading? Where am I going?" and to concerns about things left undone, remorse, brokenness, meaninglessness. Now let's add *bureaucratic pain,* with all the ensuing tests, paper forms, and multiple care providers.

But neither the story nor is the pain, is over. At the physical level, the continued barrage of pain stimuli from a tumor pressing on organs and tissues (called *nociceptive input*) or from actual damage to nerves (called *neuropathic pain*) causes dynamic changes within the spinal cord and the brain. Some of these changes are the body's internal efforts to reduce the sensation of pain (the gate-control theory). But, more often, the pain sensation is amplified, modulated, or distorted due to neuroplasticity within our central nervous system. The actual transmission and sensation of pain is altered when pain is constant and due to tissue damage. Thus, the intensity and quality of physical pain perceived by the individual changes and worsens with time if it is not relieved or if the input is blocked.

An insidious process now evolves. As physical pain increases and becomes distorted, the "other total pains" take on heightened meaning. Furthermore, other symptoms such as nausea, constipation, and fatigue impinge on and aggravate one's pain. This process of multiple symptoms; the changing and distorted nature of physical pain; and the resulting anxieties, fears, frustrations, and insomnia drive a vicious circle, creating a "monster" so to speak. The pain progressively occupies more of the patient's mental focus and limits physical activity. Immobilized by pain's unrelenting nature, neither the patient nor the family can see beyond it.

Total pain can be lessened, even relieved, but will it? Treatment of total pain or "monster" pain cannot be done by medication alone. Rather, treatment involves unraveling the various contributing factors through accurate assessment, skill, and knowledge. Each factor requires its own form of treatment as one by one the "mess" is broken down into appropriate, manageable fragments. Pain is thus unraveled, severity lessened, confidence increased, and hope restored. Some—but not all— is accomplished through drugs, radiation, or medical procedures. Excellent palliative care requires attention to all of the pain factors, not just the physical ones. With this degree of complexity, the answer lies in a team—not just professionals, but also the patient, his or her family, and their friends. Finally, three axioms within palliative care are relevant in my view:

1. Nothing stays the same for long.
2. Whatever is now "in control" will get out of control again.
3. Expect change and constantly look to prevent it or immediately relieve it.

With physical decline, whether the person is at PPS 70%, 50%, or 30%, total pain often arises. Once treated, it will arise again but, we hope, it will be less intense due to the vigilance and skill of the team in prevention and intervention. Pain does not have to spiral upward to become the monster of total pain, but can melt away in comfort with the nurture of a caring, competent, and compassionate team.

ceived loss of freedom, independence, and self-control. As the disease progresses, the roles and responsibilities formerly assumed by the patient are shifted to other people. When change happens prematurely or without consultation, as it often does with illness, some people feel angry, depressed, and unimportant. When patients are no longer able to engage with life and family in familiar and comfortable ways, living can feel pointless and unbearable (Kissane & Clarke, 2001). Some may express their desperation through questions about euthanasia or by declaring a wish to die. Others are able to adapt to these changes more easily and find positive aspects to living.

Interventions

These psychosocial interventions have been designed to specifically address the key consideration *patient grief*. There are several assessment questions that will help open up a discussion, followed by more focused comments or tips that will facilitate further exploration of the issues that frequently arise at this time; each tip is followed by a sample dialogue.

Assessment Questions

- How do you show or tell people what you are feeling? How does your family respond when you express emotion? How does that feel for you?

- When you feel hopeless about something, what do you do? How effective is that now?

- In the past, what have been sources of strength for you during troubling times?

- What religious or spiritual beliefs do you have? Are they the same as or different than those held by other people in your family? What do you think or believe happens after death?

- What legacy, gifts of love, or letters do you wish to give to your loved ones? How might you accomplish this?

Identify and explore the patient's thoughts and feelings. Often, this is a time when patients feel unable to express their thoughts and feelings with friends and family. They are concerned that, if they were to do so, people would be frightened or feel sorry for them. Supporting the patient in exploring his or her thoughts and feelings may help relieve some of the isolation and confusion that he or she feels now.

> *"I know that this can be a time when it is difficult to share your thoughts and feelings with the people closest to you. I'm wondering how you might feel talking with me about your experience. Yolanda, what is most impor-*

tant to you now? What gives you the most hope? What frightens or worries you about the future?"

Introduce and normalize the patient's grief process. Grief often begins in the anticipation of loss, and patients will grieve the losses that they encounter and anticipate as they are dying. When we acknowledge their grief, it provides another opportunity for people to understand and express their experience.

> *"I know that this time can be particularly challenging for people. You might be starting to think seriously about what lies ahead and how different your life feels from the way it used to be. All of the changes you've been through have been losses, and it is common for people to feel really sad and angry now."*

Provide opportunities for life review. When you engage dying people in self-reflection, you are helping them with a very important developmental concern: finding and making meaning of their lives. Life review gives people a sense of purpose and helps them to notice what feels unfinished or incomplete.

> *"When you think about your life, what events stand out for you? What role did you and other people play in them? What were your greatest achievements?"*

Encourage people to make choices and take action. Support the completion of unfinished business while patients still have enough energy to address or complete outstanding and important concerns. Dealing with interpersonal estrangements or conflicts may be very important now and may provide patients with a renewed sense of purpose.

> *"I often hear you talking sadly about your relationship with your son, Merv. Is there anything that you need or want to do about this now?"*

Emotions

> When John asked about his prognosis, he was told it was not good. He and Louise were shocked to find out that the disease had progressed.

Although he was experiencing some symptoms, John thought it was just indigestion from his renewed appetite for Louise's Cajun-style cooking. He has recently had nightmares about drowning but says they are too upsetting to discuss. John asked Louise not to discuss his prognosis with their friends and family.

Latimer asserted that "family members will be experiencing a number of powerful emotions" (2000, p. 82). Perhaps adjusting to the withdrawal of, or shift in, treatment and the increasing burden of disease, family may find their emotions are exhausting, intense, and unpredictable. Strong feelings arise in response to the disabilities and realities of advanced disease. Anger, fear, hope, and denial compete for the diminished energy of patients and families. It may be hard for patients and families to comprehend, after months or years of investigation and treatment, that cure is no longer possible. They have often made tremendous personal, physical, and financial sacrifices, expecting that their lives would be spared. The shock and denial that is normal now may make it difficult for people to even identify what they feel. This difficulty is further complicated when family members have different needs for emotional openness and expression. One study pointed out, "The best level of communication for one role may not be optimal for the other" (Hinton, 1998). Without safe, acceptable ways to express emotion, people may become isolated and estranged.

Patients and families may feel powerlessness, as well as anger toward themselves and/or each other, imagining that treatment failed because of something they did or didn't do. Past arguments, advice given, and decisions made may be scrutinized in the search for a legitimate reason for this terrible state. The anger may be directed at the health care system, physicians, or a higher power. This can be deeply confusing and distressing for families, as this is a time when they strive to be close and supportive. People who are uncomfortable with anger will carefully avoid topics and situations that cause it to flare.

Underneath anger there is often fear. Fears about the unknown are enormous now. Patients and families fear the dying process, uncertain whether they can tolerate the frailty, dependence, and responsibility that they anticipate. Pessagno asserted that "patients and families may seek miracle cures because of fear" (p. 105). Patients may have fears about pain, suffering, and indignity and may worry that their wishes will not be respected. Patients may also fear they will be an unbearable burden on their families, and this may lead them to withhold information about their level of discomfort or pain. They may consider extended, hospital, or hospice care in order to protect family members from the demands of caregiving.

LIFE REVIEW

For people who are facing death, the opportunity to look back over a lifetime and to highlight events, qualities, places, and people that have been most influential is especially valuable. Life review is a "way to evaluate where one has been in relationship to where one is and where one wants to go" (Pickrel, 1989, p. 127). This structured remembering enables patients to recover aspects of themselves, their identity, and their self-worth, which can be damaged or destroyed by disease progression. Reminiscing may help people to better understand and recognize themselves within their present circumstances and to clarify what is most important for the time they have left. When suggesting or facilitating life review with patients, one must be aware that past trauma and hurtful memories may also surface and that this activity may be unpleasant or inappropriate for some.

Four primary forms of life review may be particularly effective with palliative patients and their families. Several examples of activities are included for each form.

1. Structured Activity

   - Oral history interviews: Using this technique the listener takes on the role of interviewer and asks key questions on a particular topic such as, "Tell me about how you and [the patient or family member] met? Where were you? When? What were your first impressions?"

   - Family tree or genogram: Both provide a visual map of the family history. The family tree is less formal but shows who married whom and what children were born. The genogram is more detailed, often using symbols to identify estrangements, alliances, divorces, gender, and deaths, as well as marriages and children.

   - Life line: This is a simple time line with the beginning signifying birth, and the end, death. The task is to "travel" from birth to the present, naming and dating important events.

2. Family Activity

   - Review memorabilia: Patient and family get together and look through family photographs, correspondence, and mementos.

   - Family stories: Several generations of the family are invited to come together and tell their favorite family story. Stories may be funny, sad, personal, or inherited.

   - Pilgrimage or family reunion: Patients and families return to important places, such as a birthplace, or gather several generations of the family together in one place.

3. Anecdotes

   - Career or life's work: Focus on one area and recall significant milestones and achievements.

- "This is Your Life": Create an audiotape or videotape account of the patient's life story.

4. Mind Travel

- Relive an experience: Ask patient to recall and describe a favorite or difficult event. Attend to sights, smells, sounds, tastes, thoughts, and feelings.

- Dreams: Ask patients to complete a thought such as, "I always wanted to—" or "I wish I had—."

Tip: When you are doing a life review with someone, notice any themes that surface and reveal them to that person. Point out any coping strengths and strategies that emerge in your discussions.

Copyright © 1989. From Tell Me Your Story: Using Life Review in Counseling the Terminally Ill *by J. Pickrel. Reproduced by permission of Taylor & Francis, Inc., http://www.routledge-ny.com.*

According to Vachon, "Caregivers fear they will not provide the right care or will not know what to do in case of emergency" (1998, p. 52). They fear the patient will experience some kind of crisis and they will "freeze" and not be able to help or that they will even do something harmful. Caregivers may also fear that they cannot maintain or fulfill the patient's wishes or preferred care plan.

The Role of Denial

Maintaining hope may manifest itself in denial about the severity or reality of the illness. Abiven explained, "It is quite possible to live with these [opposing] realities at the same time—imminent death and remission" (1995, p. 30). People may accept that the illness is terminal and still actively hope for remission or cure. Denial may be a useful short-term coping strategy for people in unbearable circumstances. It can give people the time and space to reclaim control of their lives by choosing which facts to believe or accept, and which ones to ignore or overlook. It can help people regain a sense of hope and purpose for the future, and allow patients and families to investigate and integrate earth-shattering truths at their own pace.

Denial, though useful for coping, can also be harmful. It can prevent people from talking to each other about what is most important to them. When complete denial is maintained until death, it may interfere with the process of life review, resolution, and closure. It can also make decision making and planning for care difficult.

When the patient and/or family are not talking directly about dying, it is difficult for health care providers to assess needs and provide information (see Figure 4.1).

Interventions

These psychosocial interventions have been designed to specifically address the key consideration *emotions*. There are several assessment questions that will help open up a discussion, followed by more focused comments or tips that will facilitate further exploration of the issues that frequently arise at this time; each tip is followed by a sample dialogue.

Assessment Questions

- How do you deal with difficult feelings when they surface?
- Is this different than how other people in your family deal with feelings?
- What feelings are strongest for you now? Is this causing you any difficulties in your relationships? Your work? Your health?

Normalize feelings. When some people experience intense and difficult emotions they have an automatic impulse to stifle or minimize them. This

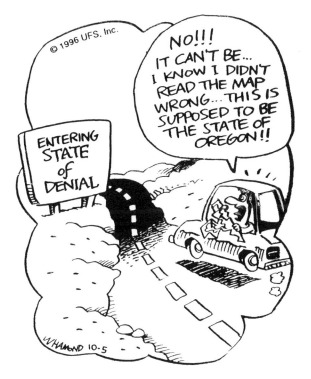

Figure 4.1. This cartoon takes a lighter look at people when they are in a state of denial. REALITY CHECK reprinted by permission of United Feature Syndicate, Inc.

behavior may well cause increased isolation, tension, and volatility. When you identify and describe typical emotions, people will feel understood and more comfortable expressing what they really think and feel.

> *"This is often a time of intense and unpredictable emotions, Beth. You may find that you are impatient and have a short fuse with the people who matter the most to you. This often happens when people are feeling powerless and exhausted. It may help to let people close to you know how you're really doing and to find other ways to release emotion."*

Identify and teach useful coping strategies. Many people facing death and bereavement will be going through this for the first time. They may not have the kind of skills and techniques that can be helpful now. Use your knowledge and expertise with others to provide people with ideas and options that they can apply to their own situations.

> *"Some people find that meditation or prayer is helpful, while others express emotion through movement or exercise. Some people benefit from creative projects such as journaling, painting, or building something. Talking with a spiritual advisor, friend, or palliative care provider may also be very helpful at this time."*

Challenge, probe, or reframe. This will be a time when layers of feelings and ways of dealing with them will compete with and contradict each other. It may look to you as if people are preventing themselves from getting what they need. It may help if you name the inconsistency that you see and check out how that behavior is or isn't meeting the person's needs.

> *"Leah, you said earlier that you are comfortable with emotions. Yet I notice that whenever your friend starts to cry or talk about how sad he feels, you change the subject or leave the room. I'm wondering what's going on?"*

Communication

John asked Louise not to discuss his prognosis with their friends and family. Louise, however, wants and needs to talk to someone. She has contacted the palliative care provider she saw when her first husband died, but she hasn't told John.

Communication is influenced by people's sense of safety and control. People coping with a recent diagnosis are usually feeling fearful, betrayed, and exhausted. One of the ways that people cope in this state is to keep conversations light and easy. Connor (2000) suggested that most people avoid talking about death out of the mistaken belief that doing so will make matters worse. People may want to talk with each other about what is really going on but may feel awkward bringing up the topic. They may fear that they won't say or do the right thing, or that they may be inviting the worst by acknowledging the possibility of death. Unfortunately, however, "It is not talking about the obvious reality that causes people to withdraw or to miss important opportunities for healing" (p. 261).

Communication also occurs in indirect ways. For example, a family may decide to host a birthday party for the patient and invite many long-lost friends and relatives, without openly acknowledging that this birthday may be the patient's last. Similarly, they may plan to have a Christmas celebration in November. Patients may want to review photo albums with their grandchildren, or talk a lot about special family times. Focusing on happy or meaningful events can be a way to remind dying individuals that they are loved and will be missed.

Sometimes people are able to talk more openly with those outside the immediate family, such as close friends, extended family, or professionals. Health care providers may be seen as experienced and neutral and therefore able to give informed, objective advice and support. It may, however, be unsettling for the patient and family to find themselves sharing their deepest concerns with strangers. This may prompt some people to find ways to open these difficult topics with each other.

UNDERSTANDING DENIAL

- Understand the patient and family context and identify how denial may be a positive force that helps them cope. Is this a new diagnosis? Does the patient and/or family have a support system? Are there multiple losses or other major issues affecting the family?

- Ask the patient and family what they understand or believe about their current situation and what they hold as most important now. What do they see as their strengths and struggles? Find out what they most hope for and fear.

- Assess prior knowledge of and experiences with illness and palliative care. What experiences have people had with illness prior to this? Have they had any involvement with hospice care before? If so, what happened? How would they characterize what happened, positive or negative?

Interventions

These psychosocial interventions have been designed to specifically address the key consideration *communication*. There are several assessment questions that will help open up a discussion, followed by more focused comments or tips that will facilitate further exploration of the issues that frequently arise at this time; each tip is followed by a sample dialogue.

Assessment Questions

- Who is talking with whom, and about what? Also, who is the family spokesperson and who is excluded from discussions?

- How do you communicate with your family? How is that for you?

- When you need to talk, whom do you talk to? Is this person aware of what's going on in your life right now? When was the last time you spoke with this person? How was it for you?

- Have you religious or spiritual beliefs that differ from those held by your family or friends?

Normalize differences. We know that, even within close families, each person may have very different perspectives on the same issue. Many people feel strongly that their way is the right way and, under stress, these beliefs may become even more rigid and entrenched. It helps to diffuse conflict when you are able to normalize differences and reframe distressing attitudes or behaviors.

> *"Mina, I hear you say that you find it is very difficult to talk with your father when he's being closed, as you put it. It is not unusual for each person in a family to communicate about this painful experience in different ways. Instead of sharing his sadness with you, perhaps your father is trying to protect you from it by pushing you away with his apparent indifference and anger. Sometimes, people don't want to burden or concern anyone with the depth of their suffering. How does this fit with who your dad is?"*

Model and teach ways to initiate difficult conversations. Often, people get hung up on the words. When you are able to coach them by providing examples or role-playing, this can help to ease people's discomfort.

> *"I know that you feel you can't tell your sister that you resent her for taking over your responsibilities. Sometimes it helps to rehearse these conversations a bit ahead of time. Perhaps we could work on this together. I could be*

you, and demonstrate some ways that you might talk about this, and you could be your sister. Would that help you to feel more comfortable?"

Family Issues

John has been trying to contact his son, Jeff, against the family's advice. Jeff and John have not spoken for 6 years. Jeff has a 2-year-old son whom he sees sporadically, but whom John has never met. John puts a lot of faith in the vitamin and ozone therapy regimes that he's using, but Louise doesn't feel they can afford to continue with them much longer.

This is a time when patients and family members can have very different needs, hopes, expectations, and coping strategies. Longstanding family rules and patterns are tested. Often, what worked well before doesn't work any longer. Smith stated, "accepting that the patient will die creates a crisis that forces the family to consider new ways of doing things" (1990, p. 129), which may contribute to painful arguments about changing priorities and roles. When people are feeling fatigued and fragile, changing roles and responsibilities is not easy. Individual family members may have very different reactions to change. Longstanding, but quiet, family issues may resurface now and generate conflict as the patient strives to complete unfinished business and resolve family rifts and feuds.

Although at this point the burden of patient care is not so much physical as emotional, families are anticipating heavy care needs in the future. Demands on the family caregiver's time and energy will increase as the patient's mobility and functioning decrease. Various family members may take time off of work and away from their own families to support the dying person. Although there are personal rewards, there are also costs. Family caregivers may experience extreme fatigue, social isolation, and financial hardship (Vachon, 1998).

MEANING AND SPIRITUALITY

Doka (2000) explained that when patients receive a terminal diagnosis, their basic assumptions about the world are threatened. Any previously held sense of safety, meaning, and purpose in their lives may be shattered. The dissolution of these fundamental beliefs contributes to spiritual pain. He identified three spiritual needs for people who are in the terminal phase of their disease process. These spiritual needs are

1. To die an appropriate death
2. To find meaning in one's life
3. To find hope that exists beyond the grave

Doka recommended that the "responsibility for spiritual care is shared" by all members of the team. Because the goal of spiritual care is to "witness, empower and validate the spiritual quest," it isn't necessary to be a clergyperson or other form of religious "expert" (p. 110). Life review and personal or religious rituals can help people identify and deal with unfinished business, uncover strengths, and connect with important values as they face their remaining journey.

Stadjuhar concluded that although the work of family caregiving comes with significant benefits, such as familiarity and freedom, "the physical and emotional devastation of terminal illness makes extraordinary demands upon families" (1998, p. 13).

It is not uncommon for resentment to build between in- and out-of-town family members. Relatives who live out of town often miss out on many changes and decisions. They may not be in attendance when important information about the disease process is shared with the patient and family, or when the decision to stop a particular treatment is made. They often don't understand or accept the decisions made and feel out of step with the patient and local family. For example, if they haven't witnessed an increase in symptoms or physical change in the patient, they may have trouble supporting the choices made by others. Often, the in-town family caregivers feel unsupported by the out-of-town family and the out-of-town family members feel unheard.

Interventions

These psychosocial interventions have been designed to specifically address the key consideration *family issues*. There are several assessment questions that will help open up a discussion, followed by more focused comments or tips that will facilitate further exploration of the issues that frequently arise at this time; each tip is followed by a sample dialogue.

Assessment Questions

- How has this situation changed your daily routines and lifestyle?
- How is it for you that Jackie has not been able to contribute to your father's care?
- How is this affecting your relationship?
- Have you been able to review changes and negotiate new roles in the family?
- How was it decided that you would be the primary caregiver?
- What are you most worried about for your grandmother's care now and down the road?

Acknowledge conflict. People will often persist in being angry with someone else or themselves but will not acknowledge or address it. When you name what you see, it opens up a dialogue and you may find that people are willing to move into exploring or addressing issues more directly.

> *"You seem quite angry with Cyril. Can you tell me more about what's happening for you?"*

Facilitate resolution. Conflict takes the family's focus away from the fact that someone is seriously ill or dying, and the grief that they feel about it. When you are able to help the family address the issues that they recognize, they may be more able to directly address other, deeper concerns.

> *"Sometimes living with the conflict takes up more energy than sorting it out. Have you tried to work this out? What happened? Perhaps it would help if I sat down with you and your family and helped you to express yourselves, hear each other, and identify some ways that you might be able to work better together."*

Protect patient autonomy. Challenge families to explore any tendencies to push patients into premature invalidism or protect them from risk, both of which may reduce their autonomy. It is important to find a balance between what patients are safely able to do and what others need or want to take on.

> *"Sondra, your mother thinks you are interfering with her life. You want to be loving and helpful, but your mom feels you are taking over and not allowing her to do things for herself. How might you two decide what you need to do and what she can do for herself?"*

OUR EXPERIENCE

During the shift from treatment to hospice palliative care providers aim to cultivate therapeutic relationships with the patients and families. This is based on an understanding of their strengths and most important concerns. The purpose of this effort is to develop a care plan that is holistic, ethical, and appropriate.

This is often the time when we first meet patients and families in our palliative care program. They come to us with the scars and skills of their life experience, and the history of this illness. We are witnesses to their anguish, despair, and fatigue, and endeavor to help them find meaning, dignity, and hope as they journey toward death and bereavement. We accompany patients and families into the domain of unknown limitations and losses, theirs and our own, and find ways to continue the journey forward into living with dying. Our experience tells us that these things are possible, in spite of the shades of fear and loss of faith that are provoked by encounters with decline and dying. At this time, we attend to the whole person, listening for the cues that inform as to what matters most to them spiritually, emotionally, socially, and physically. We help patients and families change their focus from *what is no longer to what may be.*

We recognize that people entering our system may be unfamiliar with its philosophy and language, and so we provide information and educate people about what, exactly, it entails. We help to unearth the questions that may lie under the surface so that we can help people make informed decisions about treatments, medications, and care options. What has happened to patients and families prior to coming to palliative care is an important part of their story, and so we gather information about their experiences. We know that this is a time when patients and families may hold different perspectives, and so we explore how the illness is affecting their lives and relationships with each other.

We believe that it is important for patients and families to move through this time in a way that is congruent with their own lives, not imposed by us. We empower them to do what feels true for them by building on their strengths, providing relevant information and emotional support, and teaching practical skills. Our experience guides them to understanding their emotions, thoughts, and behaviors. Sometimes this means staying out of the way when we feel most compelled to "fix" them or show them the "right" way.

TEAM ISSUES

Bad news can be broken very well or very poorly. When the latter happens, it creates distress and confusion for patients, families, and/or palliative care providers who feel the need to justify this behavior in some way. Although it may be tempting to judge peers harshly, the successful resolution to this problem lies in closer relationships with colleagues, not further division. This may result in opportunities to discuss the issue and help all team members find better ways to share bad news.

The impulse to rush in and rescue people with a lot of options and information must be monitored when patients and families are entering palliative care. Palliative care providers may perceive or identify needs that people have not yet seen and may attempt to intervene too quickly. Basing actions on knowledge or skill rather than on understanding the uniqueness of a situation makes it easy to misjudge families and miss the essence of whom they are and what they need. It is as important to let the patient and family set the pace as it is to give them choices. They need time to absorb information and make decisions; our time pressures should be secondary.

Working with the simultaneous manifestations of hope and denial can be challenging for team members. This is especially true when one or some family members demonstrate a need to talk directly and realistically when others do not. As health care providers, team members must work carefully to identify and accept the role denial plays in helping people bring hope and meaning to their lives and circumstances. This may involve finding ways to talk about needs and goals without focusing directly on the reality of death itself.

ABOUT CHILDREN

Adults may be tempted to exclude children during times of dying and death, out of fear, convenience, or oversight. Parents typically want to protect their children from the confusion, sadness, and grief that surface when someone special is dying or dies. They may believe that the children are better off remembering the person who died when he or she was well. Sometimes, parents with younger children believe that their children are too young to fully understand or too fragile to be with adults who are sad or crying. They may fear that too much information could scare or harm their children and worry that they don't really know the right or correct things to say. These normal concerns and fears of parents should be respected.

Parents may need or choose to take on caregiving duties that keep them away from home, and they may feel out of touch with their children's needs. They may have asked trusted friends or other family members to care for their children and feel worried about how this will affect them and uncertain about how much or what information to share. It may also be true that parents are struggling with their own grief and don't know if they can manage the intensity of their children's grief as well. They may expect to be too distracted with caregiving to have their children present or to be able to take care of them.

Parents, however, may not realize how much their children do, in fact, know and understand. Whether or not the children have been told, they usually sense the adult family members' sadness, worry, and absence. Left to their imaginations and resources, children often draw their own conclusions about what is happening. Depending on their age and maturity, these conclusions may or may not be accurate.

Key Points

- Children's and teens' reactions to someone who is dying and to death are highly influenced by the reactions of significant adult role models (e.g., parents, grandparents, teachers, coaches).

- Children and teens do frequently want to know when, how, and why the person will die or has died, often in detail. Young children may not ask if they sense the adults don't want to talk about it, and teens may be uncomfortable asking outright.

- Children and teens may fare better if they are included with the family through this time. For this to happen, they need clear and ongoing information, adequate preparation, and appropriate support.

Interventions

These psychosocial interventions have been designed to specifically address the needs of children. There are focused comments or tips that will facilitate further exploration of the issues that frequently arise at this time; each tip is followed by a sample dialogue.

Check patients' and families' comfort level. Find out how comfortable children are with the way the adults in the family are expressing their thoughts and feelings. Ask about their personal thoughts and feelings.

> *"Jill, I notice that your mom is crying a lot. How is that for you? What are you feeling about your dad's illness and how things are going?"*

Ask children or teens if they want to be included in discussions or activities. Be sure to involve children in family gatherings or visits before the death and inquire if they want to see the person who died. Identify ways that they can do this comfortably.

> *"Samantha, would you like to visit your grandma? Is there anything you want to know before you do? What do you think she will look like?"* Or, *"Derrick, would you like to write a note, draw a picture, or give me something to take to your brother when I see him today?"*

Ask if the child was present at the death. Identify gaps or misconceptions in their understanding.

> *"Were you there when your mom died? What did you see? What was that like for you?"* Or, *"What were you told about your mom's death? Is there anything else that you would like to know about it or her?"*

SUMMARY

Many people are not cured after diagnosis and treatment. For them, the journey toward death continues, down unfamiliar and ill-favored roads. When patients and families are told the illness is terminal, they must make the transition from acute treatment to palliation (see Table 4.1). Those who transfer to hospice care undergo a significant shift in health care systems. They will not only encounter different people but also different places, choices, and perspectives. Much of health care today is conducted with an active, aggressive approach, oriented toward cure. For most people, the concept of palliation or comfort care is foreign.

> "Death is ultimately personal; to respond to the fears and human condition of the dying always involves responding to ourselves."
>
> —(Mansell Pattison, 1977)

Patients and families entering into palliative care may be newly diagnosed or may have known about the disease for a long time. They may have had many curative treatments or none at all. Some people choose to avoid aggressive treatments that may have a negative impact on their quality of life, while others opt for other healing modalities, such as naturopathy, meditation and prayer, or homeopathy. Often, the decision to stop or withhold curative treatment is made when the doctor indicates that nothing more can be done to achieve a cure or remission.

This transition triggers intense feelings of grief, anger, fear, and denial. People will try to protect each other from these feelings and so communication about the illness may be indirect, infrequent, or nonexistent. Difficulties in communication may create isolation, misperceptions, and conflict. Whatever the journey prior to palliation has been, hospice care usually delineates a painful departure from the path that patients and families would have preferred.

Table 4.1.   Palliative Performance Scale (PPSv2) 60%–50%

PPS Level	Ambulation	Activity and evidence of disease	Self-care	Intake	Conscious level
60%	Reduced	Unable to do hobby/housework Significant disease	Occasional assistance necessary	Normal or reduced	Full or confusion
50%	Mainly sit/lie	Unable to do any work Extensive disease	Considerable assistance required	Normal or reduced	Full or confusion

REFLECTIVE ACTIVITY

The Loss Boxes

The following activity (Rothstein, 1997) can be useful for health care providers, volunteers, or students to stimulate their personal reactions to death and to discern the themes that arise for people as they are dying. It is important for people to pay attention to whatever thoughts and feelings surface as they complete each box (see Figure 4.2). This activity can be done alone or, more effectively, in a group setting.

Facilitator Script

Step 1: "Think of your life as it is now and in the space of the largest box, write words or phrases that reflect what is most important to you at this moment. Don't think too much about it; whatever comes to mind is fine (people, things,

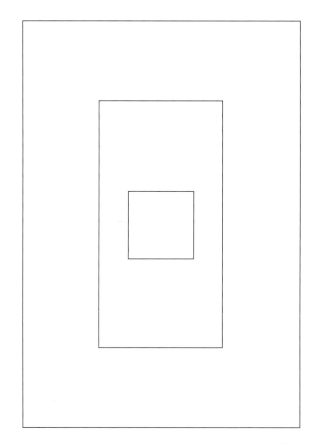

Figure 4.2. The Loss Boxes are a tool for reflecting on what has value in a person's life as he or she approaches death.

feelings, thoughts, and so forth). Take approximately 1–2 minutes for this part of the exercise."

Step 2: "Imagine that you have just received a diagnosis of a life-threatening illness. Using the second-largest box, write words or phrases that reflect what you imagine would be most important for you to have in your life at this time. Again, don't think too much about it; whatever comes to mind is fine. Take approximately 1–2 minutes for this box."

Step 3: "Finally, move to the smallest box. Imagine that you are now close to your death and write the words or phrases that reflect what you imagine would be most important now. Again, take 1–2 minutes for this."

Step 4: "Debrief the exercise with a partner. Notice what is most important to you and how that changes (or fails to change) as you imagine yourself moving closer to death. Talk about common needs, wishes, and any surprises. Also, consider the differences between you and discuss how those differences might impact the relationship, if you were to be a support for one another."

RESOURCES

Bender, M., Bauckham, P., & Norris, A. (1999). *The therapeutic purposes of reminiscence.* London: Sage Publications.

Burgess, D. (1994). Denial and terminal illness. *The American Journal of Hospice and Palliative Care, 11*(2), 46–48.

Byock, I. (1996). Beyond symptom management. *European Journal of Palliative Care, 3*(3), 125–130.

Copp, G. (1998). A review of current theories of death and dying. *Journal of Advanced Nursing, 28*(2), 382–390.

Davidhizar, R., & Giger, J. (1998). Patient's use of denial: Coping with the unacceptable. *Nursing Standard, 12*(43), 44–46.

Davies, B. (1990). Families in supportive care—Part 1: The transition of fading away: The nature of the transition. *Journal of Palliative Care, 6*(3), 12–20.

Haight, B., & Burnside, I. (1993, April). Reminiscence and life review: Explaining the differences. *Archives of Psychiatric Nursing, 2,* 91–98.

Liossi, C., & Mystakidou, K. (1997). Heron's theory of human needs in palliative care. *European Journal of Palliative Care, 4*(1), 32–35.

Mount, B. (1996). Morphine drips, terminal sedation, and slow euthanasia: Definitions and facts, not anecdotes. *Journal of Palliative Care, 12*(4), 31–37.

Nekolaichuk, C., & Bruera, E. (1998). On the nature of hope in palliative care. *Journal of Palliative Care, 14*(1), 36–42.

Quill, T., Lo, B., & Brock, D. (1997). Palliative options of last resort: A comparison of voluntarily stopping eating and drinking, terminal sedation, physician-assisted suicide, and voluntary active euthanasia. *Journal of the American Medical Association, 278*(23), 2099–2104.

Sales, E. (1991). Psychosocial impact of the phase of cancer on the family: An updated review. *Journal of Psychosocial Oncology, 9*(4), 1–18.

Smith, E. (1995). Addressing the psychospiritual distress of death as a reality: A transpersonal approach. *Social Work, 40*(3), 402–413.

Street, A., & Kissane, D. (1999–2000). Dispensing death, desiring death: An exploration of medical roles and patient's motivation during the period of legalized euthanasia in Australia. *Omega, 40*(1), 23–248.

Watson, M. (1994). Psychological care for cancer patients and their families. *Journal of Mental Health, 3,* 457–465.

Wilbur, K. (1988). Attitudes and cancer: What kind of help really helps? *The Journal of Transpersonal Psychology, 20*(1), 49–59.

Williams, T.T. (2001). *Refuge: An unnatural history of family and place.* New York: Vintage Books.

REFERENCES

Abiven, M. (1995). The crisis of dying. *European Journal of Palliative Care, 2*(1), 29–32.

Connor, S. (2000). Denial and the limits of anticipatory mourning. In T.A. Rando (Ed.), *Clinical dimensions of anticipatory mourning: Theory and practice in working with the dying, their loved ones, and their caregivers* (pp. 253–265). Champaign, IL: Research Press.

Doka, K. (2000). Re-creating meaning in the face of illness. In T.A. Rando (Ed.), *Clinical dimensions of anticipatory mourning: Theory and practice in working with the dying, their loved ones, and their caregivers.* (pp. 103–113). Champaign, IL: Research Press.

Greisinger, A., Lorimor, R., Aday, L., Winn, R., & Baile, W. (1997). Terminally ill cancer patients: Their most important concerns. *Cancer Practice, 5*(3), 147–154.

Hannicq, M. (1995). Family care: New principles. *European Journal of Palliative Care, 2*(1), 21–24.

Hinton, J. (1998). Open communication between people with cancer, caring relatives, and others. *Journal of Palliative Care, 14*(3), 15–23.

Kissane, D., & Clarke, D. (2001). Demoralization syndrome: A relevant psychiatric diagnosis for palliative care. *Journal of Palliative Care, 17*(1), 12–21.

Latimer, E. (2000). Helping families through a life-threatening illness. *The Canadian Journal of Diagnosis, 17*(6), 80–90.

Mansell Pattison, E. (1977). *The experience of dying.* New York: Prentice Hall.

Pessagno, R. (1998). Hope, fear and "miracle" cures. *Clinical Journal of Oncology Nursing, 2*(3), 105–106.

Pickrel, J. (1989). "Tell me your story": Using life review in counseling the terminally ill. *Death Studies, 13*(2), 127–135.

Rando, T. A. (2000). Anticipatory mourning: What it is and why we need to study it. In T.A. Rando (Ed.), *Clinical dimensions of anticipatory mourning: Theory and practice in working with the dying, their loved ones, and their caregivers* (pp. 307–378). Champaign, IL: Research Press.

Rothstein, J., & Rothstein, M. (1997). *The caring community: A field book for hospice palliative care volunteer services.* Vancouver: British Columbia Hospice Palliative Care Association.

Smith, N. (1990). The impact of terminal illness in the family. *Palliative Medicine, 4,* 127–135.

Soelle, D. (1975). *Suffering.* Philadelphia: Fortress Press.

Stadjuhar, K. (1998). Death at home: Challenges for families and directions for the future. *Journal of Palliative Care, 14*(3), 8–14.

Vachon, M. (1998). Psychosocial needs of patients and families. *Journal of Palliative Care, 14*(3), 49–56.

$$perspective$$

DYING CHILDREN
AND ADOLESCENTS

Most palliative care providers seldom work with dying children or adolescents. When they do, they look for ways to improve their knowledge, skills, and confidence. Personal and professional struggles and ethical conflicts commonly arise as questions about the appropriateness of treatments, interventions, decision making, and palliation are encountered. Often, when a child or teen is dying, the team is large and faced with multiple issues. Health care providers wrestle with boundaries and self-care and get hooked by particular individuals and choices. A brief snapshot of some of the main considerations, interventions, and issues involved follows.

THINGS TO KNOW ABOUT PALLIATIVE CARE FOR CHILDREN

The diseases fatal to children and adolescents are often different from those fatal to adults, with different illness trajectories and treatment options. Children may live with a terminal illness for a long time. A few diseases, such as some forms of leukemia, can now be cured. Although others, such as cystic fibrosis, cannot be cured, survival has greatly increased, and some individuals may be diagnosed as children but live into adulthood.

Decisions can be difficult. Any decisions about treatment, including its withdrawal, are stressful and difficult for both families and health care providers. The role of decision making is dependent on parenting style, family dynamics, and the child's ability to understand and participate.

The care provided is family driven. Parents are the primary decision makers; they make their decisions with strong, consistent, and optimistic intentions. Children are dependent on others for basic care and support. Children rely on their parents to make decisions and tend to their physical and emotional needs. Their parents are indispensable to them.

Sick children usually have a large professional care team that requires sophisticated equipment. This team usually includes both hospital and community-based services. Consistency of care and communication among the services and care team are challenging for patients, parents, and the professionals.

Parents may be providing highly intricate and technological nursing care that requires sophisticated equipment. Already stressed parents may be expected to manage highly complicated and time-consuming treatment regimes at home with minimal support.

What Helps Parents When Children Are Terminally Ill and Dying

- Respite care at home, or in facilities, to provide relief for family care-givers

- Reliable, convenient access to practical, spiritual, and psychosocial resources

- A consistent, community-based person or team to be a guide and advocate within the health care system

- Health care providers who are caring, connected, and responsive to parents' needs and requests

What Helps Children Who Are Terminally Ill and Dying

- Clear, age-appropriate information about the illness and its progression

- Opportunities to grow and develop through education, play, and social interaction

- Being supported to participate in decisions about care, including the time, place, and type of treatment

- Psychosocial interventions that use art, poetry, journaling, music, physical activity, and play

TEAM ISSUES

Team members almost invariably struggle to understand and accept the dying or death of a child. It is contrary to our thinking about children to accept that any child will not grow and mature to live a full lifetime. Health care providers may be deeply saddened or angered by the untimeliness and unfairness of this harsh reality. They may also feel they have failed the child or family in their effort to find a cure. Personal and organizational opportunities for spiritual growth and development should be identified and nurtured.

Often, health care providers get to know and care deeply about the children with whom they work, and letting go may be difficult. Fellow team members may become judgmental or unsupportive when they believe someone is too involved. The anticipatory grief and bereavement of professional caregivers who have been involved with a child, perhaps over several years, is significant and legitimate, however. Team meetings, group and individual support, and rituals must be created to honor and acknowledge the value and meaning of each child's dying process and death and the meaning of the care provider's grief.

Parents and health care providers may have different opinions about the child's needs. This difference of opinion is probably most challenging when decisions are being made about withdrawing active treatment or life-sustaining measures. Parents may choose not to, or be unable to, include the child in the decision-making process because of the child's age, neurological, physical, or emotional state. Conferences with the family and various team members may help to increase understanding and bridge differences.

RESOURCES

Durham, E. (1998). Caring for Cody. *American Journal of Nursing, 98*(4), 42–44.

Faulkner, K.W. (1997, June). Talking about death with a dying child. *American Journal of Nursing, 97*(6), 64–69.

Frager, G. (1996). Pediatric palliative care: Building the model, bridging the gaps. *Journal of Palliative Care, 12*(3), 9–12.

Goldman, A. (1996). Home care of the dying child. *Journal of Palliative Care, 12*(3), 16–19.

Liben, S. (1996). Pediatric palliative medicine: Obstacles to overcome. *Journal of Palliative Care, 12*(3), 24–28.

Liben, S. (1998). Home care for children with life-threatening illness. *Journal of Palliative Care, 14*(3), 33–38.

Papadatou, D. (1997). Training health professionals in caring for dying children and grieving families. *Death Studies, 21,* 575–600.

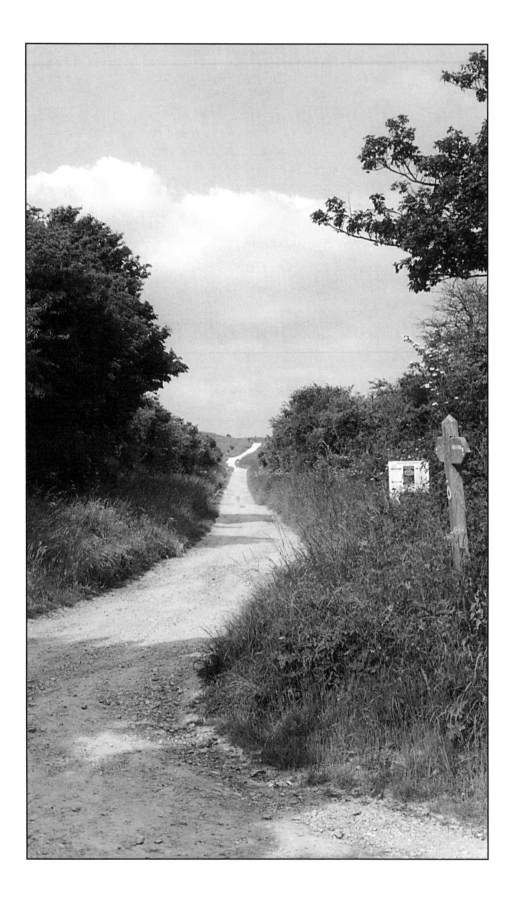

5

The Long and Winding Road

ILLNESS PREDOMINATES
(PPSv2 level: 40% to 30%)

The patient's CHANGE IN MOBILITY to a completely bed bound status marks this transition. Although the rate of progression varies with the specific disease, overall disease progression is pronounced and ongoing. The illness is at a very advanced stage, with little or no chance of improvement. Pain, nausea, or dyspnea may worsen or occur for the first time and weakness and fatigue become more evident. New palliative treatments or alternative medication routes may be introduced. Changes in care and caregiving routines occur as patients must rely on others for assistance with most of their basic needs. Alternatives to care at home may have to be considered. Patients are coming to terms with living in bed and thinking about the length and quality of their lives in this state.

This is a time of increased DEPENDENCE AND WITHDRAWAL. Patients periodically retreat into themselves, withdrawing from interactions with other people. Family members start to acknowledge the significance of the patient's decline and may feel that the person they knew is slowly disappearing. The social world of both patients and families often shrinks. The speed of the patients' decline and movement through this transition will affect dependence, coping abilities, and adaptation. This interval may last for only a few weeks, but for some with progressive chronic disease, it may last for up to 1 or 2 years. Davies (2000) characterized this phenomenon of decline as "fading away."

FAMILY STRESS and FAMILY GRIEF are heightened when the lives of family members are dramatically altered by the demands of the patient. The responsibilities of caregiving and spending quality time with the patient compete with, and take precedence over, most normal activities. Primary caregivers can be stressed by changing routines, and many have difficulty adjusting their schedules and expectations to fit each new circumstance. If the patient is deteriorating quickly and withdrawing from previous pleasures and priorities, family and friends start to understand that death is inevitable.

Depending on the rate of progression, patients may be entering the dying phase of their illness. This stage is a different and deeper expression of the grief that has followed people throughout the illness. People are thinking about the end of life as they know it. The patient may be contemplating nonexistence, heaven, hell, or life after death. Meanwhile, the family struggles to simultaneously envision and block out thoughts of life without the person who is dying.

The emotional and physical toll of this transition can be significant, especially if this is a short, and therefore intense, period. The combination of ongoing caregiving and grieving places heavy demands on people's internal and external resources during this transition. FAMILY FATIGUE is common; people become weary and exhausted and yet are not willing to lessen their involvement. Worry often keeps people from the sleep and sustenance that they require.

BOB AND MARGARET

Bob and Margaret grew up together and have been married for 38 years. Bob is a mail carrier, and Margaret is a graphic designer. They have one adult child and three young grandchildren, who live close by. Margaret, now 64 years old, was diagnosed with breast cancer 5 years ago. At that time, she had surgery and extensive treatment. The cancer recurred 3 years ago but responded well to chemotherapy. Recent tests have shown, unfortunately, that the cancer is now widespread to her bones, liver, and brain. The oncologist has explained to Margaret and Bob that her prognosis is that she has 1–2 months to live. Margaret has declined any further treatment.

Most of the time Margaret is in bed. When she is awake, she is nauseated and uncomfortable. She does not want to increase her pain medications, however, because they make her drowsy. Bob is troubled by her significant weight loss and constantly tries to en-tice her with her favorite foods. She has no ap-petite, though, and is taking in only sips of lemon-ade, water, and melted Popsicles. Margaret occasionally talks openly about dying, but only with friends.

> "The fundamental tension of opposites, I think, is the struggle—especially when you're seriously ill—between wanting to live and wishing to die."
>
> —(Schwartz, 1996, p. 48)

Margaret knows that Bob is not sleeping or eating properly and feels that she has let him down. At the same time, she also says that he is a stubborn person and that she is too tired to convince him to allow their friends and family to help out. Bob finds displays of emotion very embarrassing and unsettling and asks people not to say or ask anything that will make him cry. He says that after Margaret dies, he will have all the time and privacy that he needs to grieve, but for now his focus is on her needs. He is determined to learn the right way to do everything and puts a lot of pressure on himself to do it all. He has a hard time asking for and accepting help, although many friends and family have offered. He believes that every moment with Margaret may be her last and doesn't want her to feel alone or abandoned. He worries when he is away from her and is not interested in spending time with other peo-ple or activities.

Although she acknowledges that death will occur at some point, Mar-garet hopes to soon feel better. She feels sad about leaving her grandchil-dren and about not being there to see them grow up. She does not want them to be told that she is dying and is uncomfortable with them seeing her in her present condition. Bob feels she is distancing herself from the children and struggles with how to explain this to them.

KEY CONSIDERATIONS

Change in Mobility

Margaret, now 64-years-old, was diagnosed with breast cancer 5 years ago. At that time, she had surgery and extensive treatment. The cancer re-curred 3 years ago but responded well to chemotherapy. Recent tests have shown, unfortunately, that the cancer is now widespread to her bones, liver, and brain. Most of the time Margaret is in bed. When she is awake, she is

nauseated and uncomfortable. She does not want to increase her pain medications, however, because they make her drowsy. Bob is troubled by her
significant weight loss and constantly tries to entice her with her favorite
foods.

A number of changes in the patient's mobility and function occur between
PPS 40% and 30%. New or recurring physical symptoms such as pain, nausea,
shortness of breath, and constipation commonly surface now. These physical
symptoms often cause patients and families a great deal of fear and anxiety.
Dealing with the medical/physical issues typically becomes the primary focus for
the team, patients, and families at this time. Lamers, a psychiatrist and hospice advocate, explained that "in the absence of effective . . . symptom management, there
is little chance the dying person will be able to address . . . the social, psychological, and spiritual challenges inherent in the last phases of life" (2000, p. 291).
Patients are bed bound and unable to care for themselves. Assistance is required
for toileting, eating, and dressing. Appetite and intake vary, but are often reduced.
Because of fatigue, people require regular naps throughout the day or over several
days. There are good days and bad days, and families find unpredictability is the
norm. This is often likened to a roller coaster ride with the good days treasured
and the bad days taxing for the patient and family. Emergence of confusion can
signal medical complications such as drug side effects or, more seriously, an in-
farction or progression of a brain tumor.

Further physical changes may occur quickly over a few days, be protracted
over several weeks, or even progress over a few months, depending on the particular disease. Patients now have few reserves and their condition is fragile. The uncertainty of what and when changes will occur is quite unsettling for all. The
plateau is more like a precipice. If decline occurs quickly from PPS 40% to 30%,
patients and families may not have the time to adjust to one change before another
presents itself.

Patients' ongoing changes or high care needs will cause patients and families
to reevaluate their plans and expectations. The need for equipment and assistance
in the home increases; this can be hard for people to accept. At some point, patients and/or families may decide that care at home is not possible, triggering internal or interpersonal conflicts if there is disagreement on what should happen.

Interventions

These psychosocial interventions have been designed to specifically address the
key consideration *change in mobility*. There are several assessment questions that

will help open up a discussion, followed by more focused comments or tips that will facilitate further exploration of the issues that frequently arise at this time; each tip is followed by a sample dialogue.

Assessment Questions

- What physical, emotional, or mental changes have you experienced over the past few weeks? What do these changes mean to you? How has that been?

- What outside resources or personal strengths have been most helpful to you as you met each change?

- What kind of support and information about these changes has your family physician, home care nurse, or hospice program provided? How helpful has that been?

Provide information and referral to helpful resources. Many families will not have had much previous contact with community resources or palliative care when symptoms were minimal and manageable. Now, faced with multiple concerns, families may have many contact names and numbers but not know who does what.

> *"It seems like you have a number of questions about why all of these symptoms are happening and how you are going to care for your sister now. You are also uncomfortable with the recent increase in her pain medication. Would you be interested in discussing your concerns with her family physician or one of the home care nurses who could help you plan her care?"*

Educate people about what to expect at this time. Although we may have seen these kinds of changes before, most families and patients are going through this change in mobility for the first time. They may need to hear the same information more than once and in different ways. When you normalize what is happening, it lessens the sense that things are out of control.

> *"Unfortunately, some of the changes you are experiencing have their own timelines. It may be helpful to know that the changes you've described are expected at this point in your illness. If you or your husband have questions about this process, you could meet with the doctor, or perhaps I could organize a team conference so we could talk about this process and your wishes in more detail. Would you like that?"*

Identify and prioritize important decisions. As mobility decreases, a number of difficult decisions may arise. When the patient's and family's needs and values are understood, you will likely be more efficient and effective in your role as guide and advocate. Be sure that family caregivers are part of the decision-making process.

> *"Over the next couple of weeks, you will likely be making a number of important decisions about care at home. Can you tell me what is working or not working for you now?"*

Dependence and Withdrawal

> Although she acknowledges that death will occur at some point, Margaret hopes to feel better soon. She feels sad about leaving her grandchildren and about not being there to see them grow up. She does not want them to be told that she is dying and is uncomfortable with them seeing her in her present condition. Bob feels she is distancing herself from the grandchildren and struggles with how to explain this to them.

This may be a time of adjusting to the painful paradox between increasing physical care needs and diminishing ability to sustain social and familial bonds. New symptoms emerge, and daily life begins to revolve around dealing with patients' mobility and body functions. Medication, rest, and hygiene routines impose a rigid structure on each day. No longer able to get out of bed unassisted, patients now depend on their caregivers. This sort of dependence, in various forms, is often the thing most dreaded by patients. In real and symbolic ways, it signifies loss of control, becoming a burden, and living at the mercy of others. No longer able to fully manage personal care in areas such as dressing, eating, drinking, and toileting, many patients feel that their lives and bodies are letting them down and going out of control. They may withdraw into silence, sleep, or depression. Others are able to adjust and appreciate this time and the care being provided. A few even view each day as sacred regardless of their physical limitations.

Most patients stay connected to a partner or a very small circle of friends and family, but a few withdraw completely into themselves. Lamers (2000), in his description of grief in dying persons, stated that people will respond to this circumstance in different ways. Some may seek confirmation that death is imminent, whereas others may not be ready to recognize or acknowledge the obvious signs.

This is an ambivalent time for both patients and families. The inevitability of dying may be apparent, yet some patients and families are able to maintain their hope for a miracle or cure. Patients may express time-limited hopes such as wanting to live until Hannukah or the springtime.

Typically, this is the time when family and friends begin to discuss care and make decisions for patients, instead of with them. This can be very difficult for both patients and families. Patients may feel excluded and see their autonomy and self-determination disappearing. Many family members worry about their ability to make decisions that respect the patient's wishes. Some family members will naturally assume a decision-making role, whereas others are uncomfortable with what feels like taking over. Some patients will be clear, open, and consultative about their wishes for their care, whereas others will be silent, commanding, or inflexible. Occasionally, the patients' expectations are unrealistic, or the plan that was agreed to when the patient was healthier is no longer reasonable. The family becomes caught between the patient's wishes, financial and systemic realities, and their own resources. A compromise must be realized between plans that honor the patient's requests and those that fit within the current limitations and resources of the caregivers.

This can be a conflicted time for patients. Emotional bonds may intensify, but people may also begin to detach or disengage from each other. Patients' minds, bodies, and spirits often have different timetables. The person's body may not be ready to die at the same time as her spirit and vice versa. This dichotomy can cause tremendous anguish and spiritual pain. Patients may question the benevolence and wisdom of God or nature and feel ambivalent about life and living. With increasing fatigue and limitations, some people may no longer feel that life is worth living. Others accept life as it is for them, often feeling resigned to their current condition. They may quietly withdraw from life, with the feeling that death has become an acceptable, even welcome, alternative to living with dying. Many patients will contemplate ending their lives, but only a few will seriously consider doing so.

Developing a Death Plan

Canine suggested that death planning helps patients and families deal with the "worry and flurry that often follows a terminal diagnosis" (1996, p. 70). Following their plan, the patient and family might work toward what Worden described as an appropriate death, meaning, "a death that one might choose for oneself or a death one could live with" (2000, p. 267). A death plan is not a plan for assisted suicide or euthanasia, nor is it an advance directive that, in many communities, patients must fill out to specify their wishes in terms of potentially life-prolonging procedures, resuscitation, and treatment. Rather, it is a concrete representation of the patient's and family's unique requirements, a way to discuss their hopes or desires, and a means of providing direction for ongoing care through the process of dying, death, and bereavement (see Developing a Death Plan on p. 180).

Interventions

These psychosocial interventions have been designed to specifically address the key consideration *dependence and withdrawal*. There are several assessment questions that will help open up a discussion, followed by more focused comments or tips that will facilitate further exploration of the issues that frequently arise at this time; each tip is followed by a sample dialogue.

Assessment Questions

- How do you see things changing for you over the next few weeks and months? What do you expect?

- What are your most important needs and biggest concerns? Who needs to know about them? How might you make these needs and concerns known?

- How do you feel about depending on your family and friends? How is it for you to have nurses and volunteers now doing most of the personal care that your family was doing when you were home?

- Many people say that it's not death they fear, but dying. How do you feel about that saying?

Identify the patient's goals and priorities about his or her remaining life. They may have changed, and clarifying them will help you to focus your interventions appropriately.

> *"Wei, you've been through a lot of changes in the last couple of months. Now that you have been living in this long-term care facility for a while, I wonder if your goals have changed in any way. What's important to you now?"*

Explore thoughts and feelings about increased dependence. Past experience will affect how comfortable the person is with being dependent. When you find out what this situation is like for the patient, you will know how much attention it needs.

"Your wife mentioned that you are a do-it-yourself kind of guy who doesn't like to be fussed over. It must be hard for you to wait for her to help you get out of bed and dressed each day. How are you coping with all of this unfamiliar dependence?"

Provide necessary information and support personal choices to maintain some independence and control. When people are feeling unwell and overwhelmed, fundamental needs can be overlooked or minimized. Ensure that the patient's wishes are heard and respected.

"I know that a lot of people have suggested that you have a catheter put in because it is difficult for you to get to the bathroom, and there is a risk that you might fall and be injured. I sense that you don't really want this. Although there are some good reasons to go ahead with this option, you don't have to. What feels right for you?"

Explore the patient's thoughts and feelings about the process of living and dying. Most patients are quite aware that their disease is advanced and that they will probably die and may be quite open about it. When you demonstrate that you are comfortable with this process and open to talking about it, the patient may have a lot to say.

"Greta, you told me you don't think you will live long enough to attend your grandson's wedding. I wonder if you can tell me more about that?"

Help patients and families identify what is special or meaningful about this time. Although some patients may die within the next few weeks, many will live for an extended time. It is important to provide opportunities for people to focus on the aspects of living as well as dying.

"Although you are spending most of your time in bed, can you identify some things that still feel possible and important for you to do? What would it take for these things to happen? Who might help?"

Family Stress

Bob is determined to learn the right ways to do everything and puts a lot of pressure on himself to do it all. He has a hard time asking for and accept-

DEVELOPING A DEATH PLAN

The development of a death plan includes three parts: the reflection, the construction, and the communication.

The Reflection

As a patient or patient and family reflect on the death plan, consider these over-arching questions to help clarify their priorities, needs, and roles:

- What has been the patient's past experience with other deaths?

- What is most important to him or her about dying?

- What does he or she need to feel safe and comfortable?

This conversation might focus on what really helped or worked in past experiences as well as on what people would do differently. It is also an opportunity to think about what seems important as the patient and family look ahead. It is helpful to consult with people whose experience or expertise could enrich and inform this discussion, such as the home care nurse, palliative care team, family physician, or spiritual leader. These people may be able to provide information that keeps the planning both current and realistic. Explore with the patient and family who else might add valuable information to this process.

The Construction

Once these initial questions have been considered, the plan is constructed around several basic elements: the patient's wishes, the family's wishes, the people involved, the nature of the illness, the limitations of the available resources, and the way information will be shared. Following are some of the questions that would help patients and families construct their plans:

- Where does the patient wish to die?

- What are the family's wishes and limits about care?

- Whom does the patient want to care for him or her?

- How much do people want to know about expected physical changes?

- What are the patient's wishes around resuscitation, hydration, sedation, antibiotics, and pain control? Do they have an advance directive that deals with these issues?

- How and by whom will decisions be made?

- What does the patient fear and hope for most about dying?

- Who can be privy to information about the patient's condition?

- Who will be the patient's representative when he or she is no longer able to communicate? Is there a legal directive in place?

- If this plan is no longer feasible for any reason, what alternatives or other options have patients and families considered?

The Communication

Once the patient and family have outlined their plan, they need to decide how they would like it to be communicated. This means deciding what form it will take, whom it is for, and how it will be delivered. For some, it is helpful to write out a detailed plan in which issues and tasks are identified and assigned. Others, however, may prefer to write a letter or a list or make a personal video or audiotape.

The way that the patient and family communicate their death plan must fit their style and circumstances. If the patient plans to die at home with family members providing care, then the plan might reside in a journal that each person can read and add to. In a facility, health care providers need to be aware of patients' and families' wishes, perhaps keeping the plan in the patient's room or chart.

One of the challenges of building a plan is that patients (and families) are often reluctant to talk about death with others and each other. As Worden (2000) discovered in his study of communication patterns, patients intermittently wanted to talk about their deaths and were selective about whom they talked with. He suggested that professionals must be sensitive to when patients want to speak and with whom. It is not uncommon for patients, friends, and families to commit to a plan that later proves to be unrealistic or undesirable. Health care providers could help people struggling to uphold an untenable plan by suggesting a periodic review. Although the plan is patient centered, it needs to reflect reality so that it feels reasonable and achievable by those directly involved in care. Patients must be prepared to hear other people's perspectives and be willing to negotiate. A functional plan is one that is clear, comfortable, flexible, and realistic.

Source: Canine, 1996.

---

ing help, although many friends and family have offered. He believes that every moment with Margaret may be her last and doesn't want her to feel alone or abandoned.

When a person chooses to remain at home as long as possible, or even to die there, family caregivers must learn many new roles in addition to being a spouse, friend, son, mother, and so forth. These new roles may include nurse, advocate, confidante, and counselor. Adjusting to new roles means that previous relationships are altered. People are often pulled out of their comfort zone and forced to relate to each other in ways that may feel awkward or impossible at first. Out of necessity, or simply out of the desire to help, family caregivers may find themselves doing things that they never imagined, such as bathing a parent or injecting medications into a child. Family caregivers may find that doing, or helping,

FOCUS ON: WHEN A PATIENT ASKS TO DIE

The Oxford English Dictionary (1989) defined *euthanasia* as "a means of bringing about a gentle and easy death, or the action of inducing a gentle and easy death." Some may describe it as "ending my life," while others describe it as "killing the patient." However it is perceived, euthanasia is an action taken with the direct and immediate purpose of causing intentional death, using lethal substances or methods.

Advanced disease brings with it new realities that include dependence, frailty, and pain. At this time, patients often talk to families, volunteers, and other health care providers about ending their lives. They may be struggling with a loss of control, fear, or uncontrolled symptoms. They feel hopeless in the face of increasing physical changes and emotional or spiritual suffering. They may not know about, or have access to, care and support that can alleviate these fears. They believe choosing when and how to die helps them regain control of their lives, to avoid what they fear and ensure autonomy to the end. They may view euthanasia as a right to control their death; an extension of the right to control their life. For patients, choosing when and how to die may seem to be a quick solution to the uncertainty of what lies ahead.

It is important to note that patients may raise questions about ending their lives without actually wanting to end their lives. They may use discussions about euthanasia as a way to give voice to the many fears they are carrying about dying, pain, loss, and dependence. Expressing a desire to die may be the only way people can demonstrate how terrible they feel.

Other people may fear future suffering and loss of dignity. They may worry that their increasing needs will take a devastating toll on family and friends. As people feel that nothing can be done to slow down or change the inevitability of decline and death, they may doubt that there is any reason to continue living in this way. Feeling powerless and hopeless in the face of this situation, some people may consider euthanasia as a dignified and acceptable solution (Kissane & Clarke, 2001).

Times may occur when patients move beyond talking about their wish to die and actually begin to make concrete plans. This is often done while people are still mobile and fairly independent in preparation for a time when they are no longer able to carry out this action themselves. If euthanasia is illegal, patients are unlikely to discuss this plan with others, making it difficult for family and health care providers to understand or address the person's concerns.

Many health care providers feel anxious and uncomfortable when patients do ask to die. They try to appreciate the patient's situation and empathize with their struggle to find meaning in what's left to their lives. Although many patients think about euthanasia, most do not even consider it a serious option. Understanding that this is usually a plea for understanding and compassion, rather than a call for death, helps health care providers support patients without feeling threatened or accountable. When health care providers listen and explore the concerns and fears of patients, they can help patients to work through these fears and concerns. Providing relief for their symptoms, loneliness, and fears may leave further discussions of euthanasia unnecessary.

Although euthanasia is illegal in most countries, many health care providers still struggle with this issue, wanting to help, yet feeling unable to. Caught between personal values, professional ethics, and the law, health care providers may feel powerless, accountable, and constrained all at once. None of us are neutral observers. We must be aware of our own experience of pain and suffering as we work to address the complex issues involved with care of the dying. Here are some guidelines for ways to respond when a patient asks to die:

- Explore the physical, social, emotional, and spiritual concerns that led to this request. Refer as appropriate.
- Obtain permission to share concerns and plan with appropriate people (e.g., family members, physician, nurses, counselors, priest).
- Develop a plan with the patient to address the patient's concerns.
- Regularly revisit the plan and reassess the patient's situation.

---

with these tasks is empowering and provides them with new ways to express their love; these tasks, however, can also be burdensome and unsettling.

This changing situation affects the ways that people relate to each other. Perhaps the patient was the family referee; now that she is no longer able to do that, others may feel unprotected and unheard. Alternately, family members may have been very distant from each other emotionally and physically and now are wrestling with being caregivers together. At times, people are able to resolve their long-standing issues, or declare a truce in order to care for the patient. Often, the usual battles continue.

If admission to a facility is necessary, family members must make significant adjustments. It can be hard for family members to relinquish the role of caregiver and nurse and value being just the wife, daughter, or friend. They may feel useless once the patient is being monitored and tended by a team of nurses and doctors. It may be difficult for family caregivers to shift from the importance of doing almost everything to sitting quietly at the patient's bedside. It may also be tiresome and time consuming for family members to travel between home and the facility; take care of house, self, and family; and spend time with the patient. Others may find that this shift in care is a great relief, as they are now free of the responsibilities and burden of care.

Changes that occur for the patient precipitate many changes to the lives of families and caregivers. They often begin to disconnect from their outside world of work and social engagements. They need to take time away from their jobs, or stop other nonessential activities. Patients may be too frail to be left alone, so that family members often feel compelled to stay close at hand in case they are needed. Priorities and routines revolve around what is happening with the emotional, social, and spiritual needs of the patient. If the patient's condition is unpredictable, this makes it difficult for family caregivers to make plans and follow through with commitments.

The stress of living with advancing illness and increasing care often leaves families too weary for social interactions. They may have trouble relating to the events and concerns of other people. This lack of contact and association outside the home may result in isolation from vital activities and people who could provide much-needed comfort, respite, and a fresh perspective. Enyert and Burman (1999) reported that a potential impact of caregiving was a decline in caregivers' morale and physical and mental health due to inattention to self-care routines. Although caregiving may be a strain for some, they found that other caregivers were able to move beyond the immediate circumstances of caring for a dying person and experience a transformed appreciation and meaning for life. Davies (2000) found that very few spouses and adult children paid attention to their own needs while caring for a dying relative and that those who were inflexible about sharing roles and changing routines suffered from more isolation and resentment than those who were flexible.

Interventions

These psychosocial interventions have been designed to specifically address the key consideration *family stress*. There are several assessment questions that will help open up a discussion, followed by more focused comments or tips that will facilitate further exploration of the issues that frequently arise at this time; each tip is followed by a sample dialogue.

Assessment Questions

- Who is doing the practical, physical tasks such as giving medications, bathing, and toileting?

- Are you as involved as you want to be? Are you finding this too much?

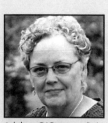

Adaline O'Gorman, B.A. in social work, M.A. in counseling psychology, art therapist, is a Victoria Hospice counselor and a former hospice volunteer coordinator.

In My Own Voice
Working with
Difficult People

Adaline O'Gorman

The topic of working with difficult people embodies an insidious assumption: "THEY" are the difficult people and I must "work with them." Before I dare to go to that stance, I need to look in the mirror to see who may be difficult for others to encounter. I believe that my attitude, my feeling state, and my actions and reactions contribute to the difficulty in a situation and that I can clean up my part of the exchange first.

We all come to this work with history and sensitivities. If I have difficulty in an encounter, it may be that the situation activates feelings of fear, helplessness, or other difficult emotions for me. There may be reminders of old family patterns and distressing past situations. A small example: I grew up in a quiet family where interruptions were nonexistent. When I am in a volatile, noisy family with several people vying for my attention, I quickly become flustered and want to run away. Colleagues with a different family experience roll with the noise easily.

Some of the people that I find difficult to work with include aggressive people who demand what seems unreasonable, people with many crippling fears, very silent people whose needs are difficult to identify, and people who seem manipulative or underhanded in their dealings with me. This list probably tells more about my skills and deficiencies than anything else because it identifies where I am likely to experience emotional triggering.

Identifying triggers is a gradual process. Often, we don't recognize until later that we have been triggered and sometimes it takes the witnessing of another to help us. Red flags for me include strong reactions, especially of fear, shakiness, frustration, helplessness, or fatigue. If I "can't get them out of my head," I suspect some trigger has occurred. I want to be aware of what triggers me so that I can deal with the "difficult person" in effective ways that override my emotional history.

I know from experience that many people who might otherwise have been difficult were cooperative when someone truly listened to them. Most of the time, it works to reflect and validate the experience of the other, but not always. So I have alternative ways to approach situations that may be difficult for me. Although there are no guarantees of effective navigating, I have found the approaches of Wade and Rosenberg very helpful.

Allan Wade (1997) has provided me with "new eyes" to see and respond to resistant people. He suggests that, in response to painful events in their lives, people develop patterns that protect them from the impact of the pain. Wade refers to resistance as "small acts of living," and he honors defiance as protecting life. If we view resistant behavior such as withdrawal, argumentativeness, suspiciousness, and so forth as a response to pain that has become habituated, it allows us to approach with more curiosity than counter resistance, and the doors to negotiation are more likely to remain open. I know that I am not so likely to take things personally when I am curious about someone. My curiosity allows me to stay connected in conversation and leads me to a better understanding of the intent underlying the "difficult" behavior.

Marshall Rosenberg's (1999) *Nonviolent Communication* provides a model of effective communication that helps to dissolve conflict. He recommended that we pay attention to ourselves and to the other person and identify four aspects of the situation:

1. Observe what is happening in the exchange or what is happening internally, such as shakiness or shallow breathing.
2. Acknowledge our feelings associated with the situation.
3. Acknowledge our need or wish that is unmet or compromised in this situation and gives rise to our emotion. Alternately, check out the other person's feelings and needs.
4. Request or invite the other person to consider another way of dealing with the situation—one more likely to get results that we both want—or offer something that the other seems to be asking of us.

Internalizing these four steps—observations, feelings, needs, and requests—is simple. Remembering to apply them when there is tension in the air is not simple. But I know it is a way to see more clearly the truth and humanity in both of us. I have come to be compassionate with myself and others who struggle to find our way in this emotional minefield, knowing that sometimes things blow up. Apologies and forgiveness have their place, as does an immense curiosity for what difficulty can teach us about ourselves and others. There is, for me, a special satisfaction in being able to find a way to resolve a challenge with a 'difficult' person, particularly when we both get what we need. I see it as a step toward wholeness for us both, with a ripple effect in the work and in our larger lives (p. 193).

- How do you find coming in to the hospital to visit your sister? How is this affecting your self-care and work routines?
- If things continue to progress as they are now, what do you envision will be your needs in the future? How might you plan for those future needs now?
- Who might be able to help you with your less important but necessary errands and duties?
- What prevents you from asking for or accepting help now?

Provide a gentle reality check. Family caregivers tend to minimize or ignore the negative outcomes of caregiving until they, or the patient, reach a crisis point. If you identify potential problems early in the process, you may help people to avoid desperate moments and family stress later on.

> *"Your mother is not sleeping well at night, and you haven't been sleeping either. You've said that you're also feeling tired and unwell. I know that you want to do this alone, Ina, but it may become unmanageable. What are your thoughts and feelings about getting some extra help?"*

Identify the dynamics that are occurring within family relationships. If there are several family members involved in care, it is likely that old issues will resurface in this new context. It is important for people to find ways to work together, in spite of preexisting issues. Although it is unlikely that

ANTICIPATORY MOURNING AND FAMILY STRESS

According to Rando in her seminal works on death and dying, anticipatory mourning is "the phenomenon encompassing grief and mourning, coping, interaction, psychosocial reorganization, planning, balancing conflicting demands, and facilitating an appropriate death that is stimulated in response to the awareness of life-threatening or terminal illness in oneself or a significant other"(2000, p. 4). She asserted that certain personal, social, and cultural factors contribute to the stress of contemporary illnesses. Among these factors are protracted illnesses and dying trajectories that have contributed to extended periods of uncertainty, disruption, and anxiety for both patients and families. She added that, today, family members live at greater and greater distances; this adds significantly to the burden and isolation of in-town relatives of the patient.

---

these will be resolved, people can still feel good about what they have accomplished together.

> *"Most families have their different points of view and long-standing issues. These often resurface and make it difficult for people to provide care. Can you identify any issues within your family that are interfering with what you are hoping for at this time? Are there ways for you to deal with these or put them aside so that everyone might find value and satisfaction in working together through this next period?"*

Explore people's feelings and thoughts about caregiving and facility placement. Some people may have adjusted to new roles and routines quite happily, whereas others may feel redundant or imposed upon. Understanding people's experience can help you to address their difficulties; you may then be able to advocate for positive change.

> *"Even though you both agreed that coming to hospice was the right thing to do, you really miss the freedom and privacy you had at home. Also, it is sometimes hard to let go of the caregiver role and go back to feeling like you are 'just the wife.' How are you coping with this change? What could make this situation more comfortable for you?"*

Educate about and emphasize the importance of self-care. As mentioned previously in this chapter, people often neglect themselves when caring for a dying person. It is as though the dying person is the only one with legitimate needs for comfort, rest, and companionship. When you talk about the importance of self-care with families, it may give them permission to recognize their own needs and take some time to tend to them.

> *"Brenda, you've been housebound for several weeks and have noticed that you are becoming irritable and short-tempered. When people aren't taking time for themselves, it affects their ability to care for someone else. How do you feel about calling a couple of friends and arranging to meet for lunch and a walk?"*

Together we're holding the
  space—like a backyard—
No longer the whole block,
  not yet shut in—
Just a small portion of time
  and opportunity.
Gently turning over rocks,
  looking under the leaves.
What needs your attention
Beyond the obvious things to
  be done?
Sitting quietly, asking—
What else? and what else?
  and what else?
When there won't be many
  more chances.

—(Adaline O'Gorman &
Moira Cairns, 2003)

Reinforce and remind people of their strengths and resilience. Families can often feel inadequate about their ability to provide good care in light of the many physical changes patients are going through. Reviewing how people have coped with other difficult times may help some people feel more capable and confident as they face the next challenges.

> *"You have been through a tremendous amount of change, and at times you've felt in over your heads. Can you remember any past challenges that you faced and what strengths helped you to get through? How is this current situation similar and how might you use these strengths to guide and inform you as things progress?"*

Family Grief

> Bob finds displays of emotion embarrassing and asks people not to say or ask anything that will make him cry. He says that, after Margaret dies, he will have all the time and privacy that he needs to grieve, but for now his focus is on her needs. He believes that every moment with Margaret may be her last. He worries when he is away from her and is not interested in spending time with other people or activities.

Until this time, death was perhaps more of a conceptual fact. Now, as people witness the patient's decline, death starts to feel real. Some family members begin to imagine life without the patient and this triggers a new level of grief. At this time, the losses that people grieve are both present and future oriented. These losses relate to current changes in the patient's physical and mental condition and also those that families anticipate as death approaches. Families may express concerns about how they see the patient and identify this as suffering. Sometimes the patient is, indeed, suffering, but in the context of his or her own grief; the intense feelings that surface may be more a reflection of the family's own pain than that of the patient.

Each change along the journey toward death and bereavement will stimulate grief. Patients and families shift between life as it was before the illness and how it is now, comparing their present situation with how life used to be. They may long intensely for things to get back to normal while sensing that things will never be the same. They grieve the lack or absence of easy communication and familiar contact with the patient and each other.

As PPS declines to the 30% level, people's bodies change significantly. Many experience dramatic weight loss and emaciation, whereas others may gain weight through fluid retention and edema. Along with physical changes, cognitive decline is a source of sorrow and grief for families. Some patients remain mentally clear during this transition, whereas others have some degree of confusion. This is caused either by disease progression or a medical complication, rather than a fundamental personality change. Whatever the reason, patients and families often feel tremendous sadness, anger, and powerlessness as this occurs.

When patients move to a facility or withdraw from decision making and family events, families begin to discover what life may be like after the person dies. People often say that it feels as if the person has already died and it is a struggle to be positive while experiencing their grief. Some suppress their emotions, not wanting to upset the patient, saying that they will do their crying when it's all over. Others discount or deny their feelings. Caregiving and grief can be all-encompassing; many people will attend to one of these, to the exclusion of the other, as a way of surviving this difficult time.

Interventions

These psychosocial interventions have been designed to specifically address the key consideration *family grief*. There are several assessment questions that will help open up a discussion, followed by more focused comments or tips that will facilitate further exploration of the issues that frequently arise at this time; each tip is followed by a sample dialogue.

Assessment Questions

- How are you feeling about the changes that you are seeing? What do these changes mean to you?

- How are you making room for your own emotional needs while caring for someone else?

SEVEN COMPONENTS OF FADING AWAY

According to Davies (2000), a transition that she termed "fading away" is triggered at this time by patients' and families' growing awareness that death is the inevitable outcome of the patient's disease process. She explained that this transition is characterized by seven interrelated, interdependent components.

1. Redefining: Patients and families reconcile themselves with what was, what will not be, what is now, and what will come. This means redefining whom the individual, other people, and family members are in relation to one another.

2. Burdening: Although patients feel like a burden, their families minimize this feeling, often by focusing on the privilege of caregiving. She suggested that patients feel they are a burden to the extent that they have not redefined themselves.

3. Struggling with Paradox: This refers to the pronounced collision between living and dying experienced by the dying person.

4. Contending with Change: Roles, relationships, and patterns change when someone in a family is dying. People adapt better to these changes when redefinition has occurred.

5. Searching for Meaning: People have an inward journey of reflecting on changes to one's life, beliefs, and relationships due to the illness. Changes can then be reframed into a meaningful context.

6. Living Day to Day: People shift their focus away from the future and into the immediate present, characterized by an attitude of "making the most of it" or "getting through it."

7. Preparing for Death: This ranges from the practical (estate and funeral plans) to the personal (granting the patient's wishes and giving assurances to the patient that surviving friends and family will be taken care of).

From Davies, B. (2000). Anticipatory mourning and the transition of fading away. In T. Rando (Ed.), Clinical dimensions of anticipatory mourning: Theory and practice in working with the dying, their loved ones and their caregivers (pp. 135–153). Champaign, IL: Research Press. Adapted by permission.

- How is life for you now that your wife has been in the hospital for the past 3 weeks?

Normalize feelings of exhaustion, stress, and grief. When people know what to expect and where they fall on the "normal" continuum, it is often very reassuring.

"The sadness and hopelessness that you are feeling is understandable. These changes are happening faster than you had expected. When this happens, people can feel quite overwhelmed. They often worry about whether they can get through this time. Ling, can you tell me how this time has been for you? It is often reassuring to talk with someone else who is going through, or who has gone through, this experience. Is there anyone who could stay with your husband so that you could attend the ALS caregivers support group next week?"

Acknowledge mixed feelings. One of the things that make anticipatory mourning/grief difficult to express is the tension between holding on and letting go.

"It is really hard to watch someone you love dying. You may be full of mixed feelings, perhaps wanting her to keep fighting, but also hoping that her suffering will soon end. These mixed feelings are often confusing. What would help you to accept and honor this ambivalence?"

Help people express both their joy and sorrow. Often at a time of loss, the source of people's deepest sadness is also the source of their greatest joy. By helping people to recall the joyful parts of what is now causing sorrow, you may help them find a healthy balance between the depths of pain and affection.

"The hardest part about losing your mom is that she has always been there when you needed her. It's scary to imagine life without her because she has been such a constant, loyal support. What are some of the bits of wisdom that you've gleaned from her that will guide you throughout your life?"
(or)
"Although you've talked about the real sorrow that you feel in seeing your mom getting sicker, are there still things that give you great joy? How might you build on this in the remaining time that the two of you have together?"

Family Fatigue

Margaret knows Bob is not sleeping and eating properly and feels that she has let him down. She also says that he is a stubborn person and that she is too tired to convince him to allow their friends and family to help out.

Stajduhar and Davies (1998) posited that chronic fatigue, physical exhaustion, sleeplessness, burnout, and ill health are a direct result of the physical and emotional burdens of caregiving. Keeping up with the patient's ongoing physical and emotional changes is exhausting to families. They often have not had time to integrate and adapt to one change before another occurs. One week the patient might require a walker to move around the house, for example, and suddenly the next week it is a wheelchair. Changes to medications, care approaches, and health care providers' schedules may occur frequently. Under the emotional strain of illness and care, these repeated adjustments could render patients and families drained and bewildered.

During this transition, patients are struggling to come to terms with their lives and their approaching deaths. They may want to reminisce, complete unfinished business, or realize some outstanding hopes or dreams in the time remaining. Final talks and heartfelt good-byes with friends and others may punctuate the days. Families may often witness and even orchestrate these important encounters and activities. Although important and meaningful for everyone, these events can be emotionally, mentally, spiritually, and physically demanding.

At this time, patients may become quite careful about expending their depleted and short-lived energy. It begins to take more and more rest to recover from less and less stimulation. This too places more demands on families. Weary and fragile, people may eventually find themselves unable to cope with the situation and a seemingly manageable problem can quickly turn into a crisis. At this time, families may or may not be aware of support options such as home support workers or hospice volunteers, and may or may not be willing to use them. Initial refusals of support could result from a number of factors such as high expectations, wanting to keep promises, denial that the patient is dying, discomfort with strangers in their home, or ignorance about what anyone could possibly do to help.

Interventions

These psychosocial interventions have been designed to specifically address the key consideration *family fatigue*. There are several assessment questions that will help open up a discussion, followed by more focused comments or tips that will facilitate further exploration of the issues that frequently arise at this time; each tip is followed by a sample dialogue.

Assessment Questions

- How has caregiving affected your normal sleeping and eating routines? Is there anyone who could help you with meal preparation or house or yard work?

ON JOY AND SORROW

Then a woman said,
Speak to us of Joy and Sorrow,
And he answered:
Your joy is your sorrow unmasked.
And the selfsame well from which your
Laughter rises was oftentimes filled with your tears.
And how else can it be?
The deeper that sorrow carves into your being,
The more joy you can contain.
Is not the cup that holds your wine
the very cup that was burned in the potter's oven?
And is not the lute that soothes your spirit,
The very wood that was hollowed with knives?
When you are joyous, look deep into your heart
And you shall find it is only that which has given you sorrow that is giving you joy.
When you are sorrowful look again into your heart, and you shall see that in truth
You are weeping for that which has been your delight.
Some of you say, "Joy is greater than sorrow,"
and others say, "Nay, sorrow is the greater."
But I say unto you, they are inseparable.
Together they come, and
When one sits alone with you at your board, remember
That the other is asleep upon your bed.
Verily you are suspended like scales
Between your sorrow and your joy.
Only when you are empty are you at a standstill and balanced.
When the treasure-keeper lifts you to weigh his gold and his silver, needs must
   your joy or your sorrow rise or fall.

—(Kahlil Gibran, 1972, p.52)

- If there are weeks or months of caregiving ahead, how long do you see your-self being able to manage in this way? How are you pacing yourself?

- What other care options have you explored that might allow you to stay healthy and yet remain actively involved with the wife's care?

- What are your thoughts and feelings about respite care? Home support? Private nursing? Facility placement? Hospitalization? Help from friends or neighbors?

Demystify and simplify the health care system(s). At this point, people are often very appreciative of the support but also feel inundated with new people and information. If you can link the family's most important needs to one or two key resources, it will save the family a great deal of time and frustration.

> *"Over the past week, you had some trouble identifying whom to call for advice about your husband's temperature and you got passed from person to person. Understandably, this was very frustrating. Would it help if we clarify what assistance is most essential? Then we should be able to trim this list down to just a couple of key contact people and their numbers. When we're done, I could write the information on bright paper that you could keep by your phone."*

Legitimize rest and relaxation. It is important that people give themselves permission to take breaks. Patients and families need time to shut out the world and convalesce.

> *"You have had a lot of visitors today, and we've given you a lot of information to digest. Although there is more that we'd like you to know, it can wait until later if you need a break. Remember that even though the hospital has very regular routines and habits, it is okay to ask for some time alone."*

Introduce, facilitate, and teach people stress reduction and relaxation techniques. Many people will have already heard about or tried some techniques. You don't have to be the expert in order to guide people to some simple tools that they can use alone or with each other, to soothe and comfort themselves.

> *"I know that it has been difficult for you to sleep at night. You said that when the lights go off, your mind turns on and you begin to worry about all the things that might happen during the night. How familiar are you with relaxation techniques? Perhaps I could show you some pressure points for calming anxiety or refer you to certain tapes or books that other people find helpful."*

OUR EXPERIENCE

Our goal is to provide people with the support and tools that will help them contend with the changeable and complex needs that are characteristic of this time. The purpose of this effort is to respect and restore people's sense of control, competence, and self-confidence.

When we see families in crisis at this time, we encounter people who feel imprisoned by the disease process. It's as though their real lives are suspended by the looming presence of illness and dying. Some patients, particularly those with a chronic condition, may linger at this transition for several months or years. Although patients endure prolonged dependence, family caregivers may question their ability to continue juggling responsibilities between the patient and themselves. For other patients, this is a time of pronounced and fairly rapid change. If patients and families find these changes emotionally and mentally exhausting, they may turn to health care providers for help. For others, this may be a quiet, comfortable time. The patient may be sleeping for longer and longer periods, waking only for brief, heartfelt chats, toileting, or medication. If we parachute into people's lives at this time, we must endeavor to be both swift and gentle. Assessment, intervention, and evaluation may need to be condensed into just one or two key questions or sentences.

This can be a very unstable time in people's lives and the disease process, and so we are careful to moderate the pace of our interventions and to communicate new information carefully. Information will be reviewed frequently, because it is easily forgotten or misinterpreted at this time. We recognize that the priorities and resources of yesterday may be discarded or obsolete tomorrow and so we keep discussions straightforward and pertinent. This expectation is congruent with Corr and Corr's guidelines for helpers, which suggest that, each time you come to offer help, "assess, reassess and reassess again" (2000, p. 217).

Once patients become bed bound, we find that a number of factors influence how people will cope with this transition. Our physical care may be changing as the disease becomes unpredictable, in terms of symptoms and nearness of death. We are also helping families adapt their care strategies as these physical care needs increase. We begin to wonder whether a patient's care can continue at home, looking at the external health care resources available and the internal strengths, abilities, and resources of family caregivers. We initiate conversations about alternate care options such as home support, respite care, or facility placement. Knowing that families are becoming tired, stressed, and sensitive to the fragility of self-care, we initiate conversations about the value of self-care now and for the future. We encourage people to examine their expectations, their boundaries, and their energy.

We believe that people have come to this illness from lives already filled with trials and triumphs, and that the wisdom gleaned from those past experiences will be their most edifying guide through this time. We struggle to uphold our faith and understanding that people can and will move through this in a way that is unique and true for them. We recognize our own needs and feelings, and know these may be quite different from those of the patient and family. Using our clinical judgment and trusting our own gut feelings, we support people to learn new

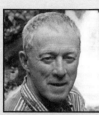

In My Own Voice
Crisis Intervention

Rae Westcott

Rae Westcott is a retired
hospice counselor, social
worker, and former
bereavement coordinator;
he has worked in the
community and on the
Palliative Response
Team (PRT).

One of my struggles in providing effective psychosocial support to palliative care patients and families is responding appropriately to the inevitable crisis situations that arise. These situations occur unexpectedly, and we have only a brief time frame in which to work. Also, although the team, especially the community nurse, has a relationship with the patient and family, I may not. The expectation is to get in there and "fix things" or at least make the situation manageable.

Crisis intervention theory, emphasizing "a little help, rationally directed and purposefully focused at a strategic time" (Sands, 1983, p. 253), is compatible with this type of brief intervention work. I believe that during crises, when coping mechanisms fail to solve the problems at hand, the patient and family are more open to interventions than at times of emotional and cognitive stability. With appropriate guidance, teaching, and support, they can manage the crisis; emerge stronger than before; and develop new, effective coping skills and greater self-esteem.

Eight crisis intervention principles have been applied to the palliative care setting (Christenson & Harding, 1985; Chung, 1993) 1) immediate intervention, 2) action, 3) limited goal, 4) hope and expectation, 5) support, 6) focused problem solving, 7) self-image, and 8) self-reliance (Puryear, 1979).

Kay, a retired nurse whose husband had lung cancer, wrote the following letter in March of 1996 about a typical crisis situation. In the following excerpt, she described the first visit from the Palliative Response Team (PRT).

I couldn't transfer John back to his chair as I had previously been able to do—my daughters were there—emotionally distraught—their behavior forced and different. The full impact of where this was going hit me suddenly, and hit me hard, and I was close to the breaking point.

Our day-to-day caseload management should include a way to respond to crises immediately. Because the crisis state is time limited, an opportunity exists to form a working relationship and have a positive impact on the patient and family. Timeliness is of the essence. Telephone contact sets up an interim plan until a visit can be arranged. In crisis situations, indirect processes do not work. The focus is on action. "Hearing the story," including ventilating and clarifying, is effective, as Kay explained:

> We had a long emotional visit in my kitchen during which I couldn't stop talking and couldn't stop crying. The PRT counselor and the nurse were caring, compassionate, and extremely supportive to me. They listened to me patiently and gently provided me with all the information I required.

Despite the fact that goals are limited to resolving the problem at hand, there is potential for a better level of functioning and for personal growth. For Kay and John, the crisis was about care at home versus hospitalization. Yet, some seeds were planted around the involvement of the grandchildren, who had not been allowed to visit for several days. Here Kay talked about how the team helped the entire family prepare for John's death.

> The counselor explained to my daughter how she could help her 4-year-old son, Duncan, accept the death of his beloved grandpa— information that was later to become so timely and so special. Duncan sat on my lap next to his grandpa and held his hand until just before he died. It was calm, it was warm, and it was very natural.

The approach that clearly states a positive expectation about problem solving generates hope. It conveys the belief that the patient and family members are capable people who are temporarily under great stress. Encouraging them to do as much as possible for themselves conveys trust that they can succeed, enhancing self-image and self-reliance. Here Kay recalled how the hospice nurse calmed her doubts.

> The nurse quietly reassured me that we were coping, and that my behavior, which was so distressing to me, was entirely normal. John was

> restless and deteriorating rapidly, and she told us what to expect. I listened to what she said—about the signs and symptoms I'd seen so many times as a nurse, but...never before as a wife. My pain was unbearable that day.

When intervening in a crisis, the method and style of support provided varies with the particular situation. We need to be perceptive enough to recognize the need for strong guidance when a "full blown" crisis exists and flexible enough to pull back once the problem is resolved. When patients and families have difficulty acknowledging the problems, information shared over time allows them to absorb and accept it in increments. Clearing up myths and misconceptions about death and the dying process allows people to focus on real problems, as Kay stated.

> I loved this man with all my heart, and with your support he died with me, in our home. I couldn't have done it without you.

As Kay's letter demonstrates, people in crisis frequently make substantial gains perhaps because they are highly motivated to learn and to do what they can. For this reason, I found work with patients and families in crisis to be professionally gratifying.

ways of coping and to keep doing what works for them. Essentially, we try to create an affirming connection between their personal journey and the information, resources, and support available to them. Once this connection is in place, our tasks are to bear witness, extend support, and stay out of the way.

TEAM ISSUES

As compassionate, empathetic people, health care providers witness the pain and suffering of patients and families and this can become a burden. Over-identification with people means clinical judgment may be affected, so that assessments and interventions are based on the provider's needs rather than those of the patient and family. This work can be intimate and personal, and palliative care providers must understand their own needs for intimacy and how these may affect the relationships formed with patients and families. Exhaustion and the compassion fatigue that comes from the continuous exposure to the vulnerability and pain of others can be the outcome when providers are not clear about their own needs and issues (Saakvitne & Pearlman, 1996).

When families are in distress and desperate, hospice workers may be tempted to move in, take charge, and take over in a way that is uncalled for and unhelpful. Although this approach may be warranted in a crisis, it is a disruptive strategy to employ with families who are doing their best to meet the demands of inevitable, progressive, natural changes.

Health care providers may have trouble supporting people who do not meet their expectations, whom they may see as noncompliant. There may be an assumption that people will accept the role and responsibilities of caregiving, without leaving them much room to refuse. The different beliefs, values, and/or priorities that cause people to follow their own plans or regimens are sometimes discounted or judged. If health care providers have an attitude about the right way of doing things, they tend to impose agendas that may make perfect sense to the professionals but are uncomfortable or impossible for others. Then when people don't comply or run into problems, the providers may feel frustrated, superior, resentful, or disappointed. For example, judgments may arise around expectations about people's ability to pay for services or their priorities in making decisions. Often female caregivers are expected to be more willing and capable than males. A male's efforts may be commended while a female's limits or abilities are criticized. When these initial reactions are not examined, judgmental, conditional, or ungenerous attitudes can develop toward particular patients and families.

SUMMARY

Advanced physical symptoms now make the reality of death difficult to deny or ignore. Patients are no longer able to care for themselves, depending on family caregivers to help with bathing, dressing, and toileting (see Table 5.1). Profes-

Table 5.1. Palliative Performance Scale (PPSv2) 40%–30%

PPS Level	Ambulation	Activity and evidence of disease	Self-care	Intake	Conscious level
40%	Mainly in bed	Unable to do most activity Extensive disease	Mainly needs assistance	Normal or reduced	Full or drowsy +/- confusion
30%	Totally bed bound	Unable to do any activity Extensive disease	Total care	Normal or reduced	Full or drowsy +/- confusion

sional health care providers also become more involved in care, and admission to a hospice or long-term care facility may occur. Patients become selective about how and with whom they expend their waning energy. Reminiscence and goodbyes may be very important or energy may be withdrawn from treasured interests and relationships as patients begin to prepare for death. Their world is shrinking and is often viewed from bed.

Stressed and fatigued, family caregivers also begin to anticipate death. This is a time of multiple losses for families, with an increasing sense of grief as they look at what has been lost and what is yet to come. When patients move quickly through this transition, each physical change represents a step closer to death and serves as a reminder that the future will not be as they had hoped and that the patient's journey through illness is drawing to a close.

REFLECTIVE ACTIVITY

This activity is designed to increase awareness about how personal attitudes and expectations shape practice. You may choose to do this alone or with a colleague. It may be especially helpful to do it with someone in your own family. This activity is a powerful teaching tool, and the questions may be changed to focus on particularly pertinent or challenging issues.

First, imagine yourself in the following situation:

Your parents live in an in-law suite in your basement. Your elderly mother is dying from chronic obstructive pulmonary disease (COPD), and you understand that she probably has only a few months to live. As long as you can remember, your mother has had difficulty breathing. She has asthma and emphysema and still smokes almost a pack of cigarettes a day. Over the past month, you have seen her condition deteriorate. She needs considerable help to get out of bed. She is scared of suffocating and wants to die. She doesn't take her medications regularly because she believes they will pro-

PROFESSIONALS' DIFFICULTY WITH DYING PATIENTS

In the late 1970s, Worden and Kubler-Ross (1978) surveyed 6,000 health care professionals, including physicians, nurses, psychologists, social workers, and clergy. One of the questions that they asked was, "Is there a kind of dying person that you have difficulty working with?" Interestingly, most of the professional groups had difficulty with dying patients who were struggling with some aspect of dying that lay outside of the health care professionals' presumed professional expertise. Physicians often had difficulty with people who were anxious, whereas nurses had difficulty with patients who were younger than they were or of the same age or gender. Social workers and psychologists had difficulty working with patients who were in pain. Clergy had difficulty working with people who were nonreligious or unknown to them. It seemed that one's inability or ability to relate to the patients' experiences made the job more or less difficult, depending on one's profession.

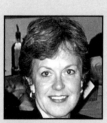

Elizabeth Causton,
M.S.W., is a counselor
with Victoria Hospice.
She works on the
Palliative Response
Team and the inpatient
unit.

In My Own Voice
The Dance

Elizabeth Causton

When we work with a conscious awareness of where we stand in relationship to patients and families, respecting their unique "dance" in response to grief and loss, we are less likely to become overinvolved or to get lost in our work.

The idea of a family dance is not new, but it works particularly well as an image that reminds us of the importance of paying attention to boundaries as we work with people who are, in Vanier's words, "vulnerable and broken." The image can also be used to describe the sense of continuity of the family dance, which has evolved over generations. It reminds us that every family dance has its own history and that every step taken on the family dance floor has a reason in the context of that shared history.

So, when one member of the family either sits down or lies down on the dance floor because of terminal illness, the dance may look quite clumsy as the family tries to modify their routine to accommodate the changes, but the new steps are not random. They, too, have meaning in the context of what has gone on before.

Still, as we watch families struggle with a difficult dance, to music that always gets faster and louder in a crisis, we may be tempted to get onto their dance floor to try and teach them a new dance, with steps from the dance that we are most familiar with—our own. Of course, this rarely works, for the obvious reason that our dance steps do not have a history or a reason in the context of another family's particular dance. Our valuable and unique perspective is lost the moment we step out onto someone else's dance floor. Regardless of our good intentions, we truly become lost in our work.

The greater value of our role is to stay on the edge of the dance floor and from that vantage point, to observe, comment on, and normalize the process that the family is going through. We may suggest options, new dance steps that the family hasn't thought of, but we do so with the recognition that they can only consider new ideas in the context of their own history. This is what it means to work from a "therapeutic distance," to work with an awareness of where we stand in relation to the people with whom we are working.

However, whereas working with this kind of clarity and respect for boundaries may be our goal, experience tells us that it is not easy. The edge of the family dance floor is often, in fact, a fluid border, as difficult to define as it is to say exactly where the sea meets the sand. In addition, each of us has "hooks": people or situations that may touch us in some deep, unconscious place. Before we even know what's happened, we find ourselves on someone else's dance floor, wondering how on earth we got there. Because we have an obligation to do this work with awareness, it is important that we do our "homework," seeking to identify our "hooks" and paying attention to signs that we may have stepped over the line.

The signs that we may be losing our perspective are 1) experiencing an extreme emotional reaction to a person or situation that (perhaps without our knowing it) resonates with an unresolved issue or a difficult relationship on our own dance floor; 2) feeling a sense of ownership, as reflected in language such as "my patients" or "my families," or difficulty letting go or sharing individuals with other team members; and/or 3) experiencing a need to influence/control patients and families by directing their options and choices or by making ourselves indispensable to them.

Despite having identified signs of over-involvement, it is also important to understand the challenges inherent in our work and be gentle with ourselves as we strive to be "good enough." We need to remember that maintaining a therapeutic distance does not preclude strong emotions and deep caring. One of the greatest advantages of knowing where we stand and being clear about what we bring to our work is being able to both feel deeply and act wisely.

"What would it be like to approach our lives, and to engage in the lives of others, knowing we are all inherently whole, intrinsically well, in need of being drawn forth into the discovery of unabashed completeness? How would this change the entire dance of practitioner and patient?"

—(Santorelli, 1999, p. 78)

long her life. Your father is home with her, but she will accept only minimal help from him. She frequently calls you at work or home to come and help. Your father is also unwell; he has diabetes and you have noticed that sometimes he is quite forgetful and confused. You wonder whether his cognitive changes are because he is worried about your mother or if something else is going on. Once a week, a community nurse visits and your mother has reluctantly agreed to have someone come twice a week to bathe and groom her.

Next, remembering that this is your family situation, answer the following questions:

What are your expectations

- Of your mother
- Of your father
- Of your siblings
- Of yourself

Who is the most responsible person? Who makes decisions about care options? Who must make sacrifices? How much? Then, consider how your responses would change if the following occurs

- You lived in a different city than your parents
- You had young children or a child with disabilities or had no children
- You worked full time or didn't work at all
- Your mother or father was mentally ill or you were
- Your mother's prognosis was 2 weeks or unknown
- You disliked your mother and/or father

Now, honestly reflect on how these personal beliefs influence or direct your interventions with patients and families. Finally, if you did this exercise with someone else, discuss your responses and insights.

RESOURCES

Cooklin, A. (1989). Tenderness and toughness in the face of distress. *Palliative Medicine, 3*, 89–95.

Corr, C. (1991–1992). A task-based approach to coping with dying. *Omega, 24*(2), 81–94.

Fainsinger, R.L., Waller, A., Bercovici, M., Bengtson, K., Landman, W., Hosking, M., Nunez-Olarte, J.M., & deMoissac, D. (2000). A multicenter international study of sedation for uncontrolled symptoms in terminally ill patients. *Palliative Medicine, 14,* 257–265.

Grande, G.E., Todd, C.J., & Barclay, S.I.G. (1997). Support needs in the last year of life: Patient and care dilemmas. *Palliative Medicine, 11,* 202–208.

Robinson, C. (1996). Health care relationships revisited. *Journal of Family Nursing, 2*(2), 152–173.

Sales, J. (2001). Sedation and terminal care. *European Journal of Palliative Care, 8*(3), 97–100.

Victoria Hospice Society. (1998). *Medical care of the dying* (3rd ed.). Victoria, British Columbia, Canada: Victoria Hospice Society.

Wilbur, K. (1988). On being a support person. *The Journal of Transpersonal Psychology, 20*(2), 141–159.

REFERENCES

Canine, J.D. (1996). *The psychosocial aspects of death and dying.* Stamford, CT: Appleton & Lange.

Cassell, E. (1982). The nature of suffering and the goals of medicine. *New England Journal of Medicine, 306*(11), 639–641.

Christensen, S., & Harding, M. (1985, June). Integrating theories of crisis intervention into hospice home care teaching. *Nursing Clinics of North America, 20*(2), 449–455.

Chung, K. (1993). Brief social work intervention in the hospice setting: Person-centered work and crisis intervention synthesized and distilled. *Palliative Medicine, 7,* 59–62.

Corr, C.A., & Corr, D.M. (2000). Anticipatory mourning and coping with dying: Similarities, differences, and suggested guidelines for helpers. In T. Rando (Ed.), *Clinical dimensions of anticipatory mourning: Theory and practice in working with the dying, their loved ones and their caregivers* (pp. 223–251). Champaign, IL: Research Press.

Davies, B. (2000). Anticipatory mourning and the transition of fading away. In T. Rando (Ed.), *Clinical dimensions of anticipatory mourning: Theory and practice in working with the dying, their loved ones and their caregivers* (pp. 135–153). Champaign, IL: Research Press.

Enyert, G., & Burman, M. (1999). A qualitative study of self-transcendence in caregivers of terminally ill patients. *American Journal of Hospice and Palliative Care, 16*(2), 455–462.

Gibran, K. (1972). *The prophet.* New York: Alfred A. Knopf.

Kissane, D., & Clarke, D. (2001). Demoralization syndrome—A relevant psychiatric diagnosis for palliative care. *Journal of Palliative Care, 17*(1), 12–21.

Lamers, W.M. (2000). Grief in dying persons. In T. Rando (Ed.), *Clinical dimensions of anticipatory mourning: Theory and practice in working with the dying, their loved ones and their caregivers* (pp. 281–305). Champaign, IL: Research Press.

Oxford English Dictionary (2nd ed.). (1989). Oxford: Clarendon Press.

Puryear, D.A. (1979). *Helping people in crisis.* San Francisco: Jossey-Bass.

Rando, T. (2000). Promoting healthy anticipatory mourning in intimates of the life-threatened or dying person. In T. Rando (Ed.), *Clinical dimensions of anticipatory mourning: Theory and practice in working with the dying, their loved ones and their caregivers* (pp. 307–378). Champaign, IL: Research Press.

Rosenberg, M.B. (1999). *Nonviolent communication, A language of compassion.* Encinitas, CA: Puddle Dancer Press.

Saakvitne, K.W., & Pearlman, L.A. (1996). *Transforming the pain: A workbook on vicarious traumatization* (pp. 41–50). New York: W.W. Norton.

Sands, R.G. (1983, Fall). Crisis intervention and social work practice in hospitals. *Health and Social Work, 8*(4), 253–261.

Santorelli, S. (1999). *Heal thy self: Lessons on mindfulness.* New York: Bell Tower Publishing.

Schwartz, M. (1996). *Letting go: Morrie's reflections on living while dying.* New York: Dell.

Stadjuhar, K., & Davies, B. (1998). Death at home: Challenges for families and directions for the future. *Journal of Palliative Care, 14*(3), 8–14.

Vanier, J. (1972). *Eruption to hope.* Toronto: Griffin House.

Wade, A.(1997). Small acts of living: Everyday resistance to violence and other forms of oppression. *Contemporary Family Therapy, 19*(1), 23–39.

Worden, W. (2000). Towards an appropriate death. In T. Rando (Ed.), *Clinical dimensions of anticipatory mourning: Theory and practice in working with the dying, their loved ones and their caregivers* (pp. 277). Champaign, IL: Research Press.

Worden, W., & Kubler-Ross, E. (1978). Attitudes and experiences of death workshop attendees. *Omega, 8,* 91–106.

perspective

ALTERNATIVE THERAPIES

"At the heart of each of us, whatever our imperfections, there exists a silent pulse of perfect rhythm, a complex of wave forms and resonances, which is absolutely individual and unique, yet which connects us to everything in the universe. The act of getting in touch with this pulse can transform our personal experience and in some way alter the world around us."
–Leonard, 1981

The phrase *alternative therapies* is used to encompass healing modalities that fall outside the realm of traditional western medicine (Downer et al., 1994). This section highlights some of the nontraditional tools and therapies that many people choose to incorporate into their care as they journey through illness, death, and bereavement. These modalities differ from more traditional forms of treatment in that they are used from the perspective of fostering and enhancing personal growth, health, balance, and well-being.

When the whole person—including mind, body, spirit, emotions, and interpersonal relationships—is held as the focus of care, the approach is usually referred to as *holistic*. Although traditional western medicine is also holistic, some patients want more than what they see as an increasingly technical, depersonalized, and fragmented approach to health care (Downer et al., 1994).

The National Institutes of Health (NIH) have categorized various healing modalities into fields of practice (Dossey, 1998):

- Mind/Body: Biofeedback; relaxation, meditation, prayer, guided imagery, yoga, psychotherapy; and music, dance, and art therapy

- Bioelectromagnetic: Explores how living organisms interact with electromagnetic fields

- Alternative Medical Practice: Traditional Chinese medicine (TCM), ayurveda, homeopathy, naturopathy, acupuncture, and shamanic healing

- Manual Healing: Osteopathy, massage, chiropractic, therapeutic touch, Reiki, and healing touch

- Pharmacologic and Biologic: Drugs and vaccines not yet accepted by mainstream medicine

- Herbal Medicine: Herbal approaches from Europe, China, Asia, India, and Native American cultures

- Diet, Nutrition, and Lifestyle: Using various food groups, vitamins, and minerals for health maintenance, disease prevention, and treatment

These various fields of practice represent an overwhelming number of alternative healing modalities. Some of these modalities are well known and might be used by palliative care providers. Some hospice palliative care programs may include various practitioners in their team. The educational backgrounds, practical training, professional standards, and clinical experiences of practitioners are diverse. They range from university degrees and clinical internships to a series of weekend workshops or simply personal interest and affinity.

Unfamiliarity with techniques, insufficient evidence of outcomes, and the wide range of education and training requirements for practitioners make it difficult for many mainstream health care providers to wholeheartedly trust and support their participation. Because many people with advanced disease will be considering these options for the first time, it is often difficult for patients and families to determine which method or practitioner is best suited to them or most appropriate for their concerns (Gray et al., 1997). Patients and their families may, however, turn to one or more alternative practices when they feel that traditional systems of health care cannot offer the hope that they want (Clover & Kassab, 1998). Some people feel that the traditional western approach is too narrow and may leave some patients feeling reduced to their diagnosis and prognosis. The language of hope inherent in holistic practices speaks to people's concerns for healing, balance, peace, integration, and well-being (Bullock, 1997).

Alternative therapies may directly or indirectly suggest that miracles are possible or offer healing when the promise of a cure fades. Miracles and healing are not the same thing. One can, indeed, die and yet be spiritually and emotionally healed and whole, but this is different than finding a cure. Some alternative therapies such as music and art therapy or therapeutic touch promote comfort and connectedness and are generally less intrusive or uncomfortable than other conventional therapies (O'Callaghan, 1996). They can restore some of the personal power, control, and independence that many patients find is lost during progressive terminal disease. Families appreciate being able to do something.

The medical literature, particularly in the cancer field, has taken an interest in identifying which people are most likely to use alternative or complementary therapies. One Canadian study (Oneschuk, Fennell, Hanson, & Bruera, 1998) looked at usage of complementary medications in the following categories: *herbal preparations, vitamins, minerals,* and *other* (e.g., shark cartilage, melatonin.) This study found that the groups most apt to use these therapies were men and women younger than 60 years of age with advanced cancer. This description identifies a fairly discrete group of people. It could be suggested that this group is the most frequent user of these medications because they are more familiar with such alternatives and are able to afford them.

The costs of these medications commonly are not covered by standard medical plans. People who use alternative therapies usually make a significant emotional and financial commitment to these practices. After making such an investment, it may be hard to stop these therapies even when they are difficult to take or no longer beneficial.

Guiding Principles for Health Care Providers

- Have a basic knowledge of alternative therapies commonly used by patients and families.

- Understand how the holistic perspective used in alternative therapies empowers people and supports the healing process.

- Be aware of potential adverse effects and drug interactions that occur between some alternative substances and the medications that a patient is already taking and/or the patient's condition.

- Be aware of the influence and limitations of any personal biases and judgments about alternative therapies.

- Ask what patients and families are doing in the way of alternative therapies and what they believe the value to be.

Ethically, health care providers cannot recommend unproven therapies that are purported to cure disease. They may, however, be supportive of those therapies that patients find helpful for their personal health and well-being. When ethically appropriate, health care providers may work with involved alternative care practitioners to provide support to patients and families. Key questions regarding alternative therapies include

- What helps you maintain a sense of health and well-being?

- What alternative therapies or treatments do you use? What do you value most about this treatment option?

- How long has this [treatment, therapy] been part of your health care routine? How is it working for you?

- How comfortable do you feel talking about your concerns with your [naturopath, massage therapist, yoga teacher, and so forth]?

- How comfortable do you feel talking about the alternative therapies that you use with your health care providers such as your physician, nurse, or counselor?

- How will you know if it is time to change or stop a particular treatment?

- Are there adverse effects from this treatment that you are finding difficult to manage or maintain?

- How are you and your family dealing with the financial cost of these treatments?

- What do you imagine would happen if you stopped using this (alternative) treatment?

- How would you know if you had been ill-advised, or not given all the facts, about a specific therapy? (For example, visit www.quackwatch.com)

RESOURCES

Astin, J.A. (1998) Why patients use alternative medicine: Results of a national study. *Journal of the American Medical Association, 279*(19), 1548–1553.

Dom, H. (2001). Ayurveda and palliative care. *European Journal of Palliative Care, 8*(3), 102–105.

Eisenberg, D.M., Davis, R.B., Ettner, S.L., Appel, S., Wilkey, S., Van Rompay, M., & Kessler, R.C. (1998). Trends in alternative medicine use in the United States, 1990–1997: Results of a follow-up national survey. *Journal of the American Medical Association, 280*(18), 1569–1575.

Kabat-Zinn, J. (1990). *Full catastrophe living: Using the wisdom of your body to face stress, pain, and illness.* New York: Bantam Doubleday Dell Publishing Group.

Mackey, R.B. (April, 1995). Discover the healing power of therapeutic touch. *American Journal of Nursing,* 27–32.

Pitchford, P. (1995). *Healing with whole foods: Oriental traditions and modern nutrition.* Berkeley, CA: North Atlantic Books.

Rykov, M., & Salmon, D. (1998). Bibliography for music therapy in palliative care, 1963–1997. *The American Journal of Hospice and Palliative Care, 15*(3), 174–180.

Wilkinson, S. (1996, August). Get the massage. *Nursing Times, 92*(34), 61–65.

REFERENCES

Bullock, M. (1997). Reiki: A complementary therapy for life. *The American Journal of Hospice and Palliative Care, 14*(1), 31–33.

Clover, A., & Kassab, S. (1998). Complementary medicine for patients with cancer. *European Journal of Palliative Care, 5*(3), 73–76.

Dossey, B.M. (1998, June). Holistic modalities and healing moments. *American Journal of Nursing, 98*(6), 44–47.

Downer, S.M., Cody, M.M., McClushey, P., Wilson, P.D., Arnott, S.J., Lister, T.A., & Slevin, M.L. (1994). Pursuit and practice of complementary therapies by cancer patients receiving conventional treatment. *British Medical Journal, 309,* 86–89.

Gray, R.E., Fitch, M., Greenburg, M., Voros, P., Douglas, M.S., Labreque, M., & Chart, P. (1997). Physician perspectives on unconventional cancer therapies. *Journal of Palliative Care, 13*(2), 14–21.

Leonard, G. (1981). *The silent pulse: A search for the perfect rhythm that exists in each of us.* New York: Bantam Books.

O'Callaghan, C. (1996). Pain, music creativity and music therapy in palliative care. The *American Journal of Hospice & Palliative Care, 13*(2), 43–49.

Oneschuk, D., Fennell, L., Hanson, J., & Bruera, E. (1998). The use of complementary medications by cancer patients attending an outpatient pain and symptom clinic. *Journal of Palliative Care, 14*(4), 21–26.

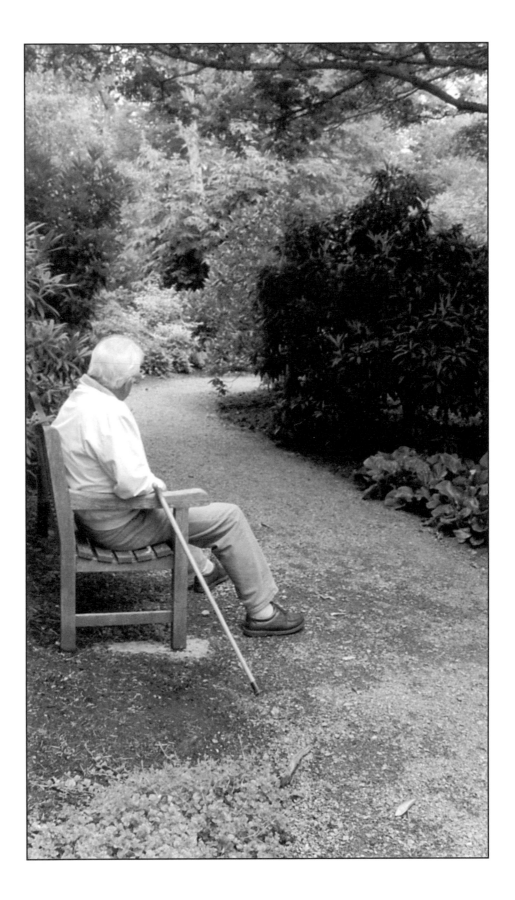

6

Watching and Waiting

As Death Approaches
(PPSv2 level: 20% to 10%)

*T*he transition from PPS 20% to 10% is very different than other transitions. Previously, the patient was directly at the center of activity and decisions; things shift as the patient progressively moves to unconsciousness and becomes disconnected from others. The familiar things that normally sustain life and connection are juxtaposed with the unfamiliar closeness of death. This space of time, hiatus, or period of limbo can be experienced as a time of quiet, peaceful closure or be turbulent and unsettling. Patients have usually fought to assert their will to live, but now a quality of relaxation may begin to emerge. According to Singh, "There [may be a] sense of the end of the struggle, a surrender, an allowing of one's contracted self to relax and melt. There is a feeling of sinking into safety, finally, after all the intensity of resistance" (2002, p. 270).

At this transition, families must shift from DOING TO BEING. Most often, patients are unresponsive and their care concerns are comparatively fewer. Personal care such as dental hygiene, bathing, and changes of clothing may be all the hands-on care that is required. Many medications are stopped and others given, such as oral solutions, patches, and subcutaneous injections. For families giving these treatments at home, it may feel like less work when compared to earlier levels of caregiving. Time spent with the patient now shifts from predominantly task-oriented activity to a quieter pace of sitting and providing companionship.

As the patient becomes unresponsive, COMMUNICATION between the patient and family is more challenging. Family members often feel disconnected, helpless, and frustrated when patients no longer can say what they need or want. Patients often don't speak or respond at all to the touch or voice of family and friends. Sometimes their words are unclear and disjointed or, at other times, seem very clear. They may speak of travel, going home, or getting ready, using journey metaphors or other words that bear some relevance to their lives.

As the patient no longer has the strength or capacity to participate, family are now MAKING DECISIONS WITHOUT THE PATIENT. This responsibility falls to the next of kin or appointed decision maker who may be the spouse, partner, adult child, sibling, or friend. Some families work as a team and make all decisions together, whereas others expect a certain person to do this alone. When the patient's wishes are known, this task is much easier. It is not, however, uncommon for patients to become unconscious or die without indicating their concerns and preferences. When this happens, family members must still make decisions based on their understanding of what the patient would have wanted. This responsibility can leave families feeling overwhelmed and uncertain.

Now that death is imminent, families start to focus on the time of death. Most people have not actually seen a person die before but many will have EXPECTATIONS ABOUT DYING. Often, these are based on misconceptions and fear. People without any prior experience of death may not know what to expect or do when the patient dies. Those with prior experiences may mistakenly feel prepared or be frightened, depending on the kind of death that they have experienced before.

One symptom experienced by patients close to death that is particularly difficult for families and health care providers is RESTLESSNESS. Patients may struggle to get out of bed and seem to be trying to go somewhere. This restlessness, stemming from several causes, occurs with varying degrees of severity, from mild to extreme agitation. Patients may shift around in bed, looking unsettled or perturbed, and it is difficult for families and health care providers to comfort or calm them. Issues and questions about sedation to relieve this discomfort may arise.

IAN AND GUS

Ian is 42. After 12 years of living with human immunodeficiency virus (HIV), he is now dying from AIDS. His partner of 15 years, Gus, is also HIV positive. Gus has an 18-year-old son, Mark, who has lived with Gus and Ian since he was 3. Earlier in the year, Ian had pneumonia, and everyone thought he was dying.

Now, Ian is completely bed bound and sleeps all of the time. He has ongoing difficulty breathing and has frequent incontinence. Despite Gus' devoted care, bedsores have developed on Ian's heels and tailbone. Movement and changes in position cause Ian some pain. Although sex was a major source of comfort to both him and Ian until recently, Gus feels he can no longer touch Ian without causing him pain. He misses the affection and interaction that he and Ian shared. Although he realizes that there may be other ways to create intimacy, he feels despondent.

> "An old man once cut some wood and was walking along carrying it. As he grew weary, he put down his load and called Death to come. When Death appeared and asked why he had called for him, the old man said, 'To get you to take up my burden.'"
>
> —Aesop (Cotter, 1999, p. 259)

Ian has had several restless nights. During these times, he pulls at his clothing and tries to get out of bed. Once, he fell, hitting his head on a table. If Gus tries to hold Ian's hands, Ian yells, "Don't hurt me." This is very upsetting to Gus and Mark. He has been mumbling intermittently about a report or project that he must finish. This is very confusing to Gus because Ian hasn't been well enough to work for 2 years. Ian has also talked about going to a cabin that his family owned when he was a child.

Several years ago, Gus and Ian invited a dying friend to live with them. Gus has horrible memories about that friend's death. He remembers his friend being blue and gasping for air when he died. Exhausted and afraid of reliving that experience, Gus has decided to admit Ian to the hospice to die, against Ian's earlier wishes. Even though Gus knows Ian didn't want to see his family, he wonders if he should call and let them know what is happening. Gus feels ambivalent about some of the choices he has made, but he didn't know what else to do. He doesn't want to burden Mark with these questions, and, although he knows that Ian would understand, he wishes they could talk about these things one more time.

KEY CONSIDERATIONS

Doing to Being

Now Ian is completely bed bound and sleeps all of the time. Movement and changes in position have started to cause him pain. Gus feels he can no

longer touch Ian without causing him pain. He misses the affection and interaction that he and Ian shared. Although he realizes that there may be
other ways to create intimacy, Gus feels despondent.

Perhaps the most difficult part of this transition is that, after months or weeks
of ongoing busyness and activity, the pace has settled down and there is less to do.
Up to this point, family members have usually been very involved in the hands-on
provision or coordination of care. The give and take between patients and families
characteristic of earlier transitions is often much less or absent altogether. It is difficult for families just to be with people and watch as they die. At the same time,
"just being there, in a centered way . . . allows for a level of deep and essential sharing that most of us do not normally get to experience" (Singh, 2000, p. 270).

Some caregivers will be relieved that the intense activity of earlier times is past.
This relief may generate a sense of calm and quiet waiting, or it may open a flood of
pent-up grief. Some people use this quiet time to reminisce or review what has happened, while others keep very busy, focusing on details such as physical attention to
the patient, making tea for family, telephoning, or arranging funeral plans. If family members are exhausted by the length or burden of care, they may fall apart at
times, or start to irritate and challenge each other (Rueth & Hall, 1999).

The reasons for these different responses are as varied and unique as the people who exhibit them; they depend on people's personalities, beliefs about themselves, and spiritual or religious beliefs, as well as their definitions of quality of
life, quality time, and dying with dignity. Behaviors and reactions may be further
influenced by the nature of people's relationships with the patient.

Many people believe that the patient should not die alone and so a vigil is
kept. Often, this belief reflects the caregiver's preferences and not necessarily the
patient's. Sometimes, a vigil is very reverent, involving a single person in silence
or prayer. Sometimes, many family members or friends gather around, sharing stories and laughter. At other times, family are attentive but also allow the patient
time to be alone. Whatever shape the vigil takes, it usually offers caregivers something meaningful to do, when nothing else need, nor can, be done.

Interventions

These psychosocial interventions have been designed to specifically address the
key consideration *doing to being*. There are several assessment questions that will
help open up a discussion, followed by more focused comments or tips that will
facilitate further exploration of the issues that frequently arise at this time; each
tip is followed by a sample dialogue.

Assessment Questions

- How are you finding ways to be close now that you aren't providing so much of John's physical care?

- How do you think he would want you to spend your time with him now?

- What is most important about this time for you?

- How are you feeling emotionally? Physically?

"When we honestly ask ourselves which persons in our lives mean the most to us, we often find it is those who instead of giving advice, solutions or cures, have chosen instead to share our pain. The friend who can be silent with us in an hour of grief, who can tolerate not knowing, not curing, not healing, and face with us the reality of our powerlessness, is the friend that cares."

—Henri Nouwen, 1974

Help people adjust to changes in the patient's condition. After the intensity of earlier transitions, it can be difficult for people to slow down, stop doing, and simply witness this time.

> *"You say that you are comfortable with the staff and the care that Alex is receiving at hospice. After all the devoted care that you gave him when he was home, I'm wondering how you are doing and what you might need and want from hospice at this time?"*

Encourage people to take regular breaks from the vigil. Normalize the fact that some patients will die when they are alone. No one knows if patients choose to do this, but the possibility may help family members to feel less disappointed or guilty if they aren't present at the time of death.

> *"Alice, I know that you are committed to being with your daughter when she dies. I want you to know, however, that sometimes patients die in those brief moments when family members leave the room to answer the phone or take a nap. We don't know if there is a reason why this happens, but we often wonder if some people choose to die in that way. What do you think?"*

Identify ways to be with patients when they are not responsive. When people feel they have a purpose, spending time with someone who doesn't speak becomes more comfortable.

> *"It is really hard to get used to talking to someone who doesn't talk back. Finding something to do with Neil at his bedside may help you feel more at ease. Perhaps listening to a favorite piece of music or reading passages out of a familiar religious text would be comfortable. What might you do when you are with him that would help you feel supportive?"*

Normalize changes in caregiver's mood or ability. The letdown that happens when patients become unresponsive may trigger unexpected reactions. People may be relieved to know these reactions are common.

> *"Up until now, you have been keeping a lot of exhaustion and sadness inside while you cared for Christine. Now that she doesn't need your constant attention, you say that you are crying all the time and struggling with simple decisions. Going from primary caregiver back to friend is a big shift. Would it be helpful to talk about how this feels for you?*

Communication

> Ian has been mumbling intermittently about a report or project that he must finish. This is very confusing to Gus because Ian hasn't been well enough to work for 2 years. Ian has also talked about going to a cabin that his family owned when he was a child.

At this time, communication between patients and families, in its most familiar forms, stops. Family members may feel that patients are already gone and may wonder if patients are aware of what is happening or who is present. Patients no longer have the strength or clarity needed to respond appropriately to questions or engage in conversation. Much of what they say may be inaudible or disconnected from reality. If patients are able to speak, the things they say are challenging to understand and often the observer is left to speculate. Some words appear to have no meaning; at other times, people are trying to communicate but have difficulty doing so. Although some may open their eyes if touched or spoken to, many will not respond at all at this time, even nonverbally.

Why Communication Is Hindered

In the process of dying, various physical changes happen. The brain may receive poor oxygen, vital organs may stop functioning, and drugs and toxins may build up in the blood and brain. These occurrences directly affect a patient's ability to be mentally clear and to communicate. At the same time, patients may develop delirium accompanied by restlessness, hallucinations, fears, and confusion. Eventually, these physical changes lead to stupor, coma, and death.

Although the impact of these physical changes on the patient is clear, the patient's *experience* of dying is less certain. As mentioned previously, patients who can still speak frequently talk about traveling, journeys, or familiar events or places as they move toward their deaths. It seems they are try-ing to communicate in a symbolic or metaphoric way, perhaps wanting to describe their journey. Most reli-gions and cultures have various beliefs about this journey at the end of life, but patients' messages are often discounted, ignored, or rejected by those around them (Callanan & Kelley, 1992). This type of communication, which occurs near the time of death, is referred to as symbolic communication. Singh ex-plained that at this time "communication moves be-yond words born of logic and reason" (2000, p. 270).

VIGIL

The *Oxford English Dictionary* lists these as some of the defini-tions of the word *vigil*: a devo-tional watching; an occasion or period of keeping awake for some special reason or pur-pose; the precise time of the day in which the flowers of dif-ferent plants open, expand and shut (1989, p. 3629).

Sometimes within days or weeks of death, patients talk about going. They seem to know that death is near and they will soon be leaving. Some patients even seem to know when their death will occur and try to share that information with others (Callanan & Kelley, 1992). They may talk about planning, waiting, or going on a trip somewhere. Often, people say they are going "home." Whether home is their actual residence or a symbolic expression is often unclear or not spoken. They seem preoc-cupied with thoughts about whether they are where they need to be for their journey to begin. They are often confused and restless. Some patients seem to be waiting for or trying to make something happen. They often speak agitatedly, as if they are in a hurry. Tickets, cars, planes, people, or papers may be named. A sense of urgency is ev-ident in repeated questions about the time or whether something or someone is ready.

Often, families react to the emotional content of the words, but the symbolic meaning is too ambiguous, abstract, or vague to comprehend. When family mem-bers persist in trying to understand or make this communication rational, both they and the patient quickly feel helpless and frustrated. Trying to correct or re-orient patients may only escalate their agitation and confusion.

Callanan and Kelley (1992) believed that the symbolic communication of pa-tients nearing death gives us essential information about their experience and what they most need. For example, a person who is restless, trying to get out of bed, and saying they want to go home, may in fact be demonstrating a readiness and desire to die. Holding this perspective—that communication at this time is purposeful rather than simply delirious—offers a way to support understanding and connect-edness between patients and families when former patterns are no longer useful.

Interventions

These psychosocial interventions have been designed to specifically address the key consideration *communication*. There are several assessment questions that will

help open up a discussion, followed by more focused comments or tips that will facilitate further exploration of the issues that frequently arise at this time; each tip is followed by a sample dialogue.

Assessment Questions

- What helps you to feel connected with James? How are you communicating with him now?

- What kinds of things is your brother saying now? What meaning are you able to make of what he says?

- How do you respond when he talks about "going home"?

Educate people about symbolic communication. Sometimes, it settles people's frustration and confusion when they understand that the words spoken may be symbolic rather than literal.

> *"Monica, for the past couple of days, your friend has been talking about selling her house and going somewhere. Perhaps she may be telling you that she is getting ready to die. Do you recall other times when she has spoken indirectly or symbolically about a difficult issue?"*

Demonstrate appropriate ways to respond to changed communication. Often, it feels awkward for people to engage with someone who is not communicating in familiar ways and who may be speaking symbolically.

> *"I understand that John has been talking about going home and you are worried about what that means. It is important to speak to him in a way that is both positive for him and comfortable for you. For example, you might say, 'John, I hear that you are getting ready to go home but you're not sure when you are leaving. I believe that you'll go when the time is right for you.' How comfortable would you be with this kind of comment?"*

Help the family tailor their communication style to fit the patient's. Often, patients cannot respond at all, or only have the strength to respond to closed, yes or no, questions.

> *"Angela, when you speak with Martin, ask very simple questions that he can answer through a gesture or just a yes or no. For example, rather than asking how he's feeling, you might ask, 'Are you thirsty?'"*

SYMBOLIC COMMUNICATION

A young woman's 63-year-old father was dying. A retired police officer, he had been close to death a number of times over the course of his lifetime. For several days, he had been very restless and agitated, wanting to get the car ready and to go somewhere, though he hadn't said where. His wife had tried to assure him that the car was parked and that he was not going anywhere, but this effort only increased his agitation. His daughter, however, believed that he might be talking symbolically about his death. She knew that her father loved to take the family on long drives and it made sense to her that he'd be talking about getting the car and going now. Late in the evening when they were alone and he was talking about going, she carefully led him through what would be his last long family drive. She recounted all the preparations he would normally make with the vehicle, ensuring that the tank was full of gas, the oil had been checked, and the tires were properly inflated. She assured him that he would be safe on this journey. She explained that this was a drive he would take alone but that everyone would be with him in spirit. She encouraged him to go with the memory of her mother's perfume mixing with the ocean air and the sound of her and her sister laughing and fighting as usual in the backseat. She reminded him that he had prior experience of this journey and that he had carefully prepared all of his family and friends. She told him that he had said and done everything he needed to. She told him he was loved and said that he could leave as soon as he was ready. Hours later, he died peacefully.

Explain the uncertainty about whether a patient in a coma is able to hear or recognize the presence of family. This helps families stay connected and feel comfortable saying things to the patient.

> *"Sandy is in a light coma right now and may hear your voice but may not be able to understand what you are saying. When she goes into a deeper coma, it's unlikely she would even be aware of or hear your voice."*

Making Decisions without the Patient

Exhausted and afraid, Gus has decided to admit Ian to the hospice to die, against Ian's earlier wishes. Even though Gus knows Ian didn't want to see his family, he wonders if he should call and let them know what is happening. Gus feels ambivalent about some of the choices he has made but he doesn't know what else to do. He doesn't want to burden Mark with these questions, and, although he knows that Ian would understand, he wishes they could talk about these things one more time.

Often, patients' preferences and expectations about care change several times as new information is gained, symptoms escalate, and the severity of illness increases. Until now, these changes have happened with patients' input and direction. Now, patients may be unresponsive and unable to contribute to ongoing decision making. Some will have stated their wishes to one or more family members. Others may have outlined their wishes in an advance directive or even a death plan. Many patients come to this transition having said very little to anyone about what they definitely want or don't want. Unable to review options with the patient, families must now rely on their own judgment about what the patient would have wanted to make the important decisions that lie ahead.

Family members step into the role of decision maker with varying degrees of comfort and confidence. Having experienced a number of major changes to the plan already, it can be difficult for families to establish which of the patient's requests are etched in stone and which ones may be altered. Enyert and Burman (1999) suggested that professional support and information must be accessible to family caregivers in order for them to realize their full capacity to give competent comfort-oriented care. There may be conflict among family members about who is the best person to balance emotions, realities, and resources, or who knows the patient best and is therefore the most qualified spokesperson. These conflicts may be exacerbated or made simpler by medical and legal mandates.

The pressure to make the right choice is huge and often is not unanimous or straightforward. Sometimes, the choices offered do not match the patient's and/or the family's needs or expectations. Family members usually try very hard to uphold the patient's wishes, or at the least to do what they think the patient would want. Unfortunately, the physical realities of dying may have been too evocative, unfamiliar, or unpleasant to discuss earlier and so the patient's wishes about resuscitation, nutrition, and hydration may not have been discussed. Sometimes, families do know the patient's wishes, but agreements made days or weeks ago are no longer reasonable and unforeseen complications or extenuating circumstances make it impossible to uphold early plans.

Many of the decisions that must be made are complex and speculative in nature; they may be uncomfortable for some family and some team members. People's expectations of themselves and each other tend to be very high and sometimes unrealistic at this time. They want to be able to say that they did everything possible to ensure the patient's comfort, dignity, and safety. The uncertainty about doing the right thing and the struggle to make decisions on behalf of the patient are hallmarks of this time.

Although families feel the burden of this responsibility, it is important to remind them that final decisions do not rest solely with them. Health care providers are also integral to decision making and may have final authority in some decisions.

COME WITH ME

Both:
Listen to these words I whisper
Press your lips to mine.
Keep me in your arms
Forever entwined.

One:
Come with me, I'll show you the way
Will you follow me into the night?
Come with me, relinquish this day
And the angels will hasten our flight.

Other:
I will not follow you into the dark
Who knows what morning we'll find.
Stay with me, never depart
How can you leave your true love behind?

One:
Come with me, you promised to be
My companion through all of our days.
Come with me, it's easy, you'll see
How you just let the light slip away.

Other:
I have been faithful through heartache and tears
True, in the way that I know.
Stay with me, I'm troubled, I'm weary
But I am not ready to go.

Both:
Listen to these words I whisper
Press your lips to mine.
Keep me in your arms
Forever entwined.

One:
Come with me, darkness is falling
I've stepped from the circle of time.
Come with me, though voices are calling
I weep for to leave you behind.

Other:
For so many years I have walked by your side,
Your hand was pressed in my own.
Sail away, slip out with the tide
For someday both our hearts will be home.

—(Susan Crowe, 1996, p. 225)

Some treatments or care requests may not be possible or available, or may even be futile or harmful. This may be a source of comfort or of conflict for families.

Interventions

These psychosocial interventions have been designed to specifically address the key consideration *making decisions without the patient*. There are several assessment questions that will help open up a discussion, followed by more focused comments or tips that will facilitate further exploration of the issues that frequently arise at this time; each tip is followed by a sample dialogue.

Assessment Questions

- What do you know about your wife's wishes? What do you believe is most important to her about her care at this time?

- What degree of intervention feels reasonable to you? Have you discussed this with your family physician?

- How supportive is your family in terms of the decisions that you are making?

Diffuse the pressure to make the right choice. It may be helpful to remind people that, on some level, this plan is the one that felt most comfortable to the patient.

> *"Leo, I know that you are really struggling with the weight of responsibility you feel and that you wish your wife had told you more about what she wanted. What would it be like to consider that, perhaps, she knew things would change and trusted you to weigh the options and make the most sensible choice?"*

Support people to make informed decisions when appropriate. Sometimes, it helps to know that they don't have to make all the decisions alone.

> *"You said that you wish your mother was still alive and able to help you make this difficult decision about your father's care. It may help to ask yourself how she might support or advise you if she were here now. You could also listen to your own instincts about this problem or you could talk over the options with a member of the health care team."*

Expectations About Dying

Several years ago, Gus and Ian invited a dying friend to live with them. Gus has horrible memories about that friend's death. He remembers his friend being blue and gasping for air when he died. Exhausted and afraid of re-living that experience, Gus has decided to admit Ian to the hospice to die.

Some people have witnessed death before and memories of that experience will color their needs and expectations now. Many people, however, haven't seen anyone die before and don't know what to expect or how to interpret what they see. Family caregivers who are unfamiliar with death may misinterpret normal end-of-life symptoms, such as mottling or apnea, and make poor decisions about what to do or not do. They may misjudge how close or far away the time of death actually is. Family members want and need accurate, timely information that helps them interpret the physical signs and symptoms they observe (Singh, 2000). Misinformation or lack of information at this time can contribute to decisions that people regret forever.

Recognizing and Responding to Predeath Changes

As death approaches, patients typically undergo a series of changes, listed here. It is important to remember that although these signs are clear indications that death is imminent, they are not the only definitive factor in predicting time of death. Patients may experience some or all of these predeath changes before they die. Patients differ in their strength of will, spirit, and life force, and these things will also affect the length of the dying process.

Breathing Pattern

- Becomes irregular
- May be shallow
- May be characterized by long pauses (apnea)
- May become wet or bubbly sounding (congestion)
- Stops at time of death

Sometimes, the soft breeze created by an open window or a small fan is helpful to people when their breathing changes. At this time, apnea is an expected change, is not uncomfortable, and is a natural process. Congestion is a symptom that may warrant intervention. If breathing sounds wet, crackling, or gurgling, speak to a nurse or physician as soon as possible.

Pulse

- May be fast
- May be faint

- Becomes irregular

- Stops at time of death

Changes in the rhythm and force of the heartbeat are normal. This is not an emergency, and there is no need for intervention.

Color

- Becomes uneven (mottled)

- May be purplish, blue, or gray

- Changes to waxy whitish yellow toward death

As circulation becomes less efficient, the patient's color changes. The blood supply to places farthest from the heart such as fingers, toes, knees, nose, eyes, and lips, will be reduced. Temperature fluctuations also happen as circulation changes, or if fever and infection are present. Although people may want to add or remove blankets, this variability in temperature is generally not uncomfortable for the patient.

Awareness

- Person may become unconscious

- Person may be communicating symbolically

- Person may be seeing visions, hallucinating

- Person may sleep with eyes open

Patients may be completely unresponsive to touch or talk, yet try to say something to someone. It may help to speak in a soothing, calm voice, paraphrasing their words to provide reassurance. Ask a nurse whether eye drops would be helpful when patients have their eyes open for long periods.

Restlessness and Delirium

- Person may become agitated or active

- Person may try to get up or out of bed

- Person may be picking at the air, clothing, or sheets

- Person may be combative

When patients are not calm or peaceful, it can be exhausting and stressful for families and health care providers. Talking over this symptom with a physician, counselor, pastor, or nurse may help people identify appropriate and effective ways to help both patients and themselves to deal with agitation and restlessness.

For many people, dying is frightening. The media—news, television, newspapers, and movies—often perpetuate an impression of death as brutal, scary, and painful. These disturbing images may work on the minds and hearts of families when their loved ones are nearing death. Expectations about the time of death are steeped in a highly individual mixture of imagination, superstitions, supposition, and spiritual and cultural beliefs. Families wonder what they will see, hear, and smell at the moment of death. For example, they may expect disturbing events such as the patient bleeding profusely, gasping for air, thrashing about, or calling out for help. Families worry that the patient may need some kind of highly technical and unfamiliar intervention just before death, such as intravenous pain medication or fluids. Family members may also fear the force of their own reactions at the time of death. They may envision that, when the patient dies, they will be so shattered that they cannot function and would be unsafe alone.

When patients linger at this transition for many days, families often struggle to find meaning or comfort with this natural, but prolonged, process. For some people, watching a family member go through several days of unresponsiveness, dehydration, restlessness, or just gentle dying is agonizing (Rando, 2000). When patients are thought to be suffering, families may prefer death and bereavement rather than this seemingly prolonged dying process.

Other people, however, will find this to be a valuable, meaningful, and sacred time full of reminiscences, music, and shared moments; it is a time to come together without outside pressures, to be present for one another in perhaps a new and intimate way. Although there is sorrow about what is now happening, there can also be joy, forgiveness, and healing.

FOCUS ON: SUFFERING

The suffering of dying people is linked to the loss of critical aspects of the self, the things that are held as most important. Dying from a progressive disease may be a painful shedding of layers of the known self. As people's strength and vitality fade, they may experience suffering. The image that patients and families once held of themselves or their loved ones no longer resonates.

Once involved in the medical/illness milieu, patients and their families may lose touch with their strengths and who they are. From the outset, the health care team may come across as all-knowing and when patients and families don't hold on to who they are, they can inadvertently surrender their power and authority to the seeming expertise of the health care team. Feeling reduced to their diagnosis, vital functions, and test results, patients easily lose their sense of confidence, identity, and individuality. Emotions engendered on this journey such as doubt, fear, anger, or sadness may further contribute to patients' and families' experiences of suffering.

Physician Ira Byock (1996) observed that Buddhism, Christianity, and Judaism incorporate a stance on the issue of suffering into their core beliefs. Buddhism holds that suffering is part of existence and comes from our natural attachment to the world. The story of Jesus dying on the Cross that is part of the Christian faith presents suffering as an opportunity to sacrifice oneself for the suffering of others. And Judaism's story of Moses leading Jewish people through the desert suggests that, though suffering is inevitable, God is with those who suffer. For many patients and families, however, "suffering is assumed to be wholly adverse and devoid of value" (Sontag, 1979, p. 125). Although most religious and philosophical traditions address human suffering, many people don't hold spiritual belief systems that help them make sense of suffering (Dom, 1999). Their response to suffering tends toward fear, avoidance, or silence.

Medical literature offers many perspectives on suffering (Byock, 1996; Cassell, 1982; Cherny, 1998; Salt, 1997; Rousseau, 2001). Definitions range from the concrete to the abstract and include terms such as *intractable symptoms, pain and delirium, existential distress, anguish,* and *angst.* Suffice it to say that suffering at end of life is a complex and highly individual phenomenon. The degree of suffering felt by dying people is tied to the meaning they make (or do not make) of their life and dying. This construction of meaning is tied to people's personal and spiritual beliefs, social relationships, culture and ethnicity, and life experiences. Meaning is evident in the individual's expression of the self, which may occur through work, prayer, meditation, conversation, counseling, art, writing, and so forth.

Two physicians, Eric Cassell and Ira Byock, mentioned previously, have studied and written extensively about suffering. Cassell (1982) held that suffering results from a sense of impending threat to the integrity of the person and that the composition of the threat is unique to each person who suffers. He put forth a typology that looks at suffering through the context of the whole person. He suggested that damage or loss to any aspects of the self (e.g., individual and family history, culture, relationships, the body, spiritual beliefs) contributes to suffering. Byock (1996) proposed that dying is the final stage of growth. He suggested that relief from suffering comes when people are able to transform their identity from who they *were* to who they *are.* He explained that people who adjust this image are able to find renewed purpose and meaning in their dying.

Although palliative care comes from a holistic, patient- and family-centered perspective, the traditional medical model is still prominent in practice. The exploration and examination of the subjective, intrinsic, and social aspects of dying people's suffering are insufficient. This is a serious omission when considering the drastic ends suffering can lead to, such as suicide, euthanasia, and terminal sedation. Professionals we are reluctant to talk at length with patients and families about suffering because, in spite of their expertise and skill, they feel fundamentally powerless and mystified. Doyle proposed that doctors fear that they "shall unleash in the patient [or ourselves], something we may not be able to cope with" (1992, p. 309).

Byock (1994) said that hospice care providers must delve deeply into their "unknowing" to find ways to respond to persistent suffering. Perhaps suffering is not a problem to be solved, but rather an essential experience to be explored, shared, and honored. How often do health care providers ask people what meaning they make of their lives and deaths or of suffering? Do they help or hinder people on this personal journey? Perhaps their need to do something and their own discomfort with suffering get in the way of their intention to truly help people.

> "Your pain is the breaking of the shell that encloses your understanding. Even as the stone of the fruit must break that its heart may stand in the sun, so must you know pain"
>
> —(Gibran, 1972, p. 58)

The mandate of psychosocial care providers is to stand with people in the midst of their most distressing and vulnerable moments. This work is both a privilege and a burden. Sometimes it means listening ever so carefully. Sometimes it means facilitating the resolution of past estrangements, hurts, or misunderstandings. At other times, it is advocating with colleagues for changes to patients' care routines or caregivers; always, trusting that the best person to make sense of suffering is the one who suffers.

Interventions

These psychosocial interventions have been designed to specifically address the key consideration *expectations about dying*. There are several assessment questions that will help open up a discussion, followed by more focused comments or tips that will facilitate further exploration of the issues that frequently arise at this time; each tip is followed by a sample dialogue.

Assessment Questions

- What other experiences have you had with dying or death? How is that affecting you now?

- What are your wishes about being with your brother when he dies? How comfortable are you with your decision?

- What do you want to know about what will happen before, or at, the time of death?

Provide accurate, sensitive information about predeath changes. This information usually helps to de-escalate people's fears and helps them make timely decisions about care and their roles.

"Gerald, you are wondering if your brother is dying now and whether you should call your mom and sister to come over. Because he is still taking sips of water and breathing quite regularly, I believe that, unless something changes, he may still have a few days left. Perhaps it would help if we talked a bit about the changes that you're seeing and what they might mean."

Explore cultural and spiritual beliefs and values about suffering, dying, and death rituals. Understanding these things may help health care providers and families to work together to create the most positive and personal atmosphere possible.

"Is there anything that we should know about you or your family's cultural or religious traditions? How do you make sense of illness and dying right now? What gives you comfort?"

Restlessness

Ian has had several nights of restlessness. During these times, he pulls at his clothing and tries to get out of bed. Once, he fell, hitting his head on a table. If Gus tries to hold Ian's hands, Ian yells, "Don't hurt me." This is very upsetting to Gus and Mark.

As mentioned previously, many patients become restless in the days before they die. This restlessness is a common part of the delirium that occurs with the many physical and biochemical changes that are a part of dying; it can vary from very mild to extreme. Generally, patients seem to be trying either to get away from or go toward something. Most people who are dying are profoundly frail, weak, and drowsy and if they are restless, they will require constant supervision and physical assistance. Families and staff may fear for the patient's safety and worry that the patient is trying to express suffering, discomfort, or pain. This level of care is emotionally and physically exhausting for most family members. Some restless patients are aggressive, whereas others are panicked or fearful. The use of physical restraints is uncommon but may be required to prevent injuries to patients, family members, or health care providers. Sometimes, at home or in a facility, the only way to bring comfort and relief in these severe situations is with sedation.

A few people see restlessness as the only way that dying people can express themselves. Each patient's personality, wishes, dignity, safety, and liability must be considered when responding to restlessness. For some family members, sedation may seem like an abrupt end to their connection with the patient, whereas others may see it as a necessary response to end the patient's suffering or restore his or her dignity. With information and support, most families are able to make decisions that they find both tolerable and respectful of the patient's wishes and safety.

Interventions

These psychosocial interventions have been designed to specifically address the key consideration *restlessness*. There are several assessment questions that will help open up a discussion, followed by more focused comments or tips that will facilitate further exploration of the issues that frequently arise at this time; each tip is followed by a sample dialogue.

Assessment Questions

- What do you make of your grandmother's restlessness? What does it say to you about how she's doing?

- How are you responding to it? What have you found is most helpful?

- What sort of response seems reasonable to you? Do you think that treating her restlessness with some sedation will bring comfort and relief?

Ensure that decisions about treatment and care are based on what the patient would have wanted. It is important that decisions not be based on the family's feelings about what is happening. By keeping this in mind, family members can reflect on the patient's wishes and honor these, while still identifying their own beliefs and attitudes.

> *"Wanda, your mother has been picking at the sheets and taking her nightgown off. I know that you are uncomfortable with this and wonder if she feels constrained in her nightgown. If she could tell you, how do you think she would want to be right now? If you believe she would be okay with this behavior, then let's talk about how to keep her safe and comfortable. If you think she would be embarrassed to be like this, then we can provide a sedative. Tell me what would be best for your mom?"*

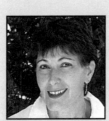

Eve Joseph is a longtime hospice counselor and poet with a B.A. in social work and an M.A. in counseling psychology.

In My Own Voice
Predeath Restlessness

Eve Joseph

I came into the unit one evening, and the nurse said to me, "There is a man who wants to know what it's like to die, so I told him you would come and talk to him." This patient was in and out of consciousness. When he was awake, he was agitated and worried. When I went in, he said, "So, you are the one who is going to tell me what death is like." "No," I replied, "you are going to tell me." He spoke about being afraid of judgment after he died. He hadn't been good enough as a father, a husband, a son, a friend, he said. He was aware of being deeply flawed, as we all are. "Death is there, by the dresser," he said, "and has been there for three nights." I don't know if he really added "and we will sleep together tonight" or if that is a trick of my memory. His restlessness wasn't fear but something else deep—some need for confession and to let something go.

Predeath restlessness, I think that this is a good term, from a counselor's perspective. It is the work of dying, or at least a big piece of the work. The term *delirium* puts the experience in the mind and in the body, but I see this as spiritual work. We cannot discount the spiritual work that is happening here.

We want to think that death is natural and peaceful and beautiful but that's not all it is. There is struggle and work in dying. It's a process, such as birth. The dying are learning how to do this. It is a struggle to get out of this world, to let go of the ties, the things not done. What I see and hear family members say is that, within predeath restlessness, they recognize times when the patient is there and times when he or she is not. My own belief about this is that the spirit goes by increments. Dying people go for a bit and come back, and in this way, they are learning how to go, how to die. We watch with eyes of the living. We don't know, can't know, and can't enter the experience of dying people. They are doing something we can't do. This is as much as I can understand—people who are dying are separate from us and we have to let them go. This is a necessary split or rift. It is not peaceful or joyful. This is enormously difficult for families. The struggle to go looks like suffering, agitation, fear, or anxiety, and the families can't do anything. They feel powerless and helpless. And family members must learn how to stay as the person who is dying learns how to go.

I think that there are some things that we can do as counselors. First, we can explore what we believe about this. We can get clear in ourselves. Then, we can help family members see another possibility for understanding what is happening. We can offer that this is the work of death and dying as opposed to terrible suffering. This doesn't mean we don't treat predeath restlessness. Treatments and medications, are very important. But offering family members language with which to understand what they see allows them to be there in a different way and to find other things to be done in response to it. Predeath restlessness forces a transition from living to dying. The patient has turned somewhere else and, often, families know that to be true. They can accept that there is enormous value and purpose in this transition. Counselors become translators, not as experts but as people who have seen this before. With enormous caution, we can share our beliefs and the possibility of something else, which is only a possibility. We can discover a language when there is no language—not to impose a language but to help people come to their own language and understanding of what they see.

Predeath restlessness is a hard place for counselors. When I am with a mother who is restless and agitated and trying to get up and I see her adult children's pain, I feel anxious, too, and I want her to be peaceful, I want her to be medicated. Even while I am frightened, anxious, powerless, and all of those things, the least I can do is stand with the patient. There is value in being calm and holding space for other possibilities and for understanding in the midst of confusion, distress, and chaos. It would be a disservice if I could take away people's suffering. The sacred is not pretty, it is bloody in moments. And our work is to stand in it, stripped to our essential humanness.

This is what we offer—all our humanity—our fear, our hope, our caring, our frailty. We are not separate; we are the same; and we are here. This is what we offer.

Provide family caregivers with considerable support to change the care plan because of restlessness or other symptoms. Care becomes exhausting and people often cannot manage alone, but they worry about no longer honoring what the patient wanted and planned.

> *"Up to now, you've been able to care for Charles at home in spite of your heart condition. Now that he is restless, his care has become quite risky for you to manage alone. How would you and your family feel if he was admitted to hospice now?"*

OUR EXPERIENCE

As the time of death approaches, our goal as palliative care providers is to help patients and families begin to prepare for death. We add to their understanding with our experience, knowledge, and support. Our purpose is to address their natural fear and anxiety and to help families engage with dying people in ways that feel comfortable, authentic, and meaningful for them.

The atmosphere around the patient feels different at this time. Although there may be more silence and more peace, the atmosphere also feels more tense and heavy. People experience feelings of anticipation and uncertainty as they realize that the next hurdle is death. Often, people's feelings are concentrated and intense. This time can seem deeply sacred.

Family members move back and forth along a continuum between attachment and release. At times, they seem to be fiercely holding on to the patient, while at other times they seem to be gently (or resolutely) letting go. Because most patients nearing death cannot communicate their thoughts and feelings verbally, families may make their own interpretations about the patient's readiness for death. It helps some families to believe that the patient is ready to go. Others say it feels like the patient has already died. Statements like this may be a reflection of the family's feelings of disconnection and loss, or a way to ready themselves for the inevitability of death.

Generally, this time seems to be easier when patients and families have come to terms with each other and the dying process. Moments of shared meaning and intimacy may help families find comfort and accept this part of the journey. Some families give the patient permission to go, and then they wait peacefully until that time comes. Others give permission, but feel impatient when death doesn't happen right away. It can be difficult for people to fathom how the patient can keep going for days without food or drink, and they may become concerned that the patient is starving. They wonder what can be done to bring relief, or how long this can go on.

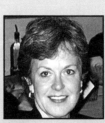

Elizabeth Causton, M.S.W., is a hospice counselor who works with dying patients and their families in the community and on the inpatient unit. She has also done extensive teaching in the field of death and dying.

In My Own Voice
The Power of Language

Elizabeth Causton

"Definitions are not neutral. They are not just the innocent tools that allow us to describe reality. Rather, they shape our perceptions of reality. They select. They emphasize. They embody a bias. Therefore, definitions constantly need redefinition" (Wathchter, 1990).

Palliative care today differs from traditional medical care of the dying in that it weaves the medical, psychosocial, and spiritual approaches to care into a holistic pattern that more closely reflects the rich, complex, textured nature of human beings. An ongoing challenge is to maintain the separate strands of interdisciplinary expertise and language, while creating a tapestry that is of one piece, an exquisite work of art and science.

Specifically, we must not lose the language that characterizes phenomena of symbolic communications and visions, so beautifully described in *Final Gifts* (Callanan & Kelley, 1992). These phenomena are now commonly understood to be a natural part of the dying process. We must not forget that the power of language, as used in a particular culture or profession, not only reflects and reinforces current belief systems but also creates images and determines, in large part, how we respond. So, for example, if symbolic communications were to be woven into our practice of palliative care under the heading of "delirium," they would take on all the medical connotations and characteristics of a "symptom." This would determine how we assess, treated and, ultimately, try to "fix" the "problem." In this assimilation, we would lose the language of health and normalcy that ought to characterize these phenomena, and we would lose the perspective that holds the mystery inherent in the dying process in a safe and sacred way.

Michael Kearney, Irish physician and author, said that the process of dying "midwifes a person into depth" (1996, p. 151). In death, it is to this place of depth that we return, and it is in this place of depth that we rediscover the essence of who we are. The language of depth is symbolism and imagery. It is the language of mystery and awe that reminds us that the experience of dying is not, primarily, a medical event, nor is it a disease or illness to be cured. Rather, it is, in the most profound sense, an experience of healing and recovery. In order to maintain our holistic approach to the care of the dying, we must continue to preserve the language that honors this perspective as we weave together a tapestry that reflects both body and soul, science and the sacred mysteries, the known and the unknowable; a tapestry that reflects in every way our true nature.

At this time, our role is to help people find a way to "just be" with patients and themselves. This means giving them the information they need to hold this time as a natural and dignified conclusion to the life of someone loved. Singh said our role is to "facilitate open-eyed participation in this profound experience" (2000, p. 271). Often, it means that we, too, must "just be" with people in their deep sorrow and sadness and support whatever is happening in front of us.

FOCUS ON: SEDATION AT THE END OF LIFE

Health care providers often hear patients' request to go to sleep. Talk of suicide, euthanasia, and other expressions of a will to die are not uncommon in people as they approach the end of life (Chater, Viola, Paterson, & Jarvis, 1998). Coyle studied the last four weeks of life for cancer patients and found that "over a quarter of these patients discussed suicide as an option at some time. Patients appeared to use discussions of suicide as means to ensure that the listener understood the depth of their suffering" (Coyle, Adelhardt, Foley, Portenoy, 1990, p. 86). These discussions may express their immense suffering rather than a request for terminal sedation, however (Coyle et al., 1990).

Sedation at the end of life is an uncommon therapy, carried out after careful ethical and medical review in response to the repeated request of patients to end their distress of symptoms that do not respond to other forms of intervention. Braun (1999), of the Calgary Regional Health Authority, described this as "the process of inducing and maintaining deep sleep for the relief of severe suffering caused by one or more intractable symptoms when all possible alternative interventions have failed." An intractable symptom is one that cannot be adequately controlled despite aggressive therapy that does not compromise consciousness (Chater et al., 1998) and is differentiated from a difficult symptom that could potentially respond within a tolerable time frame to noninvasive treatments (Cherny & Portenoy, 1994).

Sedation at end of life has been variously called terminal sedation, palliative sedation, twilight sedation, slow euthanasia, and sedation for refractory or intractable symptoms in dying people. These various terms and definitions illustrate some of the complexities of this issue and show the range of opinion and feeling on this subject. Personal beliefs, faith convictions, medical ethics, and philosophical values, especially those concerning the nature of suffering and whether it may have any purpose or value, enter into discussions of terminal sedation. Differences are likely among professionals about which symptoms might potentially respond, whether all possible alternatives have or even should be tried, and what is a tolerable time frame before considering sedation. A further challenge lies in the fact that when patients go to sleep and remain asleep in this way, their life expectancy is now foreshortened (Mount, 1996). As an evolving area of hospice palliative care, there is as yet lack of clarity or consensus about these issues and health care providers often struggle to talk together about sedation at the end of life.

The literature on terminal sedation highlights the conflicting and complex rationale for terminal sedation. It may be inferred from the literature that sedation at the end of life is more tenable when the patient's life expectancy is short and when the primary indication for sedation is physical, rather than emotional or spiritual, suffering (Hallenbeck, 2000; Rousseau, 2000). Even with patients who experience physical suffering, sympoms often include extreme emotional and spiritual distress. Some patients, however, who have received terminal sedation have experienced emotional, mental, and/or spiritual anguish without significant physical deterioration (Cherny, 1998; Rousseau, 2000). Patients sometimes feel they are in an intolerable situation and have no hope that things can improve. Some authors suggest that existential suffering is tied to a feeling of meaninglessness (Cassell, 1982; Morita et al., 2000). Cassell (1982) said that suffering occurs when people feel out of control, when the situation is dire, and when their personal integrity is threatened.

Cherny pointed out, "Uncontrolled suffering in a dying patient is a medical emergency" (World Congress on Pain, 1999). Certainly, authority and expertise on this issue reside with palliative medicine, partly because sedation requires a medical intervention. The literature on sedation at the end of life is predominantly oriented to medical definition, description, and clinical guidelines, and falls short on examining the psychosocial and psychospiritual aspects. Cherny (1998) suggests that the decision to provide sedation to a patient be made with input from those health care providers who have a well-established relationship with the patient and family. Some studies recommend that when symptoms include psychosocial factors, a skilled clinician, psychologist, or psychiatrist must assess patients before a decision on terminal sedation is made (Cherny, 1998; Morita, Tsunoda, Inoue, & Chihara, 2000). In very advanced disease, clinical depression is often difficult to distinguish from the effects of disease but, if evident, is a contraindication for sedation. Certainly nurses, counselors, social workers, volunteers, occupational and physiotherapists, or spiritual care people who have worked closely with the patient and family would have valuable perspectives and insights to contribute. How often decision making regarding sedation at the end of life utilizes this team approach is unclear.

Despite the necessity of informed consent, decisions about sedation at the end of life are sometimes made without enough exploration of the patient's and family's needs, concerns, resources, and alternatives. A 1998 survey of 59 physicians and two nurses from eight countries found that only 50% of patients and 69% of families had major involvement in making the decision to use terminal sedation (Chater, Viola, Paterson, & Jarvis, 1998). This raises a number of questions about how these important decisions are made and by what informed means. Another aspect of decision making is that information provided to patients and families is always subject to the provider's beliefs about how much and what information is necessary and to whom information should be given (Street & Kissane, 2001).

Health care providers' responses to existential pain must reflect their own deepest attempts to understand what the unique experience of pain or suffering means to each patient. This understanding takes time and a resolute commitment to providing truly holistic, patient-centered care. Hallenbeck stated, "I must recognize that not all relief comes from my black bag, but must come from the person" (2000, p. 318). Terminal sedation has tremendous psychospiritual significance for patients, families, and the team. Palliative care providers are accountable for engaging that nebulous psychospiritual part of the patient's and family's experience, even when such symptoms cannot be fixed or settled, and even when sedation at the end of life may on occasion be the last considered but most appropriate response to their distress.

TEAM ISSUES

Most palliative care providers have some idea of how they, themselves, would like to die and how they think death should be. This may be based on a combination of experience, religious or spiritual beliefs, and general personality characteristics. There are times when these beliefs are in conflict with those of the patient or family. Sometimes, death challenges health care providers' beliefs. Choices or circumstances that do not seem appropriate, safe, or fair can trigger this dissonance. When this happens, it is important to find ways to continue providing excellent, person-centered care and then to debrief the deep feelings and questions that are exposed.

When the time is very short between diagnosis and dying, the team may be meeting families just days before the patient dies. It is hard to enter people's lives as strangers and in a very short time witness one of the most important events in the family's history—a death. Work is usually intense and intimate with these patients and families. When team members find it hard to be so closely involved with patients who will be dead within days or hours, they may protect themselves by distancing emotionally. Others may choose to remain open and feel their own grief and powerlessness. Each response requires support and careful reflection.

When this final transition is long, it is hard on families and also on the team. When family members are asking about prognosis, team members frequently feel pressured about what to say. Because no one can know the exact time of death, caution and breadth need to be built into any response. If not, then professionals often feel inept and guilty when the outcome differs widely from what they have predicted.

SUMMARY

This transition is marked by major changes in mind, body, and spirit as patients and families make their final approach to death (see Table 6.1). Patients experience

Table 6.1. Palliative Performance Scale (PPSv2) 20%–10%

PPS Level	Ambulation	Activity and evidence of disease	Self-care	Intake	Conscious level
20%	Totally bed bound	Unable to do any activity Extensive disease	Total care	Minimal to sips	Full or drowsy +/- confusion
10%	Totally bed bound	Unable to do any activity Extensive disease	Total care	Mouth care only	Drowsy or coma +/- confusion

increased weakness and cognitive decline, which reduces their ability to interact with those around them. Moving through this transition, they become increasingly unresponsive, and any communication tends to be short-lived or symbolic in nature. One or more family members have now taken over decision making responsibilities, which can create tensions among them. Generally, the pace of care slows down and families often struggle to find new ways to be with the patient. If restlessness or delirium are present, there may be a time of anxiety or helplessness as families and health care providers decide the most appropriate responses.

The constant progression of the disease process, whether rapid or slow, creates an atmosphere of multiple unknowns. Patients have mostly withdrawn from life, and families are experiencing fear, guilt, isolation, anger, and sadness. A feeling of loss and disconnection leads people more deeply into grief as they begin to expect death at any moment. This is a time of watching and waiting, perhaps inviting death yet dreading its arrival.

REFLECTIVE ACTIVITY

The Johari Window model outlined in Figure 6.1. may be used as a tool to expand self-awareness (Luft, 1970). Rather than measuring personality, it offers a way to look at how personality is expressed. Its founders suggest that through self-disclosure and feedback from others, the Open Pane expands. This model can be used with teams and groups to stimulate discussion about differences, provide greater understanding, and increase trust (Trotzer, 1977).

	Known to Self	Unknown to Self
Known to Others	*Open Pane: Public Self* Attitudes, behaviors, motivation, values, and our way of life.	*Blind Pane: Blind Self* Things about ourselves that others see more clearly.
Unknown to Others	*Hidden Pane: Private Self* The feelings and thoughts we keep inside out of fear.	*Unknown Pane: Unknown Self* Things that we sense from time to time but don't know.

Figure 6.1. The Johari Window (Luft, 1970), a tool to expand self-awareness, offers a way to look at how personality is expressed.

Using the Johari Window model as a guide, explore your personal thoughts, feelings, and attitudes about dying and death. Other, less charged topics, such as illness, dependence, or caregiving may be substituted if you prefer. Do this activity with a partner or colleague. It is preferable to select someone whom you trust and feel comfortable opening up to, perhaps someone you know fairly well.

"We meet people between not yet and no longer."

—*Eugene Dufour (extracted from closing address, Canadian Hospice Palliative Care Association conference, Victoria, British Columbia, 2001)*

Step 1—Together, consider the model on p. 242. Orient yourself to each of the four panes.

Step 2—Without too much thought or rehearsal, take turns talking about how you would like to die, what you expect it to be like, and how you would like others to interact with you. Also consider what would be most important. This is the information that resides in the Open Pane.

Step 3—Invite the other person to share her thoughts about how she imagines your death. Then, do the same for her, saying how you envision this person experiencing death and dying. Notice any reluctance to speak and hear. This dialogue stimulates the Blind Pane.

Step 4—Working separately, acknowledge what you haven't said about yourself and your vision of dying. Be honest with yourself. What haven't you expressed out of fear, embarrassment, or a need for privacy? These aspects of your self reside in the Hidden Pane.

Step 5—Consider your dreams, visions, or gut feelings about dying and death. What messages do you discover there? This information lies in the Unknown Pane.

Step 6—Exchange information with your partner about, or preferably within, your Hidden or Unknown Panes. Observe what you choose to disclose or not. Consider how these choices might affect your relationship.

Step 7—Finally, reflect on what this exercise reveals to you about yourself personally and on how it might affect your practice with patients and families. Share your reflections with your partner.

RESOURCES

Barbato, M., & Reid, K. (1999). Parapsychological phenomena near the time of death. *Journal of Palliative Care, 15*(2), 30–37.

Bergevin, P., & Bergevin, R.M. (1996). Recognizing delirium in terminal patients. *The American Journal of Hospice & Palliative Care, 13*(2), 28–29.

Echaubard, M. (1999). Speaking without words. *European Journal of Palliative Care, 6*(3), 91–93.

Hutchings, D. (1998). Communicating with metaphor: A dance with many veils. *The American Journal of Hospice & Palliative Care, 15*(5), 282–284.

Kuhl, D. (2002). *What dying people want.* Toronto: Doubleday.

Longaker, C. (1997). *Facing death and finding hope: A guide to the emotional and spiritual care of the dying.* New York: Doubleday.

Nuland, S.B. (1995). *How we die: Reflections on life's final chapter.* New York: Vintage Books.

Reoch, R. (1996). *To die well: A holistic approach for the dying and their caregivers.* New York: HarperCollins.

REFERENCES

Byock, I. (1994). When suffering persists. *Journal of Palliative Care, 10*(2), 8–13.

Byock, I. (1996a). Beyond symptom management. *European Journal of Palliative Care, 3*(3), 125–130.

Byock, I. (1996b). The nature of suffering and the nature of opportunity at the end of life. *Clinics in Geriatric Medicine, 12*(2), 237–252.

Callanan, M., & Kelley, P. (1992). *Final gifts: Understanding the special awareness, needs, and communications of the dying.* New York: Bantam Books.

Cassell, E. (1992). The nature of suffering and the goals of medicine. *New England Journal of Medicine, 306*(1), 639–641.

Chater, S., Viola, R., Paterson, J., & Jarvis, V. (1998). Sedation for intractable distress in the dying—a survey of experts. *Palliative Medicine, 12,* 255–269.

Cherny, N. (1998). Commentary: Sedation in response to refractory existential distress: Walking the fine line. *Journal of Pain and Symptom Management, 16*(6), 404–406.

Cotter, A. (1999). *From this moment on: A guide for the recently diagnosed with cancer.* New York: Random House.

Coyle, N., Adelhardt, J., Foley, K., & Portenoy, R. (1990). Character of terminal illness in the advanced cancer patient: Pain and other symptoms in the last four weeks of life. *Journal of Pain and Symptom Management, 5*(2), 83–93.

Dom, H. (1999). Spiritual care, need and pain—recognition and response. *European Journal of Palliative Care, 6*(3), 87–90.

Doyle, D. (1992). Have we looked beyond the physical and psychological? *Journal of Pain and Symptom Management, 7*(5), 302–311.

Enyert, G. & Burman, M. (1999). A qualitative study of self-transcendence in caregivers of terminally ill patients. *The American Journal of Hospice and Palliative Care, 16*(2), 455–462.

Hallenbeck, J. (2000). Terminal sedation: Ethical implications in different situations. *Journal of Pain and Symptom Management, 3*(3), 313–320.

Gibran, K. (1972). *The prophet.* New York: Alfred A. Knopf.

Kearney, M. (1996). *Mortally wounded: Stories of soul, pain, death, and healing.* New York: Scribner.

Morita, T., Tsunoda, J., Inoue, S., & Chihara, S. (2000). Terminal sedation for existential distress. The *American Journal of Hospice and Palliative Care, 17*(3), 189–195.

Mount, B. (1996). Morphine drips, terminal sedation, and slow euthanasia: Definitions and facts, not anecdote. *Journal of Palliative Care, 12*(4), 31–37.

Nouwen, H. (1974). *Out of solitude: Three meditations of the Christian life.* Notre Dame, IN: Ave Maria Press.

Oxford English Dictionary. (1971). New York: Oxford University Press.

Rando, T. (2000). On the experience of traumatic stress in anticipatory and postdeath mourning. In T. Rando (Ed.), *Clinical dimensions of anticipatory mourning: Theory and practice in working with the dying, their loved ones and their caregivers* (pp. 155–223). Champaigne, IL: Research Press.

Rousseau, P. (2000). Palliative sedation: A brief review of ethical validity and clinical experience. *Mayo Clinic Proceedings, 75,* 1064–1069.

Rousseau, P. (2001). Existential suffering and palliative sedation: A brief commentary with a proposal for clinical guidelines. *The American Journal of Hospice and Palliative Care, 18*(3), 151–153.

Rueth, T.W., & Hall, S.E. (1999). Dealing with the anger and hostility of those who grieve. *The American Journal of Hospice and Palliative Care, 16*(6), 743–746

Salt, S. (1997). Towards a definition of suffering. *European Journal of Palliative Care, 4*(2), 58–60.

Singh, K.D. (2000). Spiritual "signs and symptoms": Toward an expanded understanding of dying. *The American Journal of Hospice and Palliative Care, 17*(4), 269–271.

Sontag, S. (1979). *Illness as metaphor.* New York: Vintage Books.

Street, A., & Kissane, D. (2001). Constructions of dignity in end of life care. *Journal of Palliative Care, 17*(2), 93–101.

Trotzer, J. (1977). *The counselor and the group: Integrating theory, training, and practice.* Monterey, CA: Brooks/Cole.

Wathchter, M.A.M. (1990). Keynote address. In Federation of Right to Die Societies, Eighth Biennial Conference of the World, Maastricht, the Netherlands.

BODY IMAGE, SEX, AND INTIMACY

"The need to touch and be touched is one of the greatest needs human beings have from birth to death. To touch a person is to affirm one's reality, whether the person is dying or not."

—Caruso, 1986, p. 69

Touch and intimacy are essential human needs that cut across boundaries of age, gender, marital status, sexual orientation, and wellness. Too often, the health care team ignores these concerns in dying and bereaved people (Caruso & Herman, 1989). Some of the reasons for this sad omission include unsound social, cultural, and physical assumptions (Caruso, 1986). But perhaps more restrictive is the almost universal discomfort that people feel about discussing sex and/or death (Steinhauser et al., 2000; Wasow, 1977). Paradoxically, a survey of patients, family, physicians, and other care providers indicated that, at the end of life, physical touch was one of their most important considerations (Cohen & Cohen, 1985).

Health care providers sometimes assume that dying people do not desire sex and intimacy and that bereaved people do not miss it (Cohen & Cohen, 1985; Wylie, 1997). The standard approach is that if the patient or individual doesn't bring it up, it is not an issue (Cohen & Cohen, 1985). Several professionals remind us, however, that sexual concerns and activities are an essential part of any thorough medical and psychosocial history (Caruso, 1986; Gilley, 1988). Changes in physical and sexual relationships represent substantial losses felt by dying patients and partners, from the time of diagnosis through bereavement. Without open dialogue, information, and acknowledgment from the health care team, terminally ill people may stop having sexual contact and physical intimacy a long time before they die. Some bereaved partners or spouses may question and agonize over why touch and intimacy ended so long before death.

Changes in the dying individual's body, emotions, energy, thoughts, and relationships impose unanticipated changes on people's sexual habits, routines, and preferences. Early in the disease, the stress and side effects of treatment may make touch and intimacy an unpleasant or awkward experience, or a low priority. Bodily changes affect individuals' self-image and identity and, if they feel ugly or exhausted, they are not likely to want touch or intimacy (Madioni, Morales, & Michel, 1997; Wasow, 1977). Partners and spouses may pick up on the patients' feelings and choose to respectfully withdraw. Both single and married people commonly describe feelings of loneliness, shame, guilt, fear, and regret in response to changes in their intimate sexual habits.

The social taboos about sex, death, and bereavement often inhibit discussion about these universally personal experiences (Madioni et al., 1997). Serious illness, surgery, and advancing disease may change patients' and their partners' feelings about their sexual attractiveness and appeal (Taylor, 1983). When people's sexual organs and other body parts are affected or removed by the illness, individuals' sexual identity is also significantly altered. This occurrence is likely true of people facing any life-threatening illness. Serious and/or long-term progressive diseases such as COPD, ALS, and AIDS also affect, and often limit, people's physical and sexual activities.

Single people are often assumed to be celibate, yet some single people may be just as sexually active as people in defined relationships. A person's marital status is not a reliable indication of whether sex and physical intimacy are an important part of his or her identity. Some single people have a regular sexual or intimate partner and the nature of these relationships may or may not be known to the patients' family or circle of friends. A single person may be heterosexual, gay, or lesbian. Depending on how comfortable the couple feels with the health care team, the nature of their relationship may or may not be apparent. Single people without partners may also have had an active and fulfilling sex life before the illness and now sorely miss the opportunities and means to continue it.

When someone is very ill, physical contact often becomes focused on personal care activities such as toileting, bathing, and feeding. A professional or family member may provide the patient's personal care tenderly or in an offhand manner. Spouses or partners who are also the caregivers may feel too tired to engage in other kinds of intimate touch such as cuddling, massage, intercourse, or masturbation. Patients may feel themselves reduced to their bodily functions—like public property requiring routine maintenance—rather than like sensual, sexual human beings. Patients may want sexual or intimate contact but may be embarrassed to say so (Taylor, 1983). Older couples may have had long and rich sexual lives prior to this illness but may feel very uncomfortable speaking about their ongoing intimate concerns with health care providers. They may recognize that they do not have the energy for intercourse or orgasm but still crave the tender stroking or caresses that are part of physical intimacy. Individuals who have a partner, but who are not interested in sex or intimacy, may feel extremely guilty about not fulfilling their partner's physical and sexual needs.

Spouses and partners often avoid touch and other kinds of sexual contact out of fear of harming or upsetting the patient and/or depleting vital energy reserves (Caruso, 1986). They may long for familiar intimacies but, instead, bury their desire, believing that their partners would be unwilling or unable or that their energies must be conserved for more important priorities. Some patients' partners look for alternative ways to express themselves sexually. Affairs, pornography, anonymous sex, flirting, and increased masturbation may be tried to combat grief, frustration, and loneliness. When partners choose to meet their sexual concerns outside of the primary relationship, they may experience shame, guilt, and confusion (Sarnoff Schiff, 1986).

Bereaved partners experience tremendous loneliness. They may miss sex and the physical presence of the person (Oliviere, Hargreaves, & Monroe, 1998). They long to touch, taste, smell, hold, and sleep with him or her. Some people have a reluctance to start anew and find any attempts at socializing, flirting, and dating discouraging and awkward (Palmer & Watt, 1987). Others may move into dating more quickly but still feel strange and uncomfortable. Loneliness and longing may lead people into unlikely relationships or marriages before they have found ways to live with their grief and sadness (Martin & Doka, 2000). Sex may be used as a coping strategy during grief as a way to allay loneliness, distract from the pain and sorrow of loss, or provide a physical release for complex emotions.

Well-meaning friends and family may put a considerable amount of pressure on bereaved people to start dating and find a new mate. This is especially common with young unmarried people and people with children. People have similar expectations if the bereaved person did not live with the person who died or was in a new relationship. Yet grief, like the love that triggers it, does not abide by social rules about how much time it takes or how deeply feelings might run.

Other bereaved people, such as parents or siblings, may also experience changes in their sexual interest. People often find that the grieving process can consume a lot of their physical and emotional energy, and this may decrease their interest in intimacy and sexual conduct. This is especially true with people for whom intimate contact is important. It can be difficult for partners to understand and be patient with each other during this time.

KEY POINTS

- Find out to what degree sex and/or intimacy have shaped the person's identity. People are sexual beings throughout their lifetimes.
- Remember that sexual contact includes all forms of intimacy, including massage, holding, cuddling, kissing, stroking, masturbation, and intercourse.
- Do not assume that sex and intimacy are not a concern because a person is single, sick, elderly, female, or bereaved.
- Affection and intimacy among people can be an abundant source of personal comfort, happiness, and reassurance, even close to death.
- Be wary of making assumptions. Not everyone likes, needs, or wants to be touched (by members of the health care team and/or family).
- Communicate with humor and sensitivity.
- Acknowledge cultural and religious differences in terms of what levels of intimacy are considered appropriate.

KEY QUESTIONS

- How has this illness affected your self-image?
- What impact has this illness had on your sex life or sexuality?
- Are you and your (spouse/partner/friend) managing to find ways to be intimate?
- What gives you comfort now?
- Are you currently dating anyone? Do you have a steady partner or (girlfriend/boyfriend)? How involved are you with your ex-partner?
- Since (you became ill) (your partner died), what do you miss most about your relationship?
- How do you let the staff know when you and your (spouse/partner/friend) need privacy?
- How is your grief affecting your sex life?

STRATEGIES TO ENHANCE AND SUPPORT PHYSICAL INTIMACY

- Initiate conversations with patients and partners about strategies for sex and intimacy. People may have reluctantly given up on intimate contact because they weren't able to identify satisfactory alternatives.

- Maintain patients' hygiene, beauty, and personal care routines. Does the patient want to wear aftershave or perfume on special occasions? Would a haircut, bath, or new pajamas help him or her to feel more fresh and attractive?

- Encourage people to take time outside of care routines to be alone together. Offer individuals who are in hospital a "do not disturb" sign for their doors.

- Suggest that intimate partners spend time in bed cuddling, touching, or holding each other even if sleeping together is no longer comfortable.

- Find out what concerns or problems bereaved people are having with sex and intimacy and explore alternatives.

Talking with dying or bereaved people about their physical and sexual desire requires skill and courage. Health care providers need to learn how to overcome their own discomfort with talking about sex and intimacy so that these vital, natural needs are addressed with respect and ease (Street, 2001). Dignity in death means people's lives will have integrity and meaning until the last moment. This includes acknowledging each person as a loving, physical, and sexual being.

REFERENCES

Caruso, D.M. (1986). Sexuality and the terminal patient. *Caring*, 68–71.

Caruso & Herman, D. (1989). Concerns for the dying patient and family. *Seminars in Oncology Nursing, 5*(2), 120–123.

Cohen, G., & Cohen, M. (1985). Sexual health in family medicine. *Canadian Family Physician, 31*(4), 767–771.

Gilley, J. (1988). Intimacy and terminal care. *Journal of the Royal College of General Practitioners*, 121–122.

Kearney, M. (1996). *Mortally wounded: Stories of soul, pain, death, and healing.* New York: Scribner.

Madioni, F., Morales, C., & Michel, J.P. (1997). Body image and the impact of terminal disease. *European Journal of Palliative Care, 4*(5), 160–162.

Martin, T., & Doka, K. (2000). *Men don't cry women do: Transcending gender stereotypes of grief.* Philadelphia: Brunner/Mazel.

Oliviere, D., Hargreaves, R., & Monroe, B. (1998). *Good practices in palliative care: A psychosocial perspective.* Brookfield: Ashgate Publishing Limited.

Palmer, E., & Watt, J. (1987). *Living and working with bereavement: Guide for widowed men and women.* Calgary, Alberta, Canada: Detselig Enterprises Ltd.

Sarnoff Schiff, H. (1986). *Living through mourning: Finding comfort and hope when a loved one has died.* New York: Viking Penguin.

Steinhauser, K.E., Christakis, N.A., Clipp, E.C., McNeilly, M., McIntyre, L., & Tulsky, J.A. (2000, November). Factors considered important at the end of life by patients, family, physicians and other care providers. *Journal of the American Medical Association, 284*(19), 2476–2482.

Street, A.F. (2001). Constructions of dignity in end-of-life care. *Journal of Palliative Care, 17*(2), 93–101.

Taylor, P.B. (April, 1983). Understanding sexuality in the dying patient. *Nursing,* 54–55.

Wasow, M. (1977). Human sexuality and terminal illness. *Health and Social Work, 2*(2), 105–121.

Wylie, B.J. (1997). *Beginnings: A book for widows.* Toronto: McClelland and Stewart.

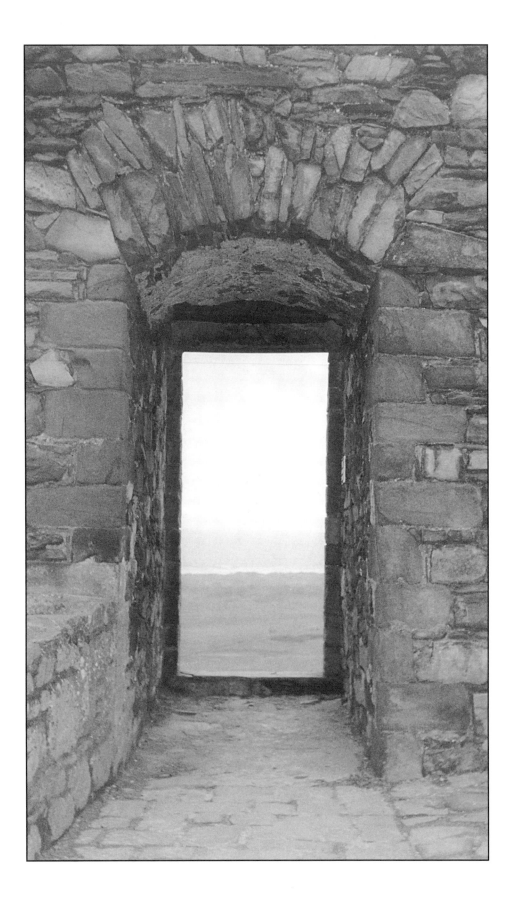

7

The Parting of the Ways

TIME OF DEATH

(PPSv2 level: 0%)

*A*t the time of death, FAMILY REACTIONS are varied. The ways that people respond will be influenced by individual and family coping styles and the events preceding the death. Often, when it comes, family members feel prepared. They have seen enough suffering and feel ready, on some level, for their loved one to die. Yet, even when families are prepared, the moment of death can feel unexpected and heartbreaking. In the time immediately after the death, family members may be highly emotional, concrete and practical, or somewhere in between.

Whether or not the family witnessed the death, they will probably need to review the NATURE OF THE DEATH. If family members were present, they may have seen or heard things that were unfamiliar to them and perhaps disturbing. As people die, they usually exhibit marked changes in breathing, heart rate, and skin color. Discussing and providing information about these changes may ease the family's memories of this time. If the family was not present during the death, they may need to know exactly what happened. People often need to re-tell or hear the story as a way to integrate this profound experience and to help them understand and accept that death has finally occurred.

When the family is ready, there are a number of AFTER-DEATH DETAILS to be considered. These details range from when the family will release the body, to making final arrangements and disposing of unused medical supplies. When the death occurs, it is helpful for the family to know how long they can keep the dead person's body with them. This gives them a chance to pay their last respects before the individual is transferred to the funeral home or morgue.

In some hospitals or other facilities, it may be difficult for families to take time to be with the body after death. There may be pressure to fill the bed quickly, or the health care team may not be comfortable keeping the body on their ward. Viewing the body immediately after death, however, is one of the ways that the family may choose to recognize that death has occurred. The family's values and beliefs about death and their feelings about the person who has died may require time for closure and the opportunity to begin to grieve and understand that this part of the journey is over. Cultural, familial, and religious traditions may suggest certain RITUALS that the family can perform at this time.

KATE

Kate, age 85, has just died. She had COPD and had been increasingly breathless and fatigued over the past few years. A single parent, she and her daughter Robin had lived together for almost all of Robin's life. Robin is married to Jeff and they have two daughters, Carrie, 10, and Mandy, 16. Kate and granddaughter Carrie were very alike; although all the family was close, these two had a special bond.

Although everyone knew that Kate's death was imminent, it still came as a shock. Robin and Jeff were disappointed that they weren't in the room with her when it happened, though it made sense to them that Carrie was there because of the bond she and Kate had shared. Robin, Jeff, and Kate thought they had prepared Carrie and Mandy for what to expect throughout Kate's decline and death. Yet, in the days leading up to the death, Mandy was clearly uncomfortable with Kate's physical and mental deterioration. She seemed frightened and embarrassed about Kate's weakness and confusion and had been spending more time away from home with her friends.

At the time of Kate's death, Carrie was holding Kate's hand and they were watching the World Series. Mandy was watching television elsewhere in the house. At first, Carrie didn't realize her grandma had died. When she realized that Kate wasn't breathing, she called to her parents in the next room. The family found it reassuring that Kate had died as her favorite team was winning. After the death, Carrie cried in short intense bursts but still wanted to stay in Kate's room, with her mother close by. She wanted to know if it was okay to touch and kiss Kate and asked how they knew for sure that Kate was dead. According to Robin and Jeff, Mandy was just the opposite of Carrie; she became hysterical when they told her that Kate had died. She screamed and immediately shut herself in her room.

"I would like to believe that when I die I have given myself away like a tree that sows seed every spring and never counts the loss, because it is not loss, it is adding to future life. It is the tree's way of being. Strongly rooted perhaps, but spilling out its treasure on the wind."

—May Sarton, 1980

With some support from the hospice nurse, Robin carefully bathed and dressed Kate while they waited for other family members to arrive. The family chose to dress her in her favorite pajamas. Carrie wrote a note to Kate and placed it in her hand, and Mandy was able to choose a flower to place next to Kate's cheek. As several family members visited, Carrie called her teacher to tell her the news, whereas Mandy stayed in her room talking on the telephone to a young cousin. When the funeral home attendants came to take Kate's body away, the family gathered together on the lawn and sadly watched her go.

KEY CONSIDERATIONS

Family Reactions

Although everyone knew that Kate's death was imminent, it still came as a shock. Robin and Jeff were disappointed that they weren't in the room with her when it happened, though it made sense to them Carrie was there because of the bond she and Kate had shared. According to Robin and Jeff, Mandy was just the opposite of Carrie; she became hysterical when they told her that Kate had died. She screamed and immediately shut herself in her room. Carrie cried in short intense bursts but still wanted to stay in Kate's room, with her mother close by.

Preparation for the moment of death is the focal point of the journey through diagnosis, illness, and bereavement. People think about it, dream about it, hope it will never happen, and fear that it will never happen. Friends and families are often surprised by how they feel and act when death finally comes. Sometimes, the time of death triggers a release of emotion and fatigue that people don't expect; this can be very unsettling. These reactions may or may not seem fitting to the people themselves and/or the situation at hand (Muller, 2000). The strength or depth of one person's response may be extremely uncomfortable for others to watch.

There is a wide range of normal behavior at the time of death. What people do is shaped by the course of the illness, the events and emotions preceding the death, and their usual coping style. Some people want to leave immediately and are uncomfortable making decisions or plans at this time. Others may be busy attending to numerous post-death details. For them, the need to move quickly and "get on with it" is the priority. They may want the body to go to the morgue or funeral home as soon as possible and may be quite uncomfortable in the presence of the person who died. Often, they are calling relatives, talking about writing the obituary, and planning the funeral or memorial service.

Others need to move much more slowly. These people may want to stay with the body for a period of time and may sit attentively at the bedside, watching over the person who died. They may invite other people to visit and see the person after the death.

At the time of death, people may cry, sob, weep, or wail. People cry to release and express emotion. Often, there is quiet and only a few tears. Friends and families may experience a deep and heavy feeling of sadness when they begin to feel the weight and emptiness of this loss. The family may be worried about their actions just before and during the time of death. They may fear, for example, that the last dose of medication killed the person, or feel guilty that they weren't present when the person actually died.

Occasionally, people go into shock at the time of death. They will be confused, panicky, or disoriented. They may be shaky, nauseated, and/or breathless. When people are in shock, they may be cold and/or sweaty, and they may pace agitatedly or stare blankly in one direction. Although shock is a natural response to overwhelming trauma, it is important that people experiencing shock receive immediate attention and care.

Interventions

These psychosocial interventions have been designed to specifically address the key consideration *family reactions*. There are several assessment questions that will help open up a discussion, followed by more focused comments or tips that will facilitate further exploration of the issues that frequently arise at this time; each tip is followed by a sample dialogue.

Assessment Questions

- Is this the way you thought or expected your mother's death would be?
- How do you feel about the way she died?
- What else are you feeling right now?

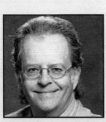

Jerry Rothstein, MA, is the Coordinator of Volunteer Services and Quality of Care for Victoria Hospice.

In My Own Voice
At the Time of Death

Jerry Rothstein

We need to take the time to say goodbye
Before the waves of emptiness wash in
To undermine the sandy bank below
And sweep us out to tidal seas alone.

We need to seek the meaning of a life
Cut short no matter what the age at death,
To share the words, smiles, memories and tears
With whatever lingers of our friend.

We need to touch the others, suffering
With us in our grief, yet still alone,
Without pretending much to understand
The cruel finality of flesh and bone.

With first reactions fumbling, rough, confused,
Begins the re-creations of our world.

Acknowledge that the timing of death often feels unexpected, even when it is anticipated. After a prolonged illness, many people are surprised by how unprepared they feel when death finally occurs; they thought they were ready and find that they are not.

> *"Even when you know that death will happen at any time and think you are prepared, it still feels unexpected, surprising, or shocking. What are you feeling about your friend's death now?"*

WORKING WITH SHOCK

Shock can be a serious condition. It is important to respond immediately. This is a crisis situation; it is appropriate to be direct about what the person needs now and later, and who will do what.

The signs of shock include cool, pale, and clammy skin; weak, rapid pulse; shallow, rapid breathing; low blood pressure; shaking, thirst, nausea and vomiting; confusion or anxiety; faintness, weakness, dizziness, or loss of consciousness (British Columbia Health Guide, 2000).

What to do

- Have the person lie down.

- Keep the person warm.

- Provide a calm and reassuring presence.

- Continue to assess reactions.

- Get medical attention if you are concerned.

Remember to

- Be calm in the center of chaos, hear the shocked person's concerns and fears, and provide safety and physical comfort.

- Normalize shock as part of their grief.

- Assess the person's support network. Ensure that someone is immediately available to support and assist the person after the death.

- Assess history of risk, such as history of mental health issues or health problems and behavioral factors such as drug or alcohol misuse.

- Plan for follow up. State what you will do now and over time; ask for permission to share your concerns with other appropriate professionals; and offer your services and/or referral for bereavement follow up, including counseling, when the shock passes.

Normalize the range and depth of reactions at the time of death. People naturally have different coping styles: Some primarily feel, others think, and some do both. When family members have different coping styles, they may find it difficult to understand and support each other. They may feel judged and labeled by their closest supports and they also may judge and label others.

> *"You and your husband, Craig, have had quite different responses to this death, and you are angry with him. You want to call people and invite them to come, but he doesn't want to have any visitors. His style is to with-*

draw from people when he's upset and yours is to seek out contact. How might you work together to find a solution that helps both of you?"

Respond to people in shock carefully and quickly. Orient people to your name and role and provide comfort and safety as appropriate. Asking unnecessary questions, yelling, speaking loudly, or moving too quickly may escalate feelings of anxiety or distress.

"My name is Jan, and I am the spiritual care coordinator from hospice. I understand that your husband has just died. Let's sit down. I will stay here beside you. Take a few slow breaths. When you are ready, tell me what happened."

Nature of the Death

At the time of Kate's death, Carrie was holding Kate's hand and they were watching the World Series. When Carrie realized that Kate wasn't breathing, she called to her parents in the next room. The family found it reassuring that Kate had died as her favorite team was winning. Watching baseball was a family pastime.

At the time of death, families may have questions or concerns about how and why it happened. Even though the death was expected, people often still ask, "What did she die from?" Families often need to be able to assign the eventual cause of death to something specific, such as an infection, heart attack, or "the cancer." They may once again question difficult decisions that they made earlier. For example, they may second-guess a decision not to treat pneumonia with antibiotics, wondering now if that choice contributed to the individual's death. This examination of events leading up to the death is a normal and helpful part of the grieving process.

The timing of the person's death and the events leading up to it may trouble the family. It is not uncommon for people to die soon after they are moved, bathed, or dressed. Family members may also feel uncertainty or guilt about the last dose of medication that was administered. Families may ask whether this last dose "killed" the patient or worry that the care they gave caused more harm than help.

When families have chosen not to be present at the time of death, there are a lot of feelings associated with not being there. Many people feel it is their duty to be there so that their loved one doesn't die alone. Some people believe that dying people may choose to die alone, or when a particular person is present. If family wanted to be there and weren't, this will be difficult. They may feel extremely guilty or disappointed.

While the patient is dying, families may see things they are unfamiliar with. Although dying patients are rarely distressed by changes to their breathing, it is often distressing for families. Breathing changes are usually quite audible and people may have heard wet wheezing, gasping, or gurgling sounds out of the mouth, throat, or chest of the dying person. These sounds may result in concerns that the dying person was drowning or suffocating. Dying people are often so weak that they sleep and die with their eyes and mouths wide open. Families may interpret it to mean that the dying person was fully aware or trying to communicate. When a patient bleeds from a wound, or from the mouth, nose, or rectum, and families see this happening, it is usually alarming. Families will also be distressed if they believe the patient suffered physically or emotionally at the time of death and was fighting to stay alive. They will need to review and debrief that they saw and heard prior to death to diffuse their concern about the individual's experience of death and to relieve any trauma they experienced by witnessing it.

Interventions

These psychosocial interventions have been designed to specifically address the key consideration *nature of the death*. There are several assessment questions that will help open up a discussion, followed by more focused comments or tips that will facilitate further exploration of the issues that frequently arise at this time; each tip is followed by a sample dialogue.

Assessment Questions

- What happened when your grandma died? How were you told about it?
- What was her death like for you? What did you see, hear, and do?
- Would you like to discuss anything about her death that you feel sorry about, or that you regret?
- Is there anything about the way she died that concerns you right now?
- Is there anything about the way she died that happened as you had hoped?

Review the illness and death. Families often want to go over various aspects of the illness and death. They need to integrate these experiences for confirmation and peace of mind. This review may encompass everything since

the diagnosis, or it may include only the last few weeks or days. (Note: Some people will not be ready to review at this time and will need follow-up later.)

> *"You and your son had lived with his cystic fibrosis for many years. There have been great triumphs and trials all along the way. There were other times when Sam was close to death, but he rallied. Sadly, this time he didn't survive. Tell me about this last part of his life.*

Discuss and explore the events just prior to death. Families may feel unsure about their actions prior to or during the death. Reviewing these actions may help to alleviate feelings of blame or doubt.

> *"I hear that some of you have questions and regrets about the things that you did or didn't do earlier today. Let's consider the choices you made and the places that you feel uncertain about. Where would you like to start?"*

Talk about the "gory details." When the death has been bloody or ugly or the patient seemed uncomfortable, it is important to reflect on what has happened. Allowing people to describe fully what they saw or heard and how it affected them can help people begin to come to terms with trauma. People who have witnessed a traumatic death are at risk for difficulty in their grief and may need ongoing counseling support.

"The actual moment of death comes as a shock even when expected. It is that final brutal farewell no one wishes to face. As a nurse I try to be acutely sensitive to each family's need at this time. Some wish privacy, but often one's presence is comforting. If I am there I will quietly say when I believe that death has occurred. Often the family will question that, hoping perhaps for just one more breath. Peace, quiet, and silent reverence is needed for this awesome moment of passing from one world into the next. The family usually needs guidance as to what to do next. I encourage them to be still. To take all the time they need to say their farewells. Perhaps to say a short prayer; light a candle, blow it out and let the spiraling smoke lift the spirit heavenward; or lay a flower in their loved one's hand. Honor this moment, honor the one who has gone, honor their grief and only when ready, say goodbye."

—*Angela Anscombe, Nurse, Victoria Hospice*

> *"Marissa, your aunt's death was very difficult. Images of some of the things that you have seen and heard will probably stay with you for some time. They may appear in your dreams or flash randomly in your mind's eye. I will call you regularly over the next few months and will be available if you have any problems or concerns. For now, is there any particular thing about your aunt's death that you want to talk about?"*

TIPS ON RESPONDING TO A DIFFICULT DEATH

- Identify yourself and your role.

- Minimize the family's exposure to trauma. Cover the body (not the face) of the person who died with a blanket or piece of clothing. If blood or other bodily fluid is visible, cover with a dark towel. If necessary, remove family from view of the body while you do this.

- Get people to sit or lie down. People may be light-headed and weak after seeing a difficult death. It can be difficult for them to concentrate or be still. They will be safer, though perhaps less comfortable, either seated or lying down.

- Provide comfort. Suggest that people have something small to drink and eat. A glass of water and a cookie are usually okay. Something to hold—such as a pillow or a pet—may be soothing and comforting.

- Listen a lot and talk a little. Encourage people to tell you what happened. Be patient; don't try to assuage tears or fill in long silences with unnecessary talk.

- Identify concerns and clarify misinformation. People are naturally worried about how traumatic the death was for the patient. Their worries often include whether the patient felt any pain, anguish, suffocation, or loss of dignity. Don't try to change or minimize what happened. Reframing if required can happen later.

- Review and repeat key information and follow-up plans.

Explore why the patient died alone or without certain people present. Many family members express a wish to be there when the patient dies. When this doesn't happen they may feel extremely angry, guilty, or sad. Discussing the character and personality of the person who died may help families to understand what happened.

> *"I know that you really wanted to be there when your sister died. You sat here all day and the minute you stepped out of her room, she went. We don't know why, but this seems to happen quite often. Can you think of any reason why she died when she did? Does this fit her personality at all?"*

After-Death Details

The family had never been through a death such as this before, and Carrie had many questions. She wanted to know if it was okay to touch and kiss Kate. She asked how they knew for sure that Kate was dead and what would happen to her grandma now. With some support from the hospice nurse, Robin carefully bathed and dressed Kate while they waited for other family members to arrive. The family chose to dress her in her favorite pajamas.

After a person dies, one of the most immediate tasks is the pronouncement of death. Usually, a physician or nurse examines the patient to certify that death has occurred. This examination varies, but it usually includes shining a bright light into the person's eyes (death is indicated if the pupils are dilated and do not respond) and listening and looking for breathing or a pulse. There may also be a check for response to pain. Once death is confirmed and pronounced, any needles, IVs, or catheters that remain in the person's body are removed.

Next, there are several decisions for families to make. Some of the decisions are minor and others major. Some must be made immediately, whereas others can wait. One of the biggest questions for families is what happens next with the person's body. When the person died at home, the family may want to know if they need to contact the coroner and when the funeral home should be called. When the person died in a facility, the family may want to know how long they can stay with the body, how it will be treated when they leave, and when and where it will go. Most people will be unaware of the laws and protocols that govern what is necessary and possible at this time. These regulations vary from place to place; different communities will have different resources, traditions, and expectations about what needs to happen after a death has occurred.

Some families wish to bathe or dress the person before the body is taken to the morgue or funeral home, and nursing staff may help them with this task. In some cultures or religious groups, members of the patient's community take responsibility for preparing the body for cremation or burial. This ritual of tending to the physical care of the patient is called laying out the body (see the sidebar on p. 266 called Laying Out the Body: A Final Tribute) and it offers people a final opportunity to give care to the person who has died.

Once death has been pronounced, the next step is the removal of the body to the funeral home or morgue. Many families will have made funeral arrangements prior to the death. Those who haven't can make this choice now. Occasionally, families elect to deal with transportation and burial without the use of a funeral home. This approach takes a significant amount of planning so that the legal and local requirements for certifying and registering a death, obtaining permission for burial or cremation, and the transportation of a body are fulfilled. For families who do wish to make their own arrangements, this provides an opportunity to be directly involved in a final act of caregiving. They may lay out the body or hold a viewing at home. They may choose to build the coffin or dig the grave themselves.

LAYING OUT THE BODY: A FINAL TRIBUTE

The term *laying out the body* means to prepare the body for burial or cremation. This laying out is often done right after the death when family gathers at the bedside or at the funeral home by members of the patient's religious or other community. Although not always possible or wanted (because of personal preferences, customs, or safety precautions), laying out a person's body can be a very meaningful ritual in which families or others can participate after a death. The family may complete laying out the body alone or with help from a member of the health care team (usually a nurse) or other community care provider. There are basically two parts to this process: washing the body and dressing the body. After these tasks are done, the body is, in a manner of speaking, laid out.

Although people may have a certain level of fear and uncertainty about this procedure, family members who were caregivers for the person before death often find that they are at ease with the body after death. They may have helped the patient with personal care and grown comfortable with this intimate contact. When families help the patient to wash, dress, and toilet, they become familiar with seeing and touching the person unclothed. They have learned about their own boundaries and about those of the person who died.

Laying out the body gives people a way to directly express their love for the person who has just died. When family members tend the body after death, they are able to ensure that it is treated with honor, respect, and dignity. Washing the body may be a way that family members choose to demonstrate their appreciation and gratitude for things that they shared with the person who died, and it may be viewed as a final act of caregiving (Maus-Bielders, 1995). Dressing the body in particular clothes gives families an opportunity to acknowledge the character of the person who died.

Rather than completely taking over the patient's care after death, health care providers should gently invite the family members to do for themselves as much as they are able (Maus-Bielders, 1995). If certain family members are uncomfortable with this responsibility, they may ask someone to help them. There may be smaller parts of the process that would or could be comfortable for the family members to perform. The family may, for example, be able to wash the face or hands and feet of the person who died. They may be comfortable choosing the clothes in which the person will be dressed but not actually putting them on the body. They may want to add a final touch, such as a brooch, flower, or token, once the person is dressed.

For most people, however, the body will go directly to the morgue or funeral home. Whatever the waiting period between the time of death and removal, the time will come when the body must be removed. This final leave-taking is one of the most difficult transitions for the family. If the family is not planning to hold a viewing at the funeral home, this will likely be the last time they will see the person who died. Families must carefully consider when and how they want the person's body to leave them and whether or not they wish to witness this.

In the days that follow, families will need to attend to many details, such as planning and holding a service or celebration of life, attending to financial or estate business, and so forth. Funeral homes attend to some of these details, such as acquiring death certificates. Many hospice programs and funeral homes have funeral planning guides or checklists for settling an estate to help families make necessary decisions. The sidebar When Death Has Occurred: Practical Tasks for Families lists many of the tasks families must undertake following a death. After a death, there may be medications, supplies, or pieces of equipment that are no longer needed. Usually, families are eager to remove this paraphernalia from the home but do not know what to do with it. Disposing of the medications is a practical matter, but it is also symbolic of the family's shifting focus from the illness to their own concerns (Bruno, 1995). Medications should not be put in the garbage or flushed down the toilet. Usually, hospital or community-based nurses, family physicians, and pharmacists will be willing to safely discard unused medication. Supplies and equipment that were purchased can be donated to regional or local aid charities such as the Red Cross or community lending cupboards.

Interventions

These psychosocial interventions have been designed to specifically address the key consideration *after-death details*. There are several assessment questions that will help open up a discussion, followed by more focused comments or tips that will facilitate further exploration of the issues that frequently arise at this time; each tip is followed by a sample dialogue.

Assessment Questions

- Is this the first time that you have seen someone die?
- Have you ever seen a dead person before?
- What questions do you have about what happens now?
- How will it be for you when your mother's body leaves the hospice unit? Do you plan to stay until then? Is there anyone that you want to be with you when that happens?

Inform family members arriving after the death about what they can expect to see when they enter the patient's room. Find out when their last visit was and review changes in the patient's condition since then. This may help to ease the shock and normalize changes in the person's body after death.

WHEN DEATH HAS OCCURRED: PRACTICAL TASKS FOR FAMILIES

This list of tasks is not meant to include everything to be done after a death, but rather it suggests the scope or range of practical details that families must consider. There will be further tasks over the weeks and months that follow.

On the day of the death:

- Select and contact a funeral home if you have not already done so. You may want to ask friends or family to recommend one.

- Lay out the body or give the funeral attendants clothing you wish the person to be buried or cremated in.

- Spend time with the body of the person who has died, saying goodbye, touching him or her, and reviewing the events prior to death.

- Identify a person who can call significant friends and family to inform them that the death has occurred and if/when you want people to contact or visit you.

In the days following the death:

- Visit the funeral home with support people to confirm your wishes regarding the funeral or memorial service, casket, burial/cremation, and so forth.

- Choose a date and discuss options for the service with funeral home staff and family.

- Write the obituary and submit to appropriate newspaper(s).

- Contact a minister or other person to preside over the funeral service.

- Contact your employer and inform him or her of the death. Discuss bereavement leave options and plan for time off.

- Contact the employer of the person who died and request that colleagues be informed.

- Contact appropriate government departments to cancel any benefits received by the person who died.

- Contact employer, government, banks, and insurance companies and identify sources of monies owed to the estate or beneficiaries (e.g., widow's pension, death benefits, life insurance policies).

- Begin to deal with ownership of property, bank accounts, and so forth.

- Begin the process of probate either yourself or through a lawyer.

"Monica, your friend's body changed a lot over the last month. She will probably look much smaller than you remember. She looks peaceful. She is lying on her bed, and her eyes are slightly open. All of the needles that were used to give her medications have been removed."

"Beside the body of someone you loved, stay long enough to let the body speak, to let it sing; long enough for a last farewell, a last look, a last touch, a last word; long enough to understand 'never again' and 'for ever'; long enough to be able to leave and to be able to remember."

—(Maus-Bielders, 1995, p. 28)

Demonstrate ways to be with the deceased person. This can include sitting at the bedside, looking at the person, and touching his or her hands. It may ease the family's awkwardness and hesitation if they see health care providers making contact with the person. (Note: Be sure that your touch is acceptable to the family.)

"Do you have any cultural or religious beliefs about seeing or touching a person who has died? Would you like to go into the room together and sit with Franklin for a few minutes? It is okay to talk with him and touch or kiss him. You may notice that he is cold in some places and his skin color is yellowish, but these are all normal changes."

Prepare people for the procedures that happen following a death. It may be helpful for people to know what steps will be taken before they happen. This will help family members decide how quickly they would like the process to progress and what they want to witness and/or do.

"When you are ready, the nurse will pronounce that death has occurred. This involves checking for a heartbeat or signs of breathing and looking at Miguel's eyes with a bright light. Then, when you are ready, the funeral home will be called, and their attendants will come and transport your uncle's body there. The part when he leaves will be hard. You might want to think about whether you will watch him go. It is okay for you to take as much time as you need. Do you have any questions?

Check out what funeral arrangements have been made, and provide information accordingly. Families feel overwhelmed and vulnerable at this time and may not be sure what they want to do now. Pertinent information and support may help them make decisions.

"Perhaps someone in your family or one of your friends can suggest which funeral home to use. I also have a list of reputable funeral homes and memorial societies and some information that may help you with the decisions that you face. Is there anyone who can help you with these decisions right now?"

Rituals

Although everyone knew that Kate's death was imminent, it still came as a shock. Robin and Jeff were disappointed that they weren't in the room with her when it happened, though it made sense to them that Carrie was. With help from the hospice nurse, Robin carefully bathed and dressed Kate while they waited for other family members to arrive. The family chose to dress her in her favorite pajamas. Carrie wrote a note to Kate and placed it in her hand, and Mandy was able to choose a flower to place next to Kate's cheek.

Rituals at the time of death are an important way for families to be with the person who has died and to mark this pivotal transition in their lives. Rituals give people an opportunity to honor the person and to acknowledge, symbolically, the death and its significance. Beck and Metrick said that ritual is "an attempt to return to a sense of wholeness that has been altered by transition" (1990, p. 1). They further explained that the purpose of ritual is to signify a turning point, a moving toward something new and unknown. According to Campbell, rituals concentrate your mind on the implications of what you are doing (Osbon, 1991). Rituals may be familiar and based on particular religious or cultural traditions, or they may be spontaneous and eclectic. Rituals link people to familiar, sometimes ancient, customs and traditions, which may provide comfort and perspective during times of pain and sorrow. After-death rituals may include praying, visiting, holding a vigil, placing a flower in the deceased's hand, taking a lock of hair, washing and dressing the body, reading poems, sharing stories, or just giving a final kiss or loving caress. Any and all of these acts may help surviving family members honor the significance of this person's death and let them go.

Interventions

These psychosocial interventions have been designed to specifically address the key consideration *rituals*. There are several assessment questions that will help open up a discussion, followed by more focused comments or tips that will facili-

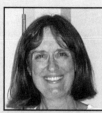

Eileen O'Donnell is a volunteer at Victoria Hospice and the daughter of a woman who died in a long-term care facility.

In My Own Voice
Between Worlds:
Diary and Reflection

Eileen O'Donnell

February 2, 2002

For weeks now, our Mum has been failing. She still has a robust desire to live, but now her body is giving up. We siblings—there are five of us—have been taking turns sitting with her through the long nights. Some nights she is clearly struggling, restless; other nights are very peaceful. Together, we are coming to terms with the fact that our Mum is leaving us.

So we decide we need to celebrate! All through our childhood years, we O'Donnell's had music; one of Mum's gifts was the gift of hospitality. So we call the aunts, the sisters and brothers, nephews and nieces, cousins and friends; we're having a party to celebrate a life! We set up the Activity Room with tablecloths, flowers, and candles and we have a great potluck; we pop casseroles in the oven and uncork the wine; we have come to say a good goodbye. We are tired from our long vigils, but there is a tenderness and joy here that is unmistakable. We raise our glasses, and sing our thanks for the gift Mum is, and for the love and friendship her life has engendered.

After the meal we gather, all 22 of us, around Mum's bed in her room. We bring the flowers, the candles, and I've already set up a little electronic piano in the corner. We start with the jolly old favorites ("It's a Long Way to Tipperary!" "Whenever I Feel Afraid"), and move later into songs of prayer and thanksgiving. Laughter, tears, the children's faces rapt as they lead us in prayer, the sounds of Mum's labored breathing as we take a moment of reverent silence to give thanks and wish her Godspeed—we tremble with the privilege of being so close to the Infinite! It is a sacred, unforgettable moment.

February 3, 2002

Last night was my sister's turn to stay with Mum; the rest of us went home. In and out of the transcendent, it's hard to deal with the mundane reality of daily life (carpools, banking, children's lessons, and homework) when your Mum lies dying. Mercifully, my husband has cheerfully taken over many of my usual chores during this time; I need and want to be present to Mum.

But today, I went to Mass, ate lunch, and took a walk around the lake before I returned to Mum's side. When I entered her room, there was a new sound to her breathing; it can't be long now, I thought. My sisters were there, and my two aunts, quiet and prayerful. We gathered around Mum and sang, again starting with old popular songs. At one point we even found ourselves singing "Oh they built the ship Titanic"—remember the part that says, "Husbands and wives—itty bitty children lost their lives!" We collapsed with laughter, giddy with the shifting from the sublime to the ridiculous. But soon we found ourselves singing the hymns we had sung as children. It grew very peaceful. Mum's breathing became shallower and less urgent. Our voices sometimes faltered, but gently entwined each other in a web of support as Mum hovered on the edge of eternity. When Mum finally breathed her last, we were singing "He Will Raise You Up on Eagle's Wings."

Oh, then, the tears, the hugs, the fervent last holding of her hands! One of my sisters reminded us that this would be the moment when Mum would be standing before her Judge, and so, conscious of the many times we all fail to be our "best," we prayed the rosary one last time with Mum, begging forgiveness for her and for our own vulnerable selves. Then another sister read the most beautiful prayer, the prayer that a priest would recite if he were present at the moment of death, a prayer full of strong and colorful images, invoking the intercession of Mary and all the Saints, and the Blessing of God on the pilgrim soul as she journeys toward the Light.

Mysteries. We had been in touch with the core mysteries of humanity. We had felt no need at that stage to call for medical intervention; just being there, with Mum and with each other, was enough. When we knew Mum was not breathing any more, we did call the nurse to document the moment of death; this, too, was accomplished peacefully.

Over the next hour or so, as family and friends arrived—my husband, my daughter, my brother, and friends—we each took a moment to whisper our last good-byes to Mum. Soon, everyone had left but one sister and me. When it was time, we chose to stay and help to wash the body. Now, this would not meet everyone's needs, but for us it was a beautiful way to accomplish the closure we needed to the phase of caring for Mum. Tenderly we sponged her still-warm skin; quietly we wept and sang again about images of her soul being raised up on eagle's wings. When the gentlemen arrived to remove the body, we stood by, then accompanied them to the door. It felt finished.

Then came the welcome moment when we fetched the homemade soup my friend had left and the good whole wheat bread, warmed it in the microwave, and gratefully ate it in Mum's room as we began to make plans for the funeral. The empty bed—our hearts knew we had to get used to this.

tate further exploration of the issues that frequently arise at this time; each tip is followed by a sample dialogue.

Assessment Questions

- What traditions or customs does your family have about how to be or what to do when someone dies?

- What could you do to honor this time and make it meaningful?

- How much time would you like to spend with your daughter-in-law's body before she goes to the funeral home?

Normalize the family's need or desire for contact with the person after death. The family may desperately want to see, touch, or feel the person but may hold back out of unwarranted fear, uncertainty, or caution. (Note: When appropriate, you could go in and see the person who died before the family does so that you can prepare them.)

"Sometimes people want to see the person after death but don't because they're not sure what to expect and feel afraid. I was with Allister when he died, and I can tell you that he looks very peaceful. Would you like to

spend some time with him? Do you want to go in alone or is there some-
one that you would like to have with you?"

Encourage people to consider and do things that they find meaningful. This
moment may be the single most important point in the journey through living and dying for families. Help the family identify gestures or activities
that symbolize their feelings about this person's death.

> *"Lottie, you have a bit of time before the orderly comes to move your
> mother's body to the morgue. Some families use this time to bathe or dress
> the person; others read a prayer, write a note, or choose a flower to place
> in the person's hand. Is there anything special that you would like to do
> with or for her before she goes?"*

OUR EXPERIENCE

Our goal is to empower and support families to respond to the death in ways that
feel safe, meaningful, and acceptable to them. We do this through our presence at
the time of death, acknowledging the death, and modeling ways to be with the
person who died.

When a death has occurred, we encounter people in their most vulnerable,
courageous, and weary moments. These moments with families are frequently
poignant, and we feel most profoundly the burden and gift of love, life, and the
work that we've chosen. This work puts us in a place where we are constantly dis-
covering, exploring, and testing our values and priorities. Perhaps more than any
other moment, the time of death forces us to reflect on who we are and what we
are doing.

Being so intimately involved with people when someone they love has just
died feels strange, intense, and blessed. It is difficult to step with caution and confidence into a family that is freshly bereft. Sometimes, we feel clumsy and exces-
sive, and at other times, helpful and adept. Families are comforted as much by our
personal gestures as they are by our professional interventions. In a speech, June
Callwood (2001) said of health care professionals in palliative care, "The kind need
to be more skilled and the skilled need to be more kind." Both are essential.

Families look to us for guidance at this time. Our manner and interaction
with the person who died creates a template for families to follow or adapt to fit
their own needs. Sometimes, we miss the importance of this aspect of our work because death is so familiar to us. We also model acceptance of all the different ways

that people may respond at this time. We show family members how to comfort each other when reactions and responses vary.

The experience that we gain and the personal growth that happens when we do this work may enable us to help families respond to death in ways that truly reflect their feelings for the person who died and for the death itself. Through gentle questions, invitations, and suggestions, we help families remember or create rituals or gestures that will help bring meaning and strength to this time of loss and sadness. With respect and curiosity, we explore the cultural, religious, and familial belief systems that families have and help them build on this opportunity for deeper bonds and connections. Through observation and reflection, we point out and acknowledge sacred moments.

TEAM ISSUES

Often, after a death, there is not enough time for health care providers to do all that they wish in order to care for families and themselves. They may be required to move on to the next patient or family, and this need to rush onward feels mechanical and disrespectful. Working within the limits and demands of an organization, this kind of pressure can adversely affect the well-being of health care providers and compromise the care that is given. At this time, people need both the skills and the organizational support to assess when and how to take time out from fixed routines and care for themselves.

Sometimes the death happens in the way the team hoped it would, and they feel reassured and satisfied with the care that was provided. Alternatively, when the death is not as expected, they often feel disappointed, responsible, or angry. When someone feels this way, it is important to review the situation with a colleague, supervisor, or the whole team. It may also be helpful to remember that death, like birth, is unique to each person. It is possible to influence or shape the dying and death experience, but ultimately health care providers are not in control of how or when it happens.

Sometimes, the death of a patient feels like a personal loss (Muller, 2000). This may happen when patients remind care providers of someone in their own lives or because, over the days or months of providing care, care providers have grown attached to this person. These losses are an inevitable, rich, and sometimes painful aspect of this work. It is possible to find the care of dying people and their families both wounding and healing. A paradox inherent in this work is that hospice and palliative care providers simultaneously learn to value life and death more intensely. It is essential to develop personal rituals that allow team members to acknowledge and grieve these special losses.

It is easy to forget how extraordinary death can be for people who have never, or rarely ever, experienced it. Palliative care providers' reactions and responses may seem casual or even heroic to the inexperienced person. The team may be surprised and impatient with people who have strong emotional reactions, such as yelling or wailing, at the time of death. They also may have difficulty with people who seem particularly numb or flat. It may be especially hard for team members to tolerate responses that differ from those of the team or from prevailing cultural norms.

SUMMARY

This final transition in someone's life marks the end of a journey that began with the investigation, diagnosis, and treatment of a life-threatening illness. This journey may have taken years to complete, or it may have only lasted a few weeks or months. Death is the much anticipated and dreaded result (see Table 7.1). People have been living with loss, change, and uncertainty. They have been searching for the meaning of this experience, and perhaps the meaning of their lives.

When a death has just occurred, time stands still for the family. Members may be in shock, feel relieved, or find themselves completely drained of energy. They may meet death with confusion, fear, sadness, or a sense of peace. Whatever has gone on before, the death of a beloved friend or family member is one of life's most defining moments. People will reflect on and remember this time for the rest of their lives.

Death brings one person's journey through life to an end. It also ushers in the next stage of the journey for those who are left behind.

REFLECTIVE ACTIVITY

The purpose of this reflective activity is to increase your awareness of how your personal experiences with death, grief, and loss may shape your work. Do this ex-

Table 7.1. Palliative Performance Scale (PPSv2) 0%

PPS Level	Ambulation	Activity and evidence of disease	Self-care	Intake	Conscious level
0%	Death	–	–	–	–

ercise when you are alone. You may want to record your responses in a journal or notebook. Later, if you wish, talk over your responses with a colleague, friend, or support person. Use what you discover from this experience to inform your practice, knowing that some people will feel as you did and some will feel differently.

Think of a death that happened in your family or circle of friends. What do you remember about the time when you first found out that this person died? (If you have not experienced a death in your family or circle of friends, choose another significant loss, such as the death of a pet, loss of a job, or end of a serious relationship.)

Think of the people who were around at the time. Were they friends and family members? Were they health care professionals? Were you alone? What did you want from them?

Think about how you responded. How did you feel and what did you do? What were you doing and feeling an hour later? Were you comfortable with the way you reacted?

Think about what you communicated to other people. What messages did you give people about how you were doing? Were they accurate?

Think about what you needed. What was the most helpful thing that someone said or did when you first found out or realized that this person had died? What was the most unhelpful?

Now think about how your experience has shaped your practice. How has this experience strengthened your practice? How has it weakened it? What are your fears and hopes about responding to a death?

RESOURCES

Legrand, M., & Gomas, J. (1998). Being present at the last moments of life. *European Journal of Palliative Care, 5*(6), 191–194.

Rinpoche, S. (1994). *The Tibetan book of living and dying.* San Francisco: HarperCollins.

Victoria Hospice Society. (1998). Death and dying. In G.M. Downing (Ed.), *Medical care of the dying* (3rd ed., pp. 437–475). Victoria, British Columbia, Canada: Victoria Hospice Society.

REFERENCES

BC health guide. (2000). Victoria, Canada: British Columbia Ministry of Health.

Beck, R., & Metrick, B. (1990). *The art of ritual: A guide to creating and performing your own ceremonies.* Berkeley, CA: Celestial Arts Publishing.

Bruno, S. (1995 July–August). The value of death attendance. *The Forum,* 11–12.

Callwood, J. (2001, October). Keynote address. Canadian Palliative Care Association Conference. Victoria, British Columbia, Canada.

Maus-Bielders, K. (1995). Saying goodbye. *European Journal of Palliative Care, 2*(1), 25–28.

Müller, M. (2000). The role of bereavement counseling in hospice work. *European Journal of Palliative Care,* 7(1), 29–31.

Osbon, D. (1991). *Reflections on the art of living: A Joseph Campbell companion.* New York: Harper Perennial.

Sarton, M. (1980). *Recovering: A journal (1978–1979).* New York: W.W. Norton.

Working with Emotions

The following story describes a situation that hospice and palliative care teams often face. As you read, note the different responses of the team members:

> *Several members of the team met with a patient's family to discuss significant changes in the patient's condition. As the conversation progressed, one of the family members began to cry. The counselor leaned toward the person, made brief eye contact, uttered a small sound of encouragement, and waited. The doctor put a box of tissues into the counselor's hands and gestured toward the crying person, indicating that she should give the tissue to the person immediately.*

This story illustrates how uncomfortable people, even skilled and compassionate professionals, can be with overt expressions of emotions. They want to provide comfort instantly, so that the person experiencing the emotion will stop crying, raging, or despairing. The story also illustrates how counselors and other health care professionals may approach emotions differently.

Psychosocial care providers value emotions as natural, healthy responses to the challenges and changes that are inherent in facing death, dying, and bereavement. Rather than offering comfort right away, they provide people with choices about the expression and exploration of emotion. This is not to say that people should be encouraged in every instance and in any setting to go with their emotion. Instead, it advocates a respectful curiosity about people's needs and wishes. At an appropriate time (now or later) and place (here or elsewhere), emotion may be expressed.

When health care providers work in hospice palliative care, powerful emotions are common and to be expected. This means finding ways to be in the presence of such emotion and do the work that is required by the situation. It requires an ability to engage with someone about a particular emotion and be both a witness and a resource as the person expresses and explores it. Also, it requires knowledge of personal emotional responses that are called forth by the work.

Working with emotion is clearly a responsibility of health care providers. The team member who is with a patient or family when emotions arise is the one to respond. Part of the counselor's role in hospice palliative care includes being a resource to other team members, reminding them that emotions do not necessarily mean the person is in trouble or that something is wrong. Counselors remind other team members that they do not have to fix an emotion or make it better. This attitude of not fixing can be challenging for those professionals who are trained to treat, alleviate, or eradicate symptoms. Listening, being present, and accepting are important and effective interventions when people are expressing emotions.

To work with emotions, empathy is needed. Empathy requires sufficient imagination to be able to put yourself in the other person's situation and imagine how you might feel or respond. Life experiences give people familiarity with emotional responses and a personal knowledge of such feelings as sadness, anger, or loneliness. This familiarity creates a connection to the person experiencing these emotions now. Courage helps health care providers walk with patients and families into their dark places as a companion, to be willing to know and feel difficult emotions again. To be empathic, it is important to not succumb to the feelings, but rather, to be able to maintain some equilibrium; to go and return.

STRATEGIES FOR WORKING WITH EMOTIONS

- **Create safety.** With privacy and time, rapport is established. A calm demeanor promotes trust and confidence. Your faith in the resiliency of the human spirit and trust in the process at hand offers an opportunity to look into challenging issues.

- **Be present and accepting.** Your willingness to hear and witness grief and suffering indicates acceptance of the associated feelings. When you don't need to fix things, people can find their own way and you can help them sort out what they feel and what they might want to do.

- **Provide permission.** People often need permission to have feelings and to express them, or to stop feeling them and rest or do something else. When you acknowledge and expect these emotions and their intensity, patients and family members begin to address the discomfort people may have about their emotions.

- **Normalize reactions.** Emotional responses may become understandable and acceptable within a framework of transitions, grief, response to an extraordinary situation, circumstances of life at this time, and personal history.

- **Teach new coping strategies.** Some people benefit from learning to express feelings, others from learning to close down feelings. Both groups should practice opening emotions for limited spans of time, thereby helping them to have some control over their emotions. Introduce other ways of expressing or releasing emotion through physical activity and creative outlets.

- **Foster positive feelings.** Self-care and techniques such as nurturing, visualization, and relaxation can help people have positive experiences in a difficult time. People may engage in personal healing activities that create some level of hope. Support from others can be appreciated as positive indicators of care and concern.

- **Explore strengths.** Information about people's past history of coping with emotion, their personal style, and the support available to them can provide reminders of capability and competence.

THE OTHER SIDE OF EMOTIONS OF GRIEF

The Other Side of Sorrow

In *The Prophet*, Kahlil Gibran says, "Your joy is your sorrow unmasked" (1972, p. 32). Once the harder part of sadness is done, there comes a sweetness in which one is able to recall the good times. Memories bring a sense of loving and being loved.

The Other Side of Hopelessness

Recognition of the natural cycles of life can bring an acceptance of oneself and one's experience of loss and grief. Being in touch with the beauty of the world can bring peace. May Sarton (1993) wrote, "Help us to be the always hopeful gardeners of the spirit who know that without darkness nothing comes to birth as without light nothing flowers."

The Other Side of Guilt

Honor guilt as a teacher of what one believes to be right and wrong. In searching for meaning in the midst of grief, one decides what one wants to hold on to and value. The remainder is forgiven and released.

The Other Side of Anger

Within one's anger, there is energy for positive action. It arises from the same source as initiative. Personal change and growth require dynamic energy.

The Other Side of Fear and Anxiety

The physical responses associated with being anxious and being excited are similar. The individual is responding to change and getting ready for the challenge. Rather than saying "I am afraid," say, "I am ready." Fear is an indicator of being at one's personal edge, where growth can happen.

AN APPROACH FOR WORKING WITH EMOTIONS

This approach demonstrates one way to help patients, families, and colleagues to acknowledge and explore their emotions, and to learn new coping strategies. Working with anger is being used as an example here. There are 12 instructions or steps outlined within this approach. Questions or suggestions about how people might achieve each step follow each instruction.

- **Identify the emotion.** What are people feeling? What triggers their anger? What issues underlie this reaction? What are the things they feel angry about?

- **Go with one's natural response.** People may need to express their anger or keep it under control. Talking, pounding, or writing an angry letter may help. Being safe with their anger (i.e., working with it apart from the source of the feeling) is important. Taking time out, distracting oneself, or taking action to make positive change are helpful.

- **Take the edge off.** Strenuous physical activity, humor, visualization, relaxation, or creative outlets all help to take the edge off, as does breaking the underlying issues into manageable pieces and addressing each separately.

- **Track how this felt.** Keeping a journal or notebook about their responses to new ways of dealing with anger helps people track their successes and challenges.

- **Normalize anger as a grief response that, as such, is likely to recur.** Expecting that the anger will be an ongoing part of grief allows people to tolerate it and be more patient with themselves.

- **Collect options for coping.** Gathering strategies that have worked for others and oneself in the past expands a person's repertoire of responses or coping techniques. There may be friends, web sites, books, handouts, or exercises that are helpful.

- **Try something new.** Trying a different way from usual practice, perhaps a strategy found in collecting options, may shift things in a positive way.

- **Track how this felt.** People need to practice this new strategy for a bit and then ask themselves what the condition or state of their anger is now.
- **Try something else new.** As people try yet another new way of dealing with their anger, they continue to build their repertoire of skills.
- **Track how this felt.** Again, this helps people know the benefits of what they are trying.
- **Look back to the beginning.** How was their anger when they started, when they took the edge off, when they tried one new thing, and so forth?
- **Identify the emotion.** Do they feel differently? How is their anger different now? What might they still want or need to do? What has changed and what has not?

QUESTIONS FOR COUNSELORS AND OTHER HEALTH CARE PROVIDERS TO ASK THEMSELVES

- How comfortable am I with emotional expression?
- Which emotions am I most comfortable with, and which challenge my comfort level? What might I do about that?
- What beliefs do I have about emotion, and how do they influence my behavior?
- How congruent is my behavior? What do I do? Do I always encourage emotion? Stop it? Sit back from it or absent myself? Hold space for emotion to come forward?
- What skills, abilities, and qualities do I have that help patients, family members, and bereaved people when they are very emotional?
- Do I trust and respect that people know what they want to do?
- How do I contribute to a climate that accepts and values emotional expression from patients, families, and other team members?

RESOURCES

Web Sites

http://www.chebucto.ns.ca/CommunitySupport/Men4Change/
anger.html
http://www.nwlink.com/~emolit/

Books

Baugher, R. (1997). *A guide to understanding guilt during bereavement.* Newcastle,
WA: Author.

Bourne, E. (1995). *The anxiety and phobia workbook.* Oakland, CA: New Harbinger
Publications.

Carson, R.D., & Rogers, N. (1990). *Taming your gremlin: A guide to enjoying yourself*
(Reprint ed.). New York: Harper Perennial.

Reeves, N. (2001). *A path through loss: A guide to writing your healing and growth.*
Kelowna, British Columbia, Canada: Northstone.

Wegela, K.K. (1996). *How to be a help instead of a nuisance: Practical approaches to
giving support, service, and encouragement to others.* Boston: Shambhala Publications.

Articles

Combs, D.C. (1993). An existential view of grief as related to aloneness. *Illness, Crisis
and Loss, 3*(2), 22–27.

Field, N.P., & Horowitz, M.J. (1998). Applying an empty-chair monologue paradigm
to examine unresolved grief. *Psychiatry, 61,* 279–287.

Neimeyer, R.A., & Stewart, A.E. (1996, June). Trauma, healing, and the narrative employment of loss. *Families in Society: The Journal of Contemporary Human Services,*
360–375.

Salka, S. (1997). Enlisting the unconscious as an ally in grief therapy: The creative use
of affirmations, metaphors, and guided visualization. *The Hospice Journal, 12*(3),
17–31.

REFERENCES

Gibran, K. (1972). *The prophet.* New York: Alfred A. Knopf.

Sarton, M. (1996). In L. Popov, *Sacred moments: Daily meditations on the virtues.* New
York: Penguin Putnam.

Sarton, M. (1980). *Recovering: A journal (1978–1979).* New York: W.W. Norton.

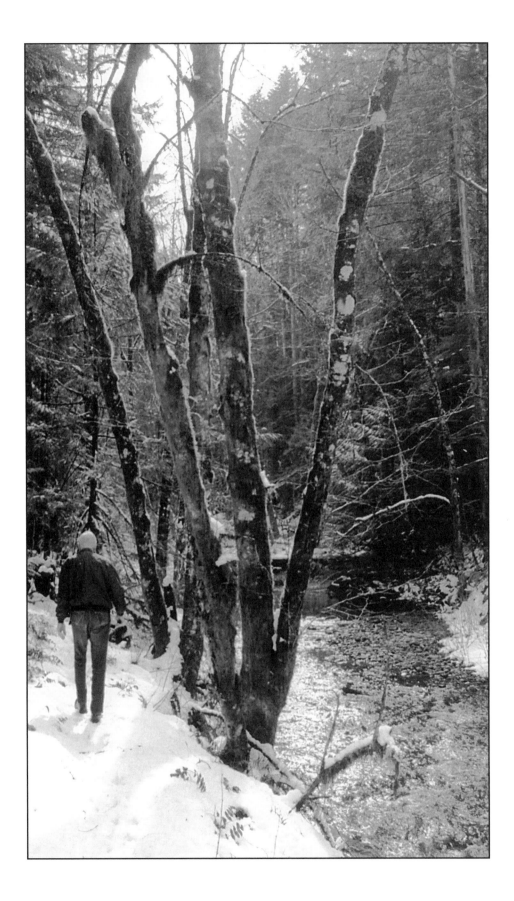

8

Walking the Edges

WHEN A DEATH OCCURS

Phase 1

*G*rief is not new for family members once the death has occurred. They have been grieving the losses that have happened along the journey through diagnosis, treatment, palliative care, and dying. The landscape of grief changes as family members make the transition from caregivers to bereaved people, however. Grief is now the path that bereaved people must travel between how things were and how they will be. The image of the labyrinth is offered as a metaphor for this journey through bereavement. Like the process of grief, a labyrinth has no dead ends or wrong turns. In it, you are always moving; it takes you inward. The journey is complex with much going back and forth over what seems to be the same territory. Finally, the path leads you to the outside world. Using this metaphor, the early phase of grief, when a death has just occurred, is like walking the edges of the labyrinth. Still struggling to grasp that the death has really occurred, people have not yet experienced the full impact of the loss and the changes it brings.

One of the first responsibilities of the family, or those acting in this capacity, will be to make arrangements for the FUNERAL, MEMORIAL, AND OTHER RITUALS. A plan or strong tradition may already be established for the family to follow, or all of the various decisions may have to be made after the death. Depending on the person, this may feel like a demanding responsibility, a loving courtesy, or both.

Families' GRIEF REACTIONS are variable in the first days following a death. Many bereaved people experience euphoria that reflects their relief that the patient who died is at peace or no longer suffering and, possibly from a caregiver's perspective, their sense of a job accomplished. Some people are overwhelmed with sadness and weep, wail, or keen with the pain of their loss. In the emptiness of this transition, many people feel numb, blank, and even shocked. They experience a sense of unreality that the death has actually happened. Often, family members will experience these emotional reactions in waves of feeling alternated with numbness. These intermittent periods seem to let people walk the edges of their grief and take reality in slowly. The death is known first in the head or the mind and only later in the heart.

At this time, the patient care team has withdrawn and the family members have limited contact with the once-regular visitors and supporters. A transition occurs from a focus on the ill and dying person and his or her supportive caregivers to the bereaved family for BEREAVEMENT FOLLOW-UP. New services may be offered at a time when bereaved people are not yet certain of their concerns and wishes. Generally, an entirely new team will provide these services. The hospice and palliative providers who have been caring for the patient and family thus far will turn care over to the bereavement care team.

This is a time of major transition. The loss of one person is deeply felt throughout the family system, leaving the family changed in many ways. Family cohesion and FAMILY INTERACTIONS are altered positively, negatively, or both. As the time and circumstances of the illness and death are reviewed, each person's behavior comes under close inspection by themselves and other family members. The sense of purpose or common goal in providing care has died with the ill patient. Each family member must learn to be a grieving person in a bereaved family. The adjustments that are called for will continue throughout the family's bereavement.

In the early days after a death, bereaved people often have much SOCIAL SUPPORT from their family, circle of friends, and community. They are busy responding to condolences and offers of help and support. Quickly, however, even supportive people may have EXPECTATIONS that bereaved friends or family members will resume their normal life. Returning to work and other routines of daily living and the activities of social life can be both exhausting and a welcome distraction.

New demands begin almost immediately following a death, as people must attend to PRACTICAL MATTERS. Funeral or memorial plans must be finalized. Services or events need to be arranged and attended. Various people and institutions must be notified of the death and a start made on settling the estate. The paraphernalia of illness—the pills and equipment—must be tidied away. Decision making can be frightening or overwhelming. After days, months, or even years of doing things for the ill person, an individual may find activity a familiar comfort and a relief from the looming emptiness that the patient used to fill.

"Grief is like a stranger who has come to stay in both the heart and the mind."

—(Staudacher, 1987, p. 4)

RICK AND JENNIFER

Rick's wife, Jennifer, was 38 when she died of breast cancer. Rick; their children Sarah, age 11, and Jesse, age 7; Jennifer's sister Judy; and Jennifer's widowed mother, Elaine, were present when she died. Rick and Jennifer shared a strong faith, which was reflected in the celebration of her life their pastor, Reverend Allen, arranged after Jennifer died. For this celebration, Rick and the children chose hymns together. Sarah asked to read a poem that she had written recently for her mother. Jesse was uncertain about going to the funeral and asked a lot of questions about what would happen. Many friends, members of the congregation, teachers, and classmates from the children's school and colleagues from Rick's work attended the service.

Over the next weeks, people called or visited the family and brought food to the home. Some normal routines returned. Though Judy stayed with Elaine at first, she soon returned to her own home, job, and family. Judy felt that she was doing fine but was concerned about her mother and Rick. Elaine continued to be anxious and dependent and didn't want to be left alone. She feared she would be unable to manage when Judy went home. She went over and over Jennifer's last day, frequently asking, "How could she die so quickly like that?" She also spoke of missing her husband, Jennifer's father, who had died some years earlier. The children played with close friends and returned to school. Jesse talked easily to friends about his feelings, but Sarah found it hard to pay attention and felt that certain classmates picked on her.

Rick felt pressured by his employer to decide when he would return to work, but he didn't know what to say. He was in a daze. He slept badly and hardly ate. He refused to go to church or to let Reverend Allen visit. He was irritated by all the advice he received from people about when and how he should proceed. He avoided the business of settling Jennifer's estate and lost his temper when someone at the bank said she would need proof of Jennifer's death. Judy offered to help Rick sort out Jennifer's things, but he wanted everything left as it was. Rick felt Jennifer's absence all the time. He missed her warmth at night in bed and hated being out in the world and seeing happy couples everywhere. This only reminded him of his loneliness and longing to see and touch her again. The hospice palliative care team had been quite close to this family and wondered how the children would cope with their mother's death. They expressed concern to the bereavement team about Rick because they had seen that he depended on Jennifer for most of the decision making in the family.

KEY CONSIDERATIONS

Funeral, Memorial, and Other Rituals

Rick and Jennifer shared a strong faith, which was reflected in the celebration of her life that their pastor, Reverend Allen, arranged after Jennifer died. Rick and the children chose hymns together. Sarah asked to read a poem that she had written recently for her mother. Jesse was uncertain about going to the funeral and asked a lot of questions about what would happen. Many friends, members of the congregation, teachers, and classmates from the children's school and colleagues from Rick's work attended the service.

Making decisions and taking care of details after someone dies can sometimes be difficult. Some families have familiar traditions to follow. Many other people, however, have little experience or connection to any tradition to guide them.

Families usually find it helpful to have some form of ritual or memorial service as a way of facing the reality that someone has died. Funerals and other memorials serve a number of purposes. They mark the transition of the person's life and offer the family an opportunity to honor and remember them. They give families and communities a time to gather together and acknowledge the importance of what has happened, the significance of this death, and the changes it brings. Friends, colleagues, neighbors, and acquaintances are able to demonstrate their respect for the person who has died as well as their caring and support for the bereaved family. Less formal gatherings, such as receptions or teas, are other ways that people may choose to gather in recognition of the death of someone.

Bereaved families may struggle with questions if they have no clear guidelines from their traditions about what to do when someone dies. They may resist going through the pain or expense of a service. Sometimes the person who died has expressed a wish that there be no service at all, or the person may have given explicit instructions concerning everything that is to take place. Typically, it is the dying person's desire to protect family members from further pain and sorrow that prompts them to make various stipulations concerning what should happen after he or she dies. Some families find this comforting, whereas others struggle to balance the wishes of the person who has died with their own beliefs or needs. Flexibility and permission to adjust the original plan can be helpful for these families. Within some families, it may be clear who will take on the primary responsibility for planning and organizing the funeral, memorial, or other gathering. For other families, painful disagreement may occur around what decisions are made and whoever makes them.

Parents often wonder whether children should attend the service or other activities related to the death. They may remember their own childhood experiences of death and funerals or be advised by others. The thought of supporting a grieving child can feel overwhelming to bereaved parents. Although these decisions need to be made on an individual basis, it is often important to reassure parents that it normally helps children to be included in the family gatherings or services (Worden, 2001). It is important for parents to explain beforehand to children what will take place and to check how they feel about attending (Wolfelt, 1990). Very young children may need some familiar and trusted person available to answer their questions or to take them if they want or need to go home. Older children may wish to have a part to play, either directly or indirectly, in the service.

Grief reactions at the time of a service or other gathering may vary greatly, from dry-eyed control to wailing and moaning. Some people may feel numb and empty, whereas others may be overwhelmed with sadness and longing—or they may display any emotion in between. Some people may be surprised at their own reactions and those of others. For many, the experience of the service or gathering is a complex mix of feelings that may include sadness, pain, comfort, and relief.

Interventions

These psychosocial interventions have been designed to specifically address the key consideration *funeral, memorial, and other rituals.* There are several assessment questions that will help open up a discussion, followed by more focused comments or tips that will facilitate further exploration of the issues that frequently arise at this time; each tip is followed by a sample dialogue.

Assessment Questions

- What are the traditions in your family, religion, or culture? How do you normally observe special events?

- What do you know about your father's wishes? Would he have wanted a funeral or memorial service? Burial or cremation? Why do you imagine those preferences were expressed?

- How can you and your family honor or mark your sister's death? What feels important for you to do? Do you imagine you might feel differently about any of those decisions 1, 5, or 10 years from now?

Help families determine what needs to be done and who will take responsibility for planning and organizing any service or memorial event. In some families, certain individuals normally assume these roles, whereas in others, it may be unclear who takes this on. This may be a new experience for family members.

> *"It sounds like there are a number of things that are important to your family at this time. How are you deciding who will attend to the various details? How do your brothers and sisters feel about this approach?"*

Invite parents to encourage children's participation in the events taking place after the person's death. Clear, age-appropriate information helps children to feel included and to make choices about what they would like to do.

> *"Megan, you sound uncertain about whether it's okay for your children to be at their grandmother's memorial service. I'm wondering what your concerns are. I'm also wondering if you have talked with your family about this? What information could help you with your decision?"*

Ensure that the decision about services suits the concerns of the family. Understanding that many options are available allows people to honor a variety of wishes and concerns.

> *"Your Aunt Mary hated funerals, and so your family is not planning a formal service. What kind of get-together do you imagine would be more appropriate? How comfortable are you with this?"*

Grief Reactions

Jennifer's mother Elaine continued to be anxious and dependent and didn't want to be left alone. She went over and over Jennifer's last day, frequently asking, "How could she die so quickly like that?" She also spoke of missing her husband, Jennifer's father, who had died some years earlier. Rick was in a daze and often sat staring into space. He slept badly and hardly ate.

Rando (1993) suggested that, in this early time of grief, bereaved people are engaged in the process of recognizing the loss. This process has two parts: 1) acknowledging that the death has occurred and 2) understanding the death itself. This is very much in keeping with Worden's (1982) task of accepting the reality of the death. In reviewing the normal responses of bereaved people, it is helpful to keep these processes in mind because they provide a view of the purpose of grieving at this transition.

In the days and weeks following a death, emotions vary widely. Generally, people feel periods of numbness that are experienced as "doing all right," "being in a fog," "being on automatic pilot," or not feeling anything at all. Bereaved people may wonder why they are doing so well and think that they did their grieving before the death. These periods of numbness are, however, usually interspersed with times of quite powerful feeling. Crying, sobbing, or wailing express deep sadness and longing. These alternating waves of feeling and numbness seem to bring the reality of the death into the bereaved person's awareness in stages. The numb times between waves are nature's way of allowing people to have a rest, do the things that need to be done, take care of business, and put one foot in front of the other without seeing too far ahead.

Bereaved people are often frustrated with how poorly their minds seem to be working. They complain of forgetfulness, poor concentration, and even confusion. In fact, their minds are often busy with constant thoughts of the person who died and the death itself. They may daydream about the person as if he or she were still alive or forget for a moment that the person has died. Generally, people catch themselves very quickly and are shaken to have forgotten. Former caregiving routines still influence bereaved family members. They may wake up suddenly, thinking that they must check on the ill person or give medications, only to realize once again that the person is gone. This sort of "denial" and the recurring awareness of loss it triggers is part of the process of beginning to assimilate the reality of this death.

As family members continue to go over the events of the person's illness and death, they are trying to understand what has happened. Despite having seen the decline, the symptoms, and the frailty, people struggle with the reality of death. They need to find an explanation or understanding that works for them. Even when people have been given good information about causes and changes at the time of death, they may need to review it again and again. It can be important to

FUNERAL BLUES

Stop all the clocks, cut off the telephone,
Prevent the dog from barking with a juicy bone,
Silence the pianos and with muffled drum
Bring out the coffin, let the mourners come.

Let aeroplanes circle moaning overhead
Scribbling on the sky the message He Is Dead,
Put crepe bows round the white necks of the public doves,
Let the traffic policemen wear black cotton gloves.

He was my North, my South, my East and West,
My working week and my Sunday rest,
My noon, my midnight, my talk, my song;
I thought that love would last forever; I was wrong.

The stars are not wanted now: put out every one;
Pack up the moon and dismantle the sun;
Pour away the ocean and sweep up the wood,
For nothing now can ever come to any good.

–(Auden, 1936)

---

re-examine any number of fears, including a fear that the person starved to death or that something could have prevented or at least forestalled the death. These repeated opportunities for review, coupled with relatively simple explanations, can go far to alleviate people's concerns. Reminders about the many physical changes that occurred at the end or reflection on how the illness had progressed so far that the body could no longer function provide reassurance that even intensive interventions could not have prevented the death.

The beliefs and values of bereaved people may be challenged as their sense of the world, fairness, and safety are shattered. People can feel quite disoriented (McGee, 1993) because their faith is shaken, or they can be angry with God for allowing this death to occur. Along with this, people may experience a loss of meaning or hope in their own lives. They may want to die, too, and be with the person who died. These are not usually suicidal thoughts, but potent expressions of longing for the person and a desire for relief from emotional pain. A search for meaning and value may emerge out of questions about this death.

Bereaved people, especially those who have been present throughout the illness and death, are often exhausted and lack energy. They can be surprised at just how exhausted they are in the aftermath of intense caregiving. People may be distressed by shortness of breath and heart palpitations. Although these are common reactions to the stress of loss, a physician should check out these symptoms. It is important that the family physician knows about the death and guides care of the bereaved person accordingly. A physician who is knowledgeable about normal grief reactions can help bereaved family members cope with their grief by providing reassurance about related health concerns and common physical reactions to grief, such as difficulty sleeping, digestive upsets, lack of appetite, and anxiety. Anti-anxiety or sleeping medication may be prescribed on a short-term basis, but a physician who understands the grief process will refrain from prescribing anti-depressants and tranquilizers for sorrow and longing. In a study by Kissane, Bloch, and McKenzie (1997), the use of psychotropic medications correlated with poor bereavement outcome. The precise relationship between medications and outcome was not explored, but the use of such medications may interfere with the normal experience and the expression of grief.

Interventions

These psychosocial interventions have been designed to specifically address the key consideration *grief reactions*. There are several assessment questions that will help open up a discussion, followed by more focused comments or tips that will facilitate further exploration of the issues that frequently arise at this time; each tip is followed by a sample dialogue.

Assessment Questions

- Tell me about Joan's death. What was your experience?

- How are the people around you responding to your grief? What is it like for you to talk about Ivan and about how you are feeling since he died?

- How are you feeling physically? What are you noticing about your patterns of eating and sleeping?

- Is there anything about your grief that you are concerned about? About other family member's grief?

Provide information about what is normal in grief at this time. The range of reactions and responses may surprise bereaved people. Written information gives them something to refer back to at a time when their memory and concentration are poor.

> *"You thought that you were doing fine until your mother's birthday last week, Marlow. Then you found yourself missing her terribly. For most grieving people, the first year can be full of calendar days that are chal-*

lenging—like your mother's birthday and, maybe, her wedding anniversary, Mother's Day, Hanukkah, and any other family celebrations that are important for you."

Name the person who died and ask what happened at the time of death. This helps people to engage with their grief and provides an opportunity to reframe misapprehensions or answer questions.

"Tell me about the time leading up to Will's death. What stands out for you? Is there anything that you wondered about at the time or has anything come up for you since?"

Give bereaved people permission to be in their present state. They can begin to recognize what is their own "normal" in grief.

"Chantelle, you tell me that you feel exhausted. I know that Allan died at home and that you nursed him, more or less 24 hours a day, for quite a while. It's not surprising that you feel so depleted. Fatigue is the most common symptom for bereaved people in the early days of grief. How might you give yourself a chance to rest and recuperate?"

Reassure bereaved people that it is all right to take care of themselves and their unique needs at this time. This reassurance allows them to limit or ask for company, or to experience the on-and-off nature of their grief.

"Your daughter seems very concerned that you should go out with friends regularly. She wants you to get on with your life. Like so many newly bereaved people, though, I get the impression that you find social gatherings too much right now and you would rather stay quietly at home. What would it be like to share these feelings with your daughter and to ask her to give you the time you need to grieve?"

Bereavement Follow-Up

The hospice palliative care team had been quite close to Jennifer's family and wondered how the children would cope with their mother's death. They expressed concern to the bereavement team about Rick because he depended on Jennifer for most of the decision making in the family. Elaine continued to be anxious and dependent and didn't want to be left alone. She feared she would be unable to manage when Judy went home. She also spoke of missing her husband, Jennifer's father, who had died some years earlier.

This is a time when the palliative care team is making decisions about who will receive bereavement follow-up and what services might be offered. The transition from the familiar patient care team to new personnel, or even a new service organization, can be hard for the family members. When services that were involved with caring for the person who died are withdrawn, family members may feel ignored and abandoned. At this time, it is important for care providers to bring closure to their relationship with the family, introduce the bereavement team, and give information about alternative supports in the community.

An assessment of the family for indicators of bereavement risk or the possibility of difficulties in grieving can be accomplished in a number of ways. The family history taken during the illness, the referrals of the patient care team, and discussions with family members following the death provide such information. Demonstrations of the family's ability to adjust to change before the death and the perception of family coping are important indicators of positive bereavement outcome (Kissane et al., 1997). Therefore, the patient care team's assessment of family functioning can guide those offering bereavement follow-up. Risk indicators (see sidebar) are well documented in bereavement and summarized in an article by Kelly et al. (1999). People who have several risk indicators apparent in their history or assessment

RISK INDICATORS IN BEREAVEMENT

- History of difficulty in the relationship with the person who died
- Challenging circumstances of the death (e.g., violent, disfiguring)
- Intensity of grief reactions, both in anticipatory grief and bereavement
- Poor quality of support network, including family, as perceived by bereaved person
- History of unresolved losses (e.g., grief, abuse, abandonment)
- Concurrent stresses (e.g., job or relationship difficulties, other caregiving roles, financial distress)
- Multiple losses
- History of drug or alcohol use
- History of illness, mental health issues, developmental problems

From Cairns, M., Johnson, A., & Wainwright, W. (1993). Bereavement care: A plan for grief support. Victoria, British Columbia, Canada: Victoria Hospice Society; *adapted by permission.*

often experience complex and powerful reactions to the death and may require a higher level of service and an early offer of support.

Because it is difficult for bereaved people to ask for help, initiating contact with them becomes an important aspect of bereavement follow-up support. A study by McLean (2000) indicated that this is the aspect of support most appreciated by bereaved people whether it comes from formal bereavement programs, family physicians, or friends and neighbors. Offering knowledgeable and compassionate follow-up provides opportunities to give normalizing information. Keeping in touch combats isolation and provides opportunities to grieve.

FOCUS ON: SUDDEN OR VIOLENT DEATH AND BEREAVEMENT FOLLOW-UP

Representatives of many hospice and palliative care programs are asked, by individuals, health care professionals, and other community organizations, to provide bereavement support services to those people in the community at large who have had a sudden or violent death in their family. Before extending services to these individuals it is important to consider the current resources and expertise within the hospice bereavement program, other resources available in the community, and the particular needs of people grieving sudden or violent deaths. It is likely that the situation or problems of these bereaved individuals will be very different from the bereaved people in hospice palliative care.

What Is Different About These Situations?

Deaths considered sudden or violent may include murder, suicide, motor vehicle accidents, drowning, and unexpected deaths from medical problems. A number of different systems, such as acute medical care, emergency response, and the justice system, will often be involved. The media may also be involved. Other problems may have been part of the picture, such as mental health issues or social issues such as prostitution or drug use.

Bereaved people in such situations have a need for consistent, skilled, and intensive support. The complexity of grief experienced by bereaved people following such a death can be overwhelming and extended. Emotions are intense, and the sense of chaos bewildering (Rando, 1993). These aspects affect resources, as the level of support needed requires more time and expertise than some hospice and palliative care programs can provide. Usually, individual counseling and/or groups with a particular focus, such as suicide bereavement groups, are required. People grieving sudden or violent deaths do not always fit into existing support groups because these individuals are particularly vulnerable and find groups overwhelming. They can take up a lot of group time with a multiplicity of issues and feelings. Also, the intensity of their reactions and the horror of their stories may be very hard for other bereaved people to hear. Conversely, the stories of supportive care and peaceful death are hard for them to hear.

Professionals and volunteers who work with people grieving sudden or violent deaths often feel out of their depth and question their competency. The depth of emotion and the traumatic aspects of the deaths can be distressing. These bereavement team members will need to debrief their work, their own feelings, and their responses with supervisors and peers. Over time, physical or professional isolation or a lack of consultation can leave bereavement care providers at risk for stress and possible burnout.

Points to Consider When Offering Bereavement Support to People Dealing with Sudden or Violent Death

- It is difficult to refuse requests for help if there is a lack of other resources in the community. Acknowledge that the time spent here may take time away from the regular palliative care work of the bereavement service.

- Be clear about your mandate and your resources. Make a conscious choice about whether you can provide staff time, expertise, and supervision to create and maintain appropriate services.

- Understand the issues of these bereaved people, the potential need in your community, and whether you can offer relevant help. Avoid overly optimistic thinking such as "It's only this one person who is in so much pain and we want to help," or "This person will fit into our existing services without any problems." You may be inundated with referrals and not have the infrastructure to respond appropriately.

- Consider whether you can refer the person to other agencies or experts in your community who could provide counseling and support. If not, perhaps you could partner with another agency in providing certain services.

- Provide your staff and volunteers with information and regular, ongoing training about common issues and interventions in grief following a sudden or violent death. Provide regular supervision to support those who are working with people grieving sudden or violent deaths.

- Know your community resources. Develop working relationships with other community services, such as mental health services, drug and alcohol services, programs for the survivors of abuse, and so forth. Refer people for issues other than grief.

- Be aware of other resources for these bereaved people (see the resources section at the end of this chapter).

Interventions

These psychosocial interventions have been designed to specifically address the key consideration *bereavement follow-up*. There are several assessment questions that will help open up a discussion, followed by more focused comments or tips that will facilitate further exploration of the issues that frequently arise at this time; each tip is followed by a sample dialogue.

Assessment Questions

- Tell me about your grief. How are you coping with your thoughts and feelings?

- How would you describe your relationship with Sidney?

- What other losses or stresses are you facing at this time? Major changes in your life, illness or health issues, recent deaths?

- How can we support you, given the services we offer?

Identify your services and the expectations that people can have in terms of follow-up. This establishes the normative nature of follow-up and allows people to make choices.

> *"I'd like to tell you about a number of services we can offer through the first year. There are bereavement volunteers who can check in with you periodically to see how you are doing. We can also mail helpful information such as tips for coping with holidays or anniversaries. What do you think might help you?"*

Assess for normal grief. Normalize that it is quite usual for people to feel that they are doing fine. Give the person permission to reach out if they wish for more support at a later time.

> *"Francine, I'm glad to hear that you are doing well. It sounds like you're having the normal ups and downs of grief and that you have good supports that you can count on. I would certainly hope and expect that you will continue to manage well through your bereavement. I would like you to know that, if you hit a tough patch, you can call us to talk things over and to see if there is any way that we might be helpful at that time."*

Assess for risk factors or indicators of difficult grief. Offer immediate and ongoing services from your organization and/or from appropriate community services.

> *"It sounds like you have a lot on your plate right now as you are grieving your mother's death and struggling in your marriage. We can certainly offer you support for your grief through some of the services we have discussed. I'm wondering, Donald, if you would like some information about marriage counseling services for you and your wife?"*

Family Interactions

> Though Judy stayed with Elaine at first, she soon returned to her own home, job, and family. She felt that she was doing fine, but was concerned about her mother and Rick. Elaine continued to be anxious and dependent and didn't want to be left alone. She feared she would be unable to manage when Judy went home. Rick continued to be in a daze. Jesse talked easily to friends about his feelings, but Sarah found it hard to pay attention and felt that certain classmates picked on her.

Many bereaved people turn to their relatives with expectations that their best support will come from within the family. Although family members may wish to provide strength and encouragement for each other, this can be complicated by the differences between and among them. One of the most difficult aspects of grief is that each family member will grieve in a unique way and on his or her own timetable. Each person's grief will be influenced by the relationship with the person who died, any previous experiences of loss, concurrent stresses, and his or her particular personal style in grief (Rando, 1993).

Not everyone has the same comfort level with expressions of emotion. This will vary with the personal style and present circumstances of the people involved. Often, families have certain patterns and tacit rules about what should or should not be expressed. Grief reactions may transgress these rules and result in discomfort among family members, or in negative judgments about how a particular family member is grieving. One person's expression of feeling may touch off another's reaction. This may provide an opportunity for deep sharing if, for example, one person's sadness puts another in touch with his or her own sadness or sense of compassion. Both people may be left feeling unsupported and vulnerable if they are unable to respond to each other in the midst of grief, however, such as when sadness in one person triggers feelings of anger in another family member.

Questions, concerns, and feelings arise that may be difficult to sort out when everyone is feeling vulnerable. It is natural in the early days of grief for bereaved people to review the illness and death of a family member. What happened, and who did what, will be gone over repeatedly and in detail. Each family member appraises his or her own behavior and that of other family members. People may worry about decisions made in the care of the person who died if they experience a sense of failure or guilt about not being good enough as caregivers. They may criticize themselves for choices made (e.g., "I should have come sooner," "I didn't understand that death was so close") or blame another for some aspect of the situation (e.g., "If you weren't so busy at work all the time, you could have been there when Dad asked for you"). Some family members may turn their heightened sense of concern onto others whom they perceive to be in trouble in their grief. This attention may not, however, be particularly welcomed by the recipient family member.

Sometimes the pain and stress of the loss is expressed through anger and recrimination. These emotions may be focused on the estate and finances as people argue about the belongings of the person who died and who gets what. Family members may think that they have certain rights and responsibilities to make decisions, or at least to be consulted, in situations that others see as their sole responsibility. The funeral or memorial service, the disposal of ashes, and the dispersal of belongings can be fraught with injured feelings. Old patterns of interaction, unresolved conflicts, and sibling rivalries may surface when families are together in stressful times, possibly in tight quarters, or perhaps for the first time since the events that caused an estrangement. Volatile sensitivities can make family decision making a minefield. As such issues are faced and dealt with, family cohesion is affected either as people come closer in understanding each other or further apart as conflict and judgment increase.

When a family member dies, the roles and responsibilities within the family are permanently altered. Sometimes the role of the person who died (e.g., the peacemaker, the mediator, the funny one) cannot be fulfilled by anyone else in the family, which leaves them experiencing empty, painful spaces. As the family struggles to adjust to these changes, some of the roles and responsibilities of the person who died may be taken on by other people. As others step into these roles (or fail to step into them), the process is not always easy because the changes feel strange and new to everyone. Expectations of who will now handle various responsibilities need to be sorted out according to what is realistic and workable. Conflict may arise as people find themselves in new relations to each other. Siblings, for example, may find that old rivalries reappear when a parent is no longer there to mediate, or a bereaved spouse may find in-laws difficult to deal with directly. Inter-relationships shift dramatically as the family strives to find a new balance among the surviving members.

Interventions

These psychosocial interventions have been designed to specifically address the key consideration *family interactions*. There are several assessment questions that will help open up a discussion, followed by more focused comments or tips that will facilitate further exploration of the issues that frequently arise at this time; each tip is followed by a sample dialogue.

Assessment Questions

- What do you miss about your stepfather? What new roles and responsibilities do you have now?

- How are members of your family handling this?

- How do you share your thoughts and feelings about the death with your family?

- How are you able to support each other?

- What other changes have happened as a result of this death?

Facilitate discussion and understanding of individual differences within the grieving family. Encourage them to communicate their particular concerns and style to others in their support network. Normalize the unique grieving pattern that each person will have and the challenges of being supportive to each other.

> *"Marjorie, you brought your mother here today because you are concerned that she is crying every day. You say that you cried together at the funeral but now you think that it is important to focus on the good memories. This works for you, but let's hear how this might be different for your mother."*

Explore and identify the new roles that the bereaved person may have. This helps to determine whether the person is willing and able to fulfill these roles and to identify choices or options.

> *"Some of your siblings are telling you that you should be keeping the family together because you are the only one who is married with children of your own. What does this mean to you? How do you feel about taking on this new role?"*

Clarify how the family is coping with making decisions, settling the estate, and distributing personal mementos of the person who died. This allows people to share challenges and disappointments and ask for help with difficult communication.

> *"Your stepson, Rob, is the executor of your husband's estate. How is he keeping you informed about what he is doing? How are you being included in the decisions that affect you? Have there been any problems?"*

Social Support and Expectations

> Over the next weeks, many people called or visited the family and brought food to the home. Some normal routines returned. The children played with close friends and returned to school. Rick felt pressured by his employer to decide when he would return to work. He refused to go to church or to let Reverend Allen visit. He was irritated by all the advice he received from people about when and how he should proceed.

The social demands during the time following a death often challenge people who are already vulnerable and exhausted. The numbers of people who attend the funeral, visit the home, or call to offer condolences can be a mixed blessing for newly bereaved people. Although appreciating the show of support, the family may be exhausted by the effort of responding to and engaging with others. Some bereaved families may choose to withdraw from their larger social circle and be close or private. Family members may be angry if they end up having to support friends and acquaintances. If bereaved people are not getting the support that they want or expect, they may feel a sense of abandonment or isolation. They can resent having to reach out and ask for support when they believe it should be forthcoming.

Within the family, each person will respond to social situations in ways that are consistent with their personality and grief. Some family members may find it very hard to be alone or to manage the day-to-day routines and will want close friends and relatives to help and to be with them. For others, time alone is imperative. These people find solace in quiet retreat where they can collect themselves. Some people will want to talk about the death and express their feelings, whereas others will want to do things and be active rather than discuss their grief (Martin & Doka, 2000).

Family and friends may be keeping a pretty close eye on a newly bereaved person: visiting regularly, providing meals, and staying for a while before returning to their own routines. Often, these well-meaning folks are impatient for the bereaved person to show signs of recovery so they themselves can get back to their life. Bereaved people may wonder themselves how soon they should be getting back to normal and returning to work, social responsibilities and so forth. People hope that a return to former, familiar activities equals a return to normal. As other people's lives return to normal, however, bereaved people find that they don't have a "normal" anymore. In fact, rather than subsiding, grief and the reality of the death are becoming more accentuated.

In North American culture, there is a "fast food" mentality that things should be done quickly. This extends to bereavement and grief. Many employers offer 3 days of bereavement leave and then expect an employee to return to work as usual. In fact, the workplace can be especially difficult for bereaved people as they are unlikely to be able to function normally. For many bereaved people, the emotional fragility and cognitive impairments that they experience as a part of grief interfere with performance of their jobs. Sometimes people are unable to work and are faced with applying for and dealing with long-term disability insurance plans. Employee assistance plans may provide a number of counseling sessions for the worker and family members. Trying to balance the need to grieve and the need to work presents a challenge to bereaved people.

On the one hand, if colleagues and supervisors are not aware of the effects of grief or do not acknowledge the loss, this can add extra pressure and exacerbate the difficulties bereaved people have with concentration and organization. On the other hand, too much interest can feel invasive and patronizing. If co-workers frequently ask about the person's bereavement, the bereaved person may not want to share the vulnerability they feel. If co-workers talk openly about the death, bereaved people may be in constant emotional turmoil and may thus be unable to work. Designating one person to discuss with the bereaved person what feels most helpful to them can resolve awkwardness on both sides and establish lines of communication that feel more supportive.

If a family belongs to a particular faith community, that community can offer support in practical, social, and spiritual forms. Bereaved people may feel judged or judge themselves about whether they are doing it right or grieving in a manner consistent with their faith. They may, therefore, avoid the support offered. When bereaved people's beliefs are challenged by a death, they may find it hard to admit this to anyone within their faith community and feel isolated, or isolate themselves, from accustomed support.

Some cultures have very clear mores about the behavior of the bereaved family and their community. Rituals and behaviors are clearly established. Everyone knows what is expected of him or her. These traditional ways may provide a haven

HELPFUL INFORMATION FOR FAMILIES AND FRIENDS OF A BEREAVED PERSON

- Acknowledge the death as soon as you can. Do not let fear that you will not say or do the right thing hold you back. Say that you are sorry to hear of the death, mention the person by name, and be willing to listen to what the bereaved person may say.

- Be genuine by being yourself. Continue your usual relationship with the bereaved person. A close friend will want and expect caring contact, but do not assume an unfamiliar intimacy.

- Listen to the bereaved person. Allow him or her to repeat his or her story. Sharing memories of the person who died can be very comforting for you and the bereaved person.

- Be willing to talk about the person who died. It is okay to reminisce and to bring up the person's name in conversation.

- Learn about grief. Ask the library for some books on grief. Check out local resources.

- Accept that you cannot take the pain away. Trying to cheer up a bereaved person denies the significance and depth of his or her grief.

- Reach out to offer support. Many bereaved people are concerned about being a burden on friends and family.

- Be patient. Mourning takes lots of time, and grief never goes away entirely. Understand that everyone grieves in his or her own way and at his or her own pace. Accept the bereaved person's evaluation of the significance of the loss and the depth of his or her feelings. Don't judge how long a person's grief appears to be taking.

- Remember that there is no right way to grieve. Avoid criticizing how someone is grieving; you cannot know what is best for them.

- Expect that your own grief may be triggered. Personal feelings of loss or grief may be related to this death or to losses that happened in your own past.

- Offer practical help. In the days after the death has occurred, help with answering the telephone, do errands and shopping, or take care of the children. Later, share a regular walk or outing and remember anniversaries, birthdays, and special holidays. When the bereaved person is ready, include him or her in social gatherings with new people, encourage the individual's growing independence, and continue to remember and talk about the person who died.

---

of comfort and safety in the time of stress and change following a death. Some family members may find these traditions awkward or restrictive, however, as expectations do not fit the reality of their concerns.

Despite any disparities between the concerns and expectations of bereaved people and the ability and willingness of their community to provide sensitive and supportive caring, social support and the perception of being supported are significant factors in how well people cope in bereavement. If a person has limited social support, or perceives it as limited, the first task in grief support is to establish connections that provide a sense of safety, acceptance, and presence.

Interventions

These psychosocial interventions have been designed to specifically address the key consideration *social support and expectations*. There are several assessment questions that will help open up a discussion, followed by more focused comments or tips that will facilitate further exploration of the issues that frequently arise at this time; each tip is followed by a sample dialogue.

Assessment Questions

- What is being with other people like for you right now?

- Do you feel well-supported? In what ways? By whom?

- In what ways has your employer (supervisor, colleague) responded to your bereavement? Has this felt supportive and understanding?

- Tell me about the traditions in your culture that guide you at this time. How are these for you?

Offer information about the range of normal responses to social situations in this phase of grief. This can be a huge relief to bereaved people as they notice their own and other's reactions.

> *"Your wife is glad to have family staying with you since your daughter Ashley died, but you wish you could just be by yourselves. Part of what distresses you about this is that you are normally a friendly and welcoming person. A lot of bereaved people find that their needs are different from their usual habits and that these needs change as they go along in their grief journey."*

Discuss people's concerns and help to identify where they may want to ask for support, patience, or privacy. This helps people to be honest in their communications with others and to take some control of their situation.

> *"You've said it's comforting to know that people are thinking about you and you are concerned that you might offend them if you don't answer*

their calls, yet you find it overwhelming to have more than one or two tele-phone calls a day. Tristan, how might you let others know what works for you at the moment?"

Identify cultural influences on the grieving process. Your openness and sensitivity establish trust and permit discussion of appropriate grief support.

"You've told me that in your nation, the elder's tradition is to remove all belongings and pictures of the person who died and store them for a year, and that you found this practice helpful since your brother's death. Tell me more about that."

Practical Matters

Rick avoided the business of settling Jennifer's estate and lost his temper when someone at the bank said she would need proof of Jennifer's death. Judy offered to help Rick sort out Jennifer's things, but he wanted everything left as it was.

Newly bereaved people are required to make a number of major decisions at a time when this is particularly challenging. They must finalize the arrangements for any service or ritual that will take place. They must begin to deal with the business of settling the person's affairs and the many details and documents involved. Many complications often arise that require patience, attention, and repeated rounds of advice, information gathering, and submission of forms and documents. These tasks bring people into contact with unfamiliar systems and with those who may unwittingly intrude on their vulnerability. Already stressed by death and loss, they may experience a sense of helplessness, frustration, or rage.

Decision making is difficult for bereaved people. Their memory, concentration, and perspective are affected by grief, so that they may have little confidence in their abilities. If their spouse or partner has died, there may be no one with whom to discuss plans, share decisions, or consider consequences. Sometimes there is no clear right or wrong decision in a particular situation. Bereaved people may find it very challenging to operate where a coin toss or leap of faith is required. It may be helpful for them to consider whether such decisions can be delayed until later. Major decisions, such as selling the house, moving closer to other family members, or investing large sums of money should be postponed, if possible. Bereaved people, especially those without close family and friendship networks, are vulnerable to being exploited at this time, as judgment about other people can be poor.

Settling the estate can be a complex and exhausting task. It may take several months to complete all the required business. Learning unfamiliar skills for dealing with financial affairs can be overwhelming for a bereaved person. The person may want and need help to probate the will, pay bills, invest money, and/or plan his or her financial future. For some people, keeping busy can be safe and comforting and an effective way to control or master feelings. If people are not comfortable expressing emotion or are not ready to acknowledge the impact of this death, keeping busy may be a significant coping mechanism for them.

Dealing with the clothes and personal belongings of the person who died can be very emotional for family members as thoughts and memories surface in relation to these material reminders. People who make speedy or rushed decisions, for whatever reasons, may regret this later. Others may delay because they lack energy, are not up to the decisions involved, or are comforted by the presence of familiar things. There is no particular time when this must be done and each person can move at his or her own pace. Some people may experience pressure from others who wish them to "get on with things," however, and sooner or later all of these practical tasks need to be done. They are concrete ways in which a bereaved person can reclaim life and create some order out of chaos.

Interventions

These psychosocial interventions have been designed to specifically address the key consideration *practical matters*. There are several assessment questions that will help open up a discussion, followed by more focused comments or tips that will facilitate further exploration of the issues that frequently arise at this time; each tip is followed by a sample dialogue.

Assessment Questions

- How are you managing to take care of the business end of things? In what ways are you getting help with this?
- Tell me about any important decisions that you are making.
- How are you pacing yourself in dealing with business affairs?

Identify the decisions that are challenging. Facilitate decision making through teaching some simple techniques. This gives bereaved people tools to use with other decisions.

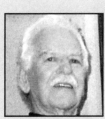

In My Own Voice
A Letter to Mel

James Dolan

James Dolan wrote this letter to a bereavement support volunteer after his partner Gordon died.

When a person dies and their loved ones are distraught, sometimes they "clear the closets." But I believe there is great spiritual comfort in having something to wear that the dead person wore. This is not just superstitious; I have found great comfort in doing this. I have a friend who is the most saintly, holy, sensitive man I have ever known. After Gordon's death, he asked for a memento or reminder. I said, "You can have anything that you would like," and he said, "Maybe a shirt."

I gave him Gordon's two "best" shirts, one almost new and one very old. He wears these shirts occasionally, and when I visited him at Christmas, he wore one on Christmas Day and the other to our New Year's dinner. I know he wore those shirts to comfort me, but he also wore them to comfort himself and his wife. I had never told him about my belief that by wearing the clothing of someone who has died we may bring their spirit closer to us. I also believe that doing this on a festive occasion reminds us of the spirit of other happy occasions that we shared. It also shows we are thinking of the person, and I believe that he will know.

Some people may think these ideas are a little odd, maybe kooky, but we must remember that our spiritual lives are not separated from our daily living, but are part of it.

The spirit is sometimes referred to as "light," so it seems to me that to light a candle and remember your loved one is a very good thing to do. I find such rituals help in my healing, whether it is during a private, quiet moment or a family celebration. I will always feel sadness on these occasions, no matter how festive they are, but this simple act will indeed help lighten the sadness and even bring me some joy.

"Julie, your partner was a talented artist and now you have a large collection of paintings. You are wondering what to do with them. Would it be helpful if we looked at your alternatives together and made a list of the pros and cons for each one?"

Provide information on dealing with practical matters. Some guidelines on settling financial and estate matters can assist bereaved people to get started with these tasks.

"You are wondering where you begin in terms of looking after your cousin's estate. This job of being executor feels pretty big. I can give you information that can help you begin. I have a list of the documents that you will need and the organizations to contact."

Encourage people to get professional help and advice on matters they feel unable to handle at this time. Normalizing this need gives bereaved people permission to do the things they want and to hand over those that they don't.

"Dealing with investments and making financial decisions is new for you. It is really hard for people to learn new skills when they are grieving. Do you have an accountant or financial advisor with whom you feel comfortable? How would it feel to get advice and guidance from such a person?"

Explore whether the demands of practical matters are obstructing the grief process. Some matters *do* need to be taken care of promptly, but other matters can be postponed.

"You've been really busy sorting out Jane's pension and insurance and so forth. You said that you have hardly had time to think about anything else. Are you finding time to talk with friends or family about Jane's death? How are you pacing yourself and deciding what's most important for you at this time?"

OUR EXPERIENCE

Our goal following the death of a patient registered with the hospice and palliative care program is to establish contact with significant family members in order to offer bereavement support. The purpose of this is to begin a relationship in which people have opportunities to learn about grief, express their unique experience, and ask for help if they need it.

Although this is a time when support for the family shifts from the hospice palliative care team to the bereavement team, we find that family members are usually quite agreeable to talking with us. Often, they have had contact with many different team members throughout the illness and death and we find that they trust that we will also give them support and compassion. Of course, if the family had a difficult experience with the patient care team, we will reap the consequences of this as well.

In our first contacts with people after the time of death, we acknowledge the impact of the loss on surviving family members. Although the patient's life has come to an end, a new chapter is beginning for the family. As we encourage people to review the illness, death, rituals, and celebrations of mourning, we are affirming that the ongoing story is theirs. We encourage them to begin to attend to themselves. We assess the bereaved family's needs for support now and in the future. We explore the current state of family members' grief and their sense of the support that is available to them within their family and social circle. Our faith in the resiliency of the human spirit allows us to trust that most people will do well with their inner strengths and social connections; however, we recognize that there are certain circumstances related to the death, the grieving person, or the person's life circumstances that make grief especially challenging. We are alert to these factors in the histories and assessments of the team and they guide our level of intervention.

Bereaved people face their future from a variety of stances, ranging from confidence to great trepidation. As previously stated, grief is an unfamiliar experience for many people and they may wonder whether they are grieving properly. We offer information about what they might expect for themselves as they progress through grief. Our belief is that this information promotes resiliency in the fluctuations of grieving and prepares people for the ongoing experience of their grief.

It is our experience that many bereaved family members will dismiss or diminish their own grief at this time. Although people may be feeling fine, our experience tells us that they have not yet felt the full impact of their grief. We discuss with people the possibility that they may feel differently at another time. In discussions with people who are not currently in touch with their grief, or who may truly not be deeply affected, we establish ourselves as nonjudgmental and available.

We discuss our range of services with bereaved individuals at this time, so that they can make informed choices about receiving support from us. We encourage people to accept some form of contact, whether through mail or telephone calls, that maintains a connection. We value both the opportunities to reassess how people are coping and the implicit invitation for bereaved people to consult with us. We encourage people to attend a weekly support group, in which they will have ample opportunity to reiterate their story and hear stories from bereaved people who are at different places along the grief journey. If family members do not feel a need for bereavement follow-up, we accept their choice and keep the door open for them to contact us at any time.

TEAM ISSUES

The reality of transferring care to a bereavement service or to other community resources is not always easy. Team members have often become closely involved with a family and have an intimate understanding of their struggles and strengths. Although health care providers might want to do the bereavement follow-up with families, this is often less than ideal for the family or the professional. The ongoing pressures of caring for those who are ill and dying will always take precedence over bereavement follow-up, and the latter will probably get postponed again and again. This creates feelings of frustration and abandonment for clients and feelings of guilt and inadequacy for team members.

Knowledge and experience lead us to believe that ongoing bereavement contact is valuable as a preventative measure. It allows people to ask questions, talk about their grief or the person who died, and discuss concerns with someone who understands bereavement. It is difficult for the bereavement care team when family members do not wish to be supported and team members are often reluctant to let people go. It is important to respect people's strength and independence and remember that most bereaved people will adjust to their loss without intervention. If bereavement care providers are not sensitive to people's wishes, they may unwittingly undermine bereaved people's confidence in their own personal and social resources. Figure 8.1 illustrates in a humorous way the reactions that bereaved people may have about overeager grief counselors. Although the bereavement team may wish to be inclusive and to offer bereavement follow-up to family members, it is important to be realistic about resource limitations. Each patient may have several family members and each of them may require some level of support. Within a formal program, this means that case loads can soon grow to unmanageable proportions. In situations in which there is no structured follow-up, health care providers such as family physicians could soon be overwhelmed by the concerns and demands of bereaved families and the ongoing support they require.

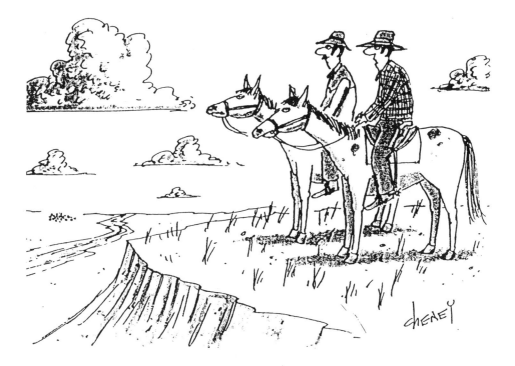

"Hard to tell from here. Could be buzzards. Could be grief counsellors."

Figure 8.1. This cartoon illustrates in a humorous way the reactions bereaved people may have about overeager grief counselors. © 2003 The New Yorker Collection from cartoonbank.com. All rights reserved. Date: April 8, 2003 Representative: Steve Urban, tech.

ABOUT CHILDREN

Children and teens will grieve in ways that reflect their developmental understanding, their previous experience with loss, and the support and information available to them. Children need opportunities to talk about the death, to ask questions, and to share memories and feelings as they journey through grief. Children want to know how their parents feel and how they grieve. They look to adults to learn what to expect and how to deal with all the troubling thoughts and feelings that may surface.

A bereaved child may be full of overwhelming emotions, particularly fear, guilt, and sadness. Often, grieving children express these feelings through behavior, which may make them seem unmanageable and demanding, displaying more sulking, clinging, or misbehaving than usual. These challenging behaviors make it difficult for parents, in the midst of their own grief, to support their children and develop or maintain ways of fostering order and respect in the family. Support from other adults who play key roles in children's lives can be crucial. It is important for the teachers to know about the loss so they can acknowledge the death, offer condolences, and provide assistance with schoolwork. Supportive adults can give the child some protection from the ignorance or discomfort of their peers and help friends understand how to be helpful.

Children's and teens' issues change with each developmental stage. Young children have a very egocentric view of the world and need help to understand that the illness or death is not their fault. Older children often worry about their own health and vulnerability and need reassurances about the health of their parents and others. Young teens, separating from parents and establishing themselves with peers, need guidance to prevent them engaging in acts of rebellion, such as skipping school, vandalism, or theft. Older teens must continue to envision themselves outside the family and plan for their independent future.

Key Points

- The ways in which children and teens express their grief change as they grow and develop. Young children grieve sporadically—in intense, brief bursts of feelings—and then move on to happier activities. In middle childhood, children often express their feelings and their grief physically through their behaviors. Early teens often withdraw and internalize their pain. By the time children are in their later teens, the expression of their grief will be quite similar to that of adults.

- Concrete, specific details that avoid euphemisms help children to comprehend what has happened. Younger children may need frequent explanations that affirm that the person who died will not be coming back to life. Older children want detailed information about the death and what follows. Information about grief reactions helps older children and teens to understand their feelings and responses.

- Children are comforted by an ongoing sense of connection with the person who died. They may want to choose a special memento, such as a photo, trinket, or an article of clothing to keep and to wear. Younger children may express their love and longing through letters, drawings, or collages. Teens may emulate the person who died or focus intensely on their positive and negative qualities and the relationship.

Interventions

Offer information to parents. Understanding grief related to the developmental stages of their children helps parents to feel competent in responding to them.

"One of the things we know is that children grieve differently at different stages in their development. What differences are you seeing between your 5-year-old and your 10-year-old?"

Work directly with families. Encourage ongoing questions and model openness and language that helps parents and children talk about their thoughts and feelings.

"I remember when my dog died. I thought it was my fault. I cried for days and kept asking my mom if he was really dead. Pat, how do you feel when you think about your Dad's death? Whom do you talk to about that?"

Normalize reactions for both parents and children. Acknowledge the challenges for parents of supporting their children while experiencing their own grief and explore alternative supports available.

"Often, parents want to protect children, so they keep their feelings inside. But children learn about how to grieve from the adults in their lives. How would it feel to let your children see you cry? What do you think would happen?" or *"When you feel unable to share your grief with Johannes, is there someone else who can support him?"*

SUMMARY

Death is the transition upon which this entire journey hinges. The patient has died, and his or her body has been taken to the funeral home. Life in the hospice unit or the routine visits of the palliative health care providers has come to an end. As families struggle to accept and understand everything that has taken place, their immediate focus will be on the person who has died, the final hours of life, and the death. Family members make the transition from being caregivers to being bereaved people. Grief is the path between how things were and how they will be. Their journey through bereavement has begun.

The early phase of grief, when a death has occurred, is like walking the edges of the labyrinth; people have not yet experienced the full impact of the loss and the changes it brings (see Table 8.1). Spiritually and emotionally, they are preparing to journey to the center of their grief. Often in a state of shock or disbelief, family members must still deal with the responsibilities, changes, and tasks that

Table 8.1. Phase 1: When a death occurs

Description	Transition and image	Grief task(s)
Immediately following a death, there is a sense of shock, numbness, and disbelief that can last hours or weeks. Panic and strong physical and emotional reactions are common. This period allows people to take information in at a slower rate and to prepare for the adjustments that lie ahead.	The patient dies and, for the family, bereavement begins. Bereaved people face grief. Image: walking the edges	To move from denial to acceptance that the death really has occurred.

Social	Physical	Emotional	Cognitive	Spiritual
On "autopilot" Withdrawal or fear of being alone Unrealistic expectations of self and others Poor judgment about relationships	Shortness of breath, palpitations Digestive upsets Physical symptoms of shock Low energy, weakness, or restlessness	Crying, sobbing, and/or wailing Indifference, emptiness Helplessness, outrage	Confusion, forgetfulness, poor concentration Daydreaming and denial Constant thoughts about the person who died and/or the death itself	Blaming God or "life" Lack of meaning, direction, or hope Wishing to die and join the person who died

are precipitated by a death. This is challenging when people are exhausted, fragile, and perhaps disoriented.

Family members begin to experience the wide range of grief reactions that will affect all aspects of their personal, family, social, and spiritual life. Many people are unfamiliar and uncomfortable with these reactions, whether they experience these themselves or witness them in others. As the numbness wears off, families encounter the powerful thoughts and feelings that accompany them as they enter the depths of the labyrinth and find ways to adjust to this enormous loss.

REFLECTIVE ACTIVITY

Personal Loss Exercise

This exercise can be used in volunteer and staff training as an introduction to grief and loss. It illustrates how much everyone knows about grief from their life experiences and what a broad range of responses and experiences there are in normal grief.

First, participants are asked to work independently to complete Parts 1 and 2. Then, their various responses are reported to the large group and recorded on a flip chart. The process and range of normal grief is introduced using the group members' experiences as illustrations. Part 3 is completed individually and, again, shared in the large group, recording the variety of ways to be helpful and the pitfalls to avoid.

Part 1

Choose a loss from your personal experience. Pick one that you will feel comfortable thinking about and discussing with others.

Part 2

Spend some time remembering your reactions to this loss, both at the time when it occurred and in the adjustment period thereafter. Write down your reactions using the prompts below.

- My behaviors
- My feelings
- My thoughts
- My physical reactions
- My spiritual responses

Part 3

Again, focus for a few moments on your loss and recall the reactions of those people around you at that time.

- What was helpful?
- What was not helpful?
- What did you need that you may or may not have received?

RESOURCES

Books

Caplan, S., & Lang, G. (1995). *Grief's courageous journey: A workbook.* Oakland, CA: New Harbinger.

Christ, G.H. (2000). *Healing children's grief: Surviving a parent's death from cancer.* New York: Oxford University Press.

Coloroso, B. (2000). *Through the rough times: Parenting with wit and wisdom in times of chaos and loss.* Melbourne, Australia: Lothian Pub.

Dershimer, R. (1990). *Counseling the bereaved.* New York: Pergamon Press.

Oliviere, D., Hargreaves, R., & Munroe, B. (1998). *Good practices in palliative care: A psychosocial approach.* Aldershot, UK: Ashgate.

Rando, T. (1984). *Grief, dying and death.* Champaign, IL: Research Press.

Shapiro, E.R. (1994). *Grief as a family process: A developmental approach to clinical practice.* New York: Guilford Press.

Wolfelt, A. (2001a). *Healing a child's grieving heart: 100 practical ideas for families.* Fort Collins, CO: Companion Press.

Wolfelt, A. (2001b). *Healing a friend's grieving heart: 100 practical ideas.* Fort Collins, CO: Companion Press.

Wolfelt, A. (2001c). *Healing a teen's grieving heart: 100 practical ideas for families, friends, and caregivers.* Fort Collins, CO: Companion Press.

Wolfelt, A. (2001d). *Healing your grieving heart: 100 practical ideas.* Fort Collins, CO: Companion Press.

Wolfelt, A. (2001e). *Healing your grieving heart for teens: 100 practical ideas.* Fort Collins, CO: Companion Press.

Web Sites

Grief Net
   http://www.griefnet.org/
Growth House Search
   http://www.growthhouse.org/search.htm
Hospice Net
   http://www.hospicenet.org/index.html
Kid Said
   http://kidsaid.com/
Widow Net
   http://www.fortnet.org/WidowNet/index.html
Parents of Murdered Children
   http://www.pomc.com
Mothers Against Drunk Driving
   http://www.madd.org
The Compassionate Friends
   http://www.compassionatefriends.org
Survivors of Suicide and related sites
   http://www.main.org/sos/
   http://www.1000deaths.com
   http://www.suicidology.org/survivors of suicide

REFERENCES

Cairns, M., Johnson, A., & Wainwright, W. (1993). *Bereavement care: A plan for grief support.* Victoria, British Columbia, Canada: Victoria Hospice Society.

Kelly, B., Edwards, P., Synott, R., Neil, C., Baillie, R., & Battistutta, D. (1999). Predictors of bereavement outcome for family caregivers of cancer patients. *Psycho-Oncology, 8,* 237–249.

Kissane, D., Bloch, S., & McKenzie, D. (1997). Family coping and bereavement outcome. *Palliative Medicine, 11,* 191–201.

Martin, T., & Doka, K. (2000). *Men don't cry... women do: Transcending gender stereotypes of grief.* Philadelphia: Brunner/Mazel.

McGee, P. (1993). *Movements in bereavement.* Unpublished doctoral dissertation, Ontario Institute for Studies in Education, University of Toronto.

McLean, L. (2000). *Expansion of bereavement support services by the Comox Valley Hospice Society.* Unpublished master's thesis.

Rando, T. (1993). *The treatment of complicated mourning.* Champaign, IL: Research Press.

Staudacher, C. (1987). *Beyond grief: A guide for recovering from the death of a loved one.* Oakland, CA: New Harbinger Publications.

Wolfelt, A. (1990). *A child's view of grief: A guide for caring adults.* Fort Collins, CO: Center for Loss and Life Transition.

Worden, W. (1982). *Grief counseling and grief therapy: A handbook for the mental health practitioner.* New York: Springer Publishing Co.

Worden, W. (2001). *Children and grief: When a parent dies.* New York: Guilford Press.

CULTURAL COMPETENCY

"Culture should not be viewed as a singular concept, but rather as incorporating institutions, language, values, religious ideas, habits of thinking, artistic expressions, and patterns of social and interpersonal relationships."

—Lum (2000)

Culture is often passed silently through generations of a family by traditions and ways of being. Everyone is a product of their family's history of experience and tradition. No one person has more or less culture than anyone else.

The title *health care provider* suggests many qualities of counselors, volunteers, nurses, and other caregivers. It implies that they are interested in health, that they care, and that they have something to offer. Most people wear this title with honor and a tremendous sense of responsibility. Health care providers think of themselves as helpers and genuinely want to help other people. Sometimes, in the context of all of this good intention and responsibility, people think that being a caring person is all that is needed to work respectfully across cultural differences. This raises questions about how health care providers view their work in terms of cultural competency. How many professionals have really examined their personal beliefs about what care, culture, or health means? How many of them are so comfortable in their chosen area of expertise that they don't need to challenge themselves to think carefully about what they don't know?

Being a nice, good person is important; being someone who understands how to work across differences in a comfortable, skilled, and competent way is invaluable. Attaining cultural competency, recognizing cultural differences, and working respectfully with people from different cultures goes beyond the mastery of one-day workshops and politically correct language. It is a lifelong process. It requires health care providers to adopt an attitude of deference, humbleness, and curiosity that may not always be supported by their role, work environment, colleagues, or the circumstances in which they find themselves. It is difficult to face people who are in distress—those looking for comfort or reassurance—and not fall back on our expertise or official roles in a way that ignores their knowledge, humanity, and ability to heal themselves. At these times, we may be tempted to direct people into choices that suit us, instead of trusting and empowering people to make their own choices.

A commitment to cultural competency requires people to look critically at themselves and discover their own racist, sexist, heterosexist, ageist, classist, and "ableist" views. Working across cultures can be exciting, threatening, inspiring, or exhausting. Regardless, it is important to remember that even nice, politically correct, caring, and skilled helpers have an inherent degree of bias and ignorance that can lead them to act with insensitivity, disrespect, or undue criticism.

SUGGESTIONS FOR CULTURAL COMPETENCY

- **Self-awareness:** It is important that health care providers reflect critically on themselves and their practice with people of other cultures. This means an ongoing commitment to identify and challenge professional biases and blind spots, as well as to address personal prejudices and limitations.

- **Cultural knowledge:** It is important that health care providers are aware of not only their own cultural background but also the cultural background of their patients and families. They should be interested in the cultural groups in their community and learn about the history, values, and traditions of these populations.

- **Individual focus and attention:** Health care providers should recognize that culturally sensitive care avoids "the cookie cutter approach" to assessment and care. People and their situations should be approached individually, without fixed assumptions or agendas. Even within cultures, it is important to remember that diversity exists and that strict adherence to one set of traditions is unlikely.

- **Institutional sensitivity:** Whenever possible, it is important that routines, programs, and systems be adapted to provide culturally sensitive care. Health care providers need to anticipate and address institutional barriers to caring for people of minority cultures and challenge their own and their colleagues' judgmental responses to differences.

- **Adaptability and flexibility:** In order to provide culturally sensitive care, norms, standards, common definitions, and assumptions should be utilized with caution. In some situations, standard approaches to communication, support, and care may be unhelpful or discriminatory. Therefore, the practice of health care providers should be adjusted to respect unfamiliar or different needs and traditions.

STEPS TOWARD CULTURAL COMPETENCY

- **Be respectful.** Find out what cultural traditions and customs are important to each family. Do not offend people through ignorance, as-

sumptions, or stereotypes. Be open and honest about your inexperi-
ence and uncertainty.

- **Determine needs.** Find out how to be supportive in ways that address the patient's and family's particular lifestyle and priorities. Know that standard expectations or assessments may not fit.

- **Identify barriers.** Find out how comfortable people will be with the way that care is usually provided. Flexibility in expectations, routines, or decision making may be important.

- **Encourage the practice of traditions.** Find out about people's cultural traditions and customs and support their continuance.

- **Educate team members.** Support team members to examine how their personal biases shape their perception of people from different cultural backgrounds. Discourage labels or judgments based on individual or cultural differences.

KEY QUESTIONS TO ASK PATIENTS AND FAMILIES

- How do you feel about being in the hospital? In hospice? At home? How comfortable are you with doctors, counselors, spiritual care providers, and nurses?

- Is there anything in particular that you do or don't want to know about your care?

- What traditions, customs, or rituals are important for you to continue at this time?

- Who are the people that you consider to be part of your family? How would you like them to be involved in your care or decision making at this time?

- Under these circumstances, what is customary for your family to be doing? How can our team help and support you to get what you need?

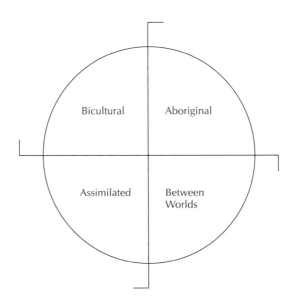

THE MEDICINE WHEEL

The Canadian Royal Commission on Aboriginal People (1996) used this medicine wheel to describe the varying degrees of cultural integration that Aboriginal youth experience. However, it aptly illustrates the struggle to converge worlds that is apparent for any person of a particular cultural heritage that is not represented by the cultural mainstream. These "other cultured" people represent a broad spectrum of variation including people who are gay or lesbian, ethnic and religious minorities, and people who have disabilities or homeless.

Some people, whose culture has been nurtured within the family, their community, and through childhood schooling, function comfortably as bicultural individuals. Bicultural individuals are at home in their traditional culture and also in that of the mainstream. Usually, they are comfortable with the predominant values and norms, and are able to speak the language of the mainstream.

Other people come from environments where their cultural heritage is peripheral to daily life. They may reject their traditional background or feel quite unfamiliar, uncomfortable, or self-conscious about it. Social scientists use the term Assimilated or Acculturated to describe this group.

In some communities, however, people have had exclusive or significant exposure to their cultural heritage and are fully grounded in the traditional cultural value systems and beliefs. These people may reject or struggle with predominant cultural expectations. They are represented by the Aboriginal section of the medicine wheel but can be found in any non-mainstream group.

The Between Worlds group on the wheel represents people who do not identify with either their traditional or the predominant culture. They feel isolated or uneasy in both worlds. When we endeavor to work sensitively across differences, it is imperative that we carefully consider the degree of assimilation that people experience with the mainstream that health care providers typically represent.

Figure 8A.1. The Medicine Wheel illustrates distinct differences in how people of a culture that is not represented by the cultural mainstream are or are not assimilated into the culture represented by health care workers. Source: Canada. Royal Commission on Aboriginal Peoples, *Report of the Royal Commission on Aboriginal Peoples,* v. 3, "Gathering Strength," p. 476, The Commission, © 1996. Reproduced with the permission of the Minister of Public Works and Government Services, 2003, and Courtesy of the Privy Council Office.

- Who is your family spokesperson? How comfortable are you with this?

- What are the customs or traditions of your family when someone is very ill or bereaved?

- Do you have any personal objects, mementos, or images that would help you feel more comfortable in this situation?

- Are there any cultural traditions, rituals, or activities that shape how your family responds right after someone dies?

CULTURAL WORLDS

The Medicine Wheel (see Figure 8A.1) has been used to demonstrate the different levels of integration of young aboriginal people into mainstream Canadian culture. It has applicability for other cultural groups.

RESOURCES

Barrett, R.K. (2001). Recommendations for culturally competent end-of-life care giving. *Virtual Mentor, 3*(12). Retrieved January 19, 2003, from www.ama-assn.org/ama/pub/category/6824.html

Hall, P., & Stone, G. (1998). Palliative care: How can we meet the needs of our multicultural communities? *Journal of Palliative Care, 14*(2), 46–49.

Kaufert, J.M., Pautsch, R.W., & Lavallee, M. (1999). End-of-life decision making among aboriginal Canadians: Interpretation, mediation, and discord in the communication of "bad news." *Journal of Palliative Care, 15*(1), 31–38.

McNamara, B., Martin, K., Waddell, C., & Yuen, K. (1997). Palliative care in a multicultural society: Perceptions of health care professionals. *Palliative Medicine, 11,* 359–367.

Neuberger, J. (1991). Judaism and palliative care. *European Journal of Palliative Care, 6*(2), 166–168.

Oliviere, D. (1991). Culture and ethnicity. *European Journal of Palliative Care, 6*(2), 53–56.

Parkes, C.M., Laungani, P., & Young, B. (Eds.). (1997). *Death and bereavement across cultures.* London: Routledge.

Sharma, K. (2000). A question of faith for the Hindu patient. *European Journal of Palliative Care, 7*(3), 99–100.

Woo, K.Y. (1999). Care for Chinese palliative patients. *Journal of Palliative Care, 15*(4), 70–74.

REFERENCES

Lum, D. (2000). *Social work practice with people of color: A process and stage approach* (4th ed.). Belmont, CA: Wadsworth/Thomson Learning.

Royal Commission on Aboriginal Peoples. (1996). Report of the Royal Commission on Aboriginal Peoples, Volume 3—*Gathering strength*. Ottawa, Ontario: Author.

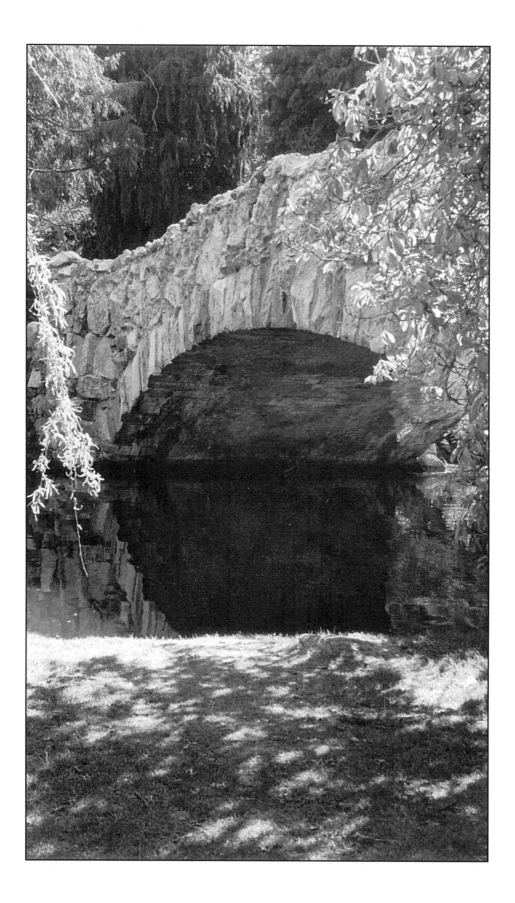

9

Entering the Depths

Adjusting to Loss
Phase 2

*A*s bereaved people begin to adjust to loss and experience the pain associated with it, they are entering the depths of grief. They are in the midst of grief, moving to the center of the labyrinth, searching for meaning and, ultimately, healing and wholeness. People are beginning to experience more intense grief feelings as the numbness of earlier days wears off. The reality of the loss moves from an intellectual recognition to an emotional experience. Most people have sufficient internal and external strengths to manage these strong emotions fairly well. Grief and bereavement are tough, but most people manage to live with their loss and grief and adapt to all of the changes that have come in the wake of the death.

Bereaved people have a whole spectrum of emotional responses, from hopelessness and despair to irritability and anger. VOLATILE EMOTIONS may surprise people because of their intensity and unpredictability. Permission and safety to express grief and vent emotions may be lacking. A few weeks after the death, social support is often less intense or consistent than it was immediately after the death. The individuals who make up these social networks may or may not know how to provide ongoing bereavement support. Bereaved people may find that others expect them to get back to typical activities and feelings when, in fact, they are beginning to feel worse. Getting support and INTERACTING WITH OTHERS can be challenging. Some people will search out alternate sources of support to augment what friends and family provide or to address the difficult issues that have arisen in their grieving.

Grief is a central item in the lives of people at this transition. As people are ADJUSTING TO GRIEF, they move from reviewing the death to reviewing the relationship they had with the person who died. All aspects of the self are affected by grief (Rando, 1993; Worden, 1982). This transition has been described as the shattering of the known world followed by the need to relearn the world (Attig, 1996). People begin to realize that their grief will go on for a while and that they will have good days and bad days.

Normal experiences of bereavement during this transition cover a huge range and will be influenced by "who people are": their age, gender, health, and relationship with the person who died. Their history of loss, the perceived quality of support available to them, and the concurrent stresses and responsibilities that they have will also affect how people grieve. The ways people express their grief and adjust and adapt differ with personality, cultural conditioning, and coping style.

As people experience the depths of their grief, spiritual issues of meaning, connectedness, and transcendence may arise. Bereaved people ask SPIRITUAL QUESTIONS about their own lives, values, and beliefs. They look appraisingly at the world and their place within it. They may seek larger meaning and purpose in something greater than themselves.

PHILIP AND KARI

Philip had suffered multiple losses. His life felt saturated with deep sadness and longing. After his wife, Kari, died he sold their large country home and moved to a small city apartment. During this time, he gave away or sold the accumulation of their 26 years of marriage. Shortly after he moved, his 14-year-old dog also died, and a few months after that, the family doctor who had cared for Kari retired from practice. Philip felt that everything he valued was gone. The funeral home had been disrespectful and insensitive in their dealings with Kari's body and with Philip. He was angry and frustrated. Philip felt emotionally and physically unable to return to work but could not sort out his long-term disability claim with the new family doctor. He contacted his union for help, but they were equally slow in responding. Philip felt isolated, unsupported, and misunderstood.

Still, Philip had some supports that were significant. After he moved to the city, he joined a small church community and felt welcomed by the congregation and the priest. Philip had long discussions with the priest about life and death, faith, and his future. He had friends who reached out to him regularly. A widowed friend told Philip that she had a vision of her husband after his death. This had been a great comfort to her, and Philip longed for some such consolation. Instead, he experienced vivid memories of the traumatic times in Kari's illness and recurring thoughts of her last day. He did not want to burden his friends with these images or his feelings of guilt and regret.

"Give sorrow words; the grief that does not speak, Whispers the o'er-fraught heart and bids it break."

—*Macbeth 4.3.242–243*

Philip felt a great deal of pressure to involve himself in social activities with old friends and with the church members. He found social outings exhausting and depressing and would spend several days in his pajamas after such events, reading on the couch. Though he didn't want to do anything or go anywhere, he felt guilty about not appreciating people's invitations and well-intended advice.

A few months after Kari's death, Philip asked for bereavement counseling though he was uncomfortable about seeking help because he felt that he should just get on with things. He criticized himself for not moving on and was unsure how much of his tears and sadness he could show to others. He was tired of being so tired. At the counselor's suggestion, he attended a bereavement group but found it extremely difficult to hear other people's stories. He felt stuck in his sadness and longing and unable to adjust to life without Kari.

KEY CONSIDERATIONS

Volatile Emotions

Philip had suffered multiple losses. His life felt saturated with deep sadness and longing. After his wife, Kari, died, he felt that everything he valued was gone. Philip was angry and frustrated. Philip felt emotionally and physically unable to return to work but could not sort out his long-term disability claim with the new family doctor. He contacted his union for help, but they were slow in responding. He felt isolated, unsupported, and misunderstood.

Although some bereaved people are comfortable with the depth of their emotions, others may experience powerful emotions or one particular emotional response that has ongoing intensity. These emotional reactions may be unexpected and/or unfamiliar. Some bereaved people can feel overwhelmed and frightened by the magnitude of their emotions. Finding ways to cope with, or even bear, such responses may be difficult due to depleted energy, worries about being "crazy," and the discomfort of friends and family in the face of these emotions.

Both Worden (1982) and Rando (1993) talked about this period as a time when people feel the pain of the loss in many ways and must confront it or work through it. Sorrow, anger, guilt, fear, and hopelessness are some of the powerful emotions that can engulf them to a degree. They may not have any previous experience with such deep emotion, and they may fear expressing these emotions in case they find themselves overwhelmed or judged and avoided by others. They may dull the pain through the use of medications, alcohol, or drugs. Struggling to control unpredictable and explosive emotion can be exhausting and unsuccessful. Often, people will say that they are afraid to start crying in case they cannot stop. Ordinary language describes deep feeling as "losing it," "falling apart," "making a spectacle of oneself," or "creating a scene." Phrases such as these, with negative connotations, make it hard for bereaved people to believe that these painful emotions are natural, normal, or healthy.

Life is full of reminders of both the loss itself and the person who died. Day-to-day existence is full of triggers for memories, and feelings arise unbidden and uncontrolled. Uncertainty about getting through the day without bursting into tears or flying off the handle can undermine a bereaved person's self-confidence. The outward manifestations of emotions, such as tears, frequent sighing, or nervous irritation, can be distressing and embarrassing for the bereaved person and the people around them. Fully expressed deep emotion, such as wailing, rage, or panic is very difficult for most people to tolerate or witness. Intense anger can threaten bereaved people's sense of self-control and the safety of themselves and others. Wailing—that terrible sound of deep despair—is like a siren; it says, "Emergency! Do something!" Most people will want to stop or contain these emotions immediately. When wailing, rage, and panic are the honest experience of a bereaved person, it becomes very difficult for him or her to find the permission and safety in which to express and deal with such emotions.

Interventions

These psychosocial interventions have been designed to specifically address the key consideration *volatile emotions*. There are several assessment questions that will

help open up a discussion, followed by more focused comments or tips that will facilitate further exploration of the issues that frequently arise at this time; each tip is followed by a sample dialogue.

Assessment Questions

- What feelings are you experiencing at this time? How do you express these or share these with others?

- How intense are your feelings? In what ways are they distressing to you? Are they interfering with your ability to maintain routines or fulfill responsibilities?

- In what ways do you try to process, manage, or control these feelings?

"My grief lies all within,
And these external manners of lament
Are merely shadows to the unseen grief
That swells with silence in the tortured soul."

—*Richard II 4.1.294–297*

Encourage people to honor their sadness. This is a natural part of experiencing loss and acknowledging its impact.

"Donna, you are really missing your mother in so many ways. How might you include sorrow as part of your life right now?"

Understand people in their ambivalence about whether life is worth living; people who are uncertain about how to go on benefit from an opportunity to express this ambivalence about life and to explore both their pain and their strengths.

"As I listen to you describe how you are feeling desperately alone since your wife's death, I wonder if life seems pretty empty right now. Bianca was your best friend and companion. What might it be like to let your children know how you are feeling? What might they have to offer you right now?"

Identify the sources of guilt and facilitate forgiveness. Guilt can feel like being stuck in an uncomfortable place in which people cannot forgive themselves for real or imagined failings.

"Jackie, right now you are feeling guilty about a number of things that happened when you were caring for your sister. You were not as kind and understanding as you would have liked to be. Which of these things might you be able to forgive yourself for and let go of now? Are there some others that you are not ready to let go of yet?"

METAPHORS FOR GRIEF AND EMOTION

Onion—As people work through the various emotions of grief, they are peeling away the layers (similar to an onion) with space in between. Also like an onion, growth begins at the center, deep inside the person.

Canal locks—The emotions of grief are similar to the water in canal locks. When bereaved people are filled up with emotion, they need to open the floodgates, to let the emotion flow out. In this way, they are able to move forward to the next stage of their journey and to find equilibrium for a while—until they come to the next lock and fill up with emotion once again and repeat the process.

Waves—Grief comes in waves. When the wave comes to bereaved people, they can be tumbled and bowled over or they can learn to ride the wave until it brings them to shore. Everyone is likely to fall many times in learning to ride.

Walls—Dealing with emotions of grief can feel like running into a wall and having to scale it to get to the other side. At first, the walls (or times of grief) are high, thick, and close together. As time goes by, they generally become smaller, farther apart, and easier to climb until a difficult event or situation creates another high wall.

Wound—Grief is like a wound, a painful open place of hurt. To heal, bereaved people must wash the wound with saline solution, tears, and protect it from further damage. Also, like a wound, grief leaves a permanent scar.

Roller coaster—The emotions of grief are like a roller coaster ride. They feel dangerous and bereaved people can't see what lies ahead. Once they are on the ride, it is more dangerous to try to get off than to stick with it until it is over.

Offer strategies for defusing anger. Holding back anger creates stress, some of which can be released through physical activity that includes big muscle movement. Safety for self and others needs to be considered.

> *"Your family tells you that you are irritable and fly off the handle pretty easily. How might you let off the steam in a way that feels safe? What physical activities do you find helpful?"*

Identify the fears. To begin to manage fears, stop and focus on them directly. A helpful aphorism: "To name it is to tame it." Knowledge about what causes fears empowers people to face them.

> *"Madeline, you are really afraid to go out at night and aren't accepting invitations from friends or family. Would it be helpful to look at the bits that feel scary and see if we can come up with ways to help you feel safe?"*

Explore strengths and strategies. Despite overwhelming emotion, people do generally find some way to keep going.

> *"You've had so much to deal with since Edward's death. We've talked about how you have been feeling sad and angry and hopeless. I'm wondering, how do you keep going? What have you found that helps?"*

Interacting with Others

> Still, Philip had some supports that were significant. After he moved to the city he joined a small church community and felt welcomed by the congregation and the priest. He had friends who reached out to him regularly. Philip felt a great deal of pressure to involve himself in social activities with old friends and with the church members. He found social outings exhausting and depressing, however. Though he didn't want to do anything or go anywhere, he felt guilty about not appreciating people's invitations and well-intended advice.

Social isolation is a common problem during this phase of bereavement, whether or not it is by choice. Some people may find social isolation thrust on them if there is little understanding of or tolerance for grief among their friends and acquaintances. Other bereaved people will withdraw from social connections or carefully choose the people with whom they interact. Interactions with others can be exhausting and frustrating for bereaved people when they are vulnerable and needy themselves. Although family, friends, and community may want to be helpful, they may be unfamiliar with how to respond to or support bereaved people. Those who are grieving may find they are expected to be patient with their acquaintances' awkwardness and expected to teach them how to be helpful.

Bereaved people may be hurt or angry in response to comments on their grief or to uninformed advice. Common misconceptions about grief and well-meant clichés affect the quality of the support that is offered. In modern Western society, there is a lack of knowledge and acceptance of grief and bereavement. For example, many people incorrectly assume that grief declines steadily over time and that it is best for bereaved people to put the person who died out of mind. Also, because grieving takes longer than most people think it should, bereaved people often hear that they should be better than they are.

Certain emotions of grief are more acceptable than others, both individually and socially. For example, anger has few, if any, expressions that are socially acceptable. Other people's discomfort with sadness and despair may lead them to try to get bereaved people to cheer up. Friends and acquaintances can effectively shut down opportunities for sharing such feelings as loneliness when they rush in with well-meaning, but misguided, advice. When bereaved people face constraints on power-fully felt emotions, they may withdraw from much of their usual social interaction.

Society has different expectations about how men and women grieve. Social pressure can create a dilemma for men regarding their emotions. On the one hand, they get the message that they should not express their emotions, as this is a sign of weakness. On the other hand, they are pressed to do so as a sign of how much they cared for the person who died. Men are expected to be strong for others and to take care of them. Bereaved men report that they are rarely asked how they are doing themselves but are asked to report on how the women and children in their families are doing (Worden, 1982). Men may receive more social support in the form of invitations and inclusion in social activities, however. Some bereaved husbands feel pressured to part-ner again long before they are ready to consider this. Women face different expecta-tions. They are expected and encouraged to express their emotions more openly than men and to share their feelings with others. Yet they often experience isolation and ex-clusion from social activities, as their emotionality is seen as a liability or an embar-rassment. Women are freer to ask for professional help with grieving. Women are given permission to grieve longer than men; for example, a bereaved mother may be supported in grieving far longer than the father would be (Staudacher, 1991).

People may wonder about how and where to get help when they are not feel-ing understood or supported and they are struggling with various aspects of their grief. Often, interacting with other bereaved people provides comforting and reas-suring connections through this difficult time. This can be more difficult than it seems, as such a search can consume the meager energy they have left. For some peo-ple, asking for help wounds their pride and sense of self-reliance. Help may come in various forms; books, Internet information and chat rooms, self-help groups, formal bereavement support groups, volunteer companioning, and professional counseling. Monroe (Oliviere, Hargreaves, & Monroe, 1998) explained the difference between bereavement support and bereavement counseling. She suggested that bereavement support bolsters bereaved people's own coping strategies and encourages them so that their personal resources and strengths come into play. Bereavement counseling focuses on resolving challenging issues, teaching new coping skills, and facilitating making changes.

Interventions

These psychosocial interventions have been designed to specifically address the key consideration *interacting with others*. There are several assessment questions that will help open up a discussion, followed by more focused comments or tips that will facilitate further exploration of the issues that frequently arise at this time; each tip is followed by a sample dialogue.

Assessment Questions

- In what ways are your family and friends responding to you? What messages are you getting from them about your grief?

- Who can listen to how you feel and be present with your pain?

- How readily do you ask for help?

Assess the strength of the support network. How supported a particular person feels is related to his or her need for support and the quality rather than the quantity of support offered.

"You come from a large family and a number of your siblings live close by. What kind of understanding and support are you getting from your family? How does this feel for you?"

"Remember that an emotion is just an emotion—neither good nor bad, right nor wrong. Emotions are not rational, but they are very real responses. Emotions or feelings can be uncomfortable but they can't hurt you. To begin, take things a little at a time and deal with each emotion as it comes. Let yourself be in the experience, be curious about it, attend to what it is like in detail, and allow the feeling to move through you and out of you. With practice, you can choose where, when, and for how long to feel your emotions. They become something you journey with rather than something you avoid."

—Lucie Mattar,
Victoria Hospice Counselor

Provide information on grief and grief support to family and friends. Family and friends can provide better support when they are informed about what is natural and what is helpful.

"You want to comfort Elsa, but she won't talk to you about her grief and this is puzzling for you because usually you are able to discuss things together. How are you responding to her tears? How would it be for you to let her cry for as long as she needs to?"

Offer opportunities to be with other bereaved people. Support groups and organizations for widows and widowers and bereaved parents and Internet chat lines bring bereaved people together. These connections are reassuring and comforting for many as affirmation of the normality and naturalness of grief.

"Norman, you are really clear that you don't want to sit around and hear other people talk about their grief. But you think you might want to know some other men who have lost their wives. I know of a walking club for bereaved spouses. What would you think about someone from the club calling you with information about it?"

Adjusting To Grief

Philip found social outings exhausting and depressing and would spend several days after such events lying on the couch in his pajamas, reading. He said that he was tired of being so tired. He felt stuck in his sadness and longing and unable to adjust to life without Kari.

Grief is the central theme in the lives of bereaved people at this transition. Family members are adjusting to being a bereaved person and to living without the person who died. They are learning to live with their grief. Their hearts and minds are full of grief. As the impact of the loss is known hour to hour, day to day, and month to month, the reality of forever is keenly felt. Time can feel like an enemy, as it does not seem to bring healing. Instead, it seems to stand still and yet rush forward. It stretches out emptily before the bereaved person.

Though the future may be impossible to face, the bereaved person reviews the past thoroughly. Memories, good and bad, arise. The whole relationship with the person who died is revisited. If a parent, sibling, or spouse of many years has died, this reviewing process may encompass most of the bereaved person's life. This process has been referred to as "tethered circling" (McGee, 1993), a circling, backward movement in which the person revisits the same thoughts, questions, and memories over and over again while holding onto something that has been found to be helpful. Reviewing is not easy, as emotions arise with the memories. Unfinished business and the difficult aspects of the relationship are identified and efforts are made to find some resolution for these. Bereaved people search for the meaning in the relationship with the person who died. They garner what was learned about life and relationships from both the nurturing and the challenging aspects of this relationship. Over time, they come to remember the person realistically, not as an angel or a devil, but as a human person.

Grief is not a constant through this time. Bereaved people experience fluctuations in their grief that they may refer to as ups and downs, good days and bad days, or waves or spells of grief. The times when grief is not so present are like holidays from grief, or a chance to catch one's breath before the next round of active grieving.

Most bereaved people find that their energy is very low. Their energy goes to grieving, at conscious and unconscious levels, which makes it unavailable for the other areas of life. Along with this lack of energy, they may experience weight gain, sleep disturbances, and exhaustion (see Figure 9.1). When bereaved people experience this profound lethargy, they often describe themselves as feeling depressed. Usually, however, this depression, or deep sadness and void that directly results from grief, is quite different from a clinical depression. It is important to know whether or not a person is depressed because that diagnosis will influence which approach or treatment would be most beneficial (see Table 9.1).

Interventions

These psychosocial interventions have been designed to specifically address the key consideration *adjusting to grief*. There are several assessment questions that will help open up a discussion, followed by more focused comments or tips that will facilitate further exploration of the issues that frequently arise at this time; each tip is followed by a sample dialogue.

Assessment Questions

- How would you describe your grief at this time? How are the ups and downs of grief affecting you?
- How is your energy level right now?
- Tell me about the relationship you had with Diana. What thoughts and memories are coming to you?

Facilitate pacing of activities and advocate self-care. Bereaved people often find it difficult to give themselves permission to grieve purposefully or to rest and rejuvenate.

> *"You are exhausted by the amount of grief you feel while having to keep going at work and at home. How are you finding time for yourself at the moment, Marlene? In what ways are you able to replenish your energy?"*

GRIEVING DIFFICULT RELATIONSHIPS

Difficult relationships with the person who died, those filled with conflict, pain, or mixed feelings, affect how bereaved people grieve. Rando (1993) identified five main problems that bereaved people may face in the aftermath of an ambivalent relationship with the person who died:

1. Reluctance to acknowledge the ambivalence
2. Opposing emotions experienced simultaneously
3. Failure to appreciate the degree of attachment
4. Strong guilt feelings
5. Generalized anger, mistrust, or alienation as a result of the relationship

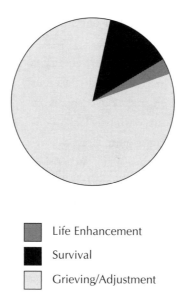

■ Life Enhancement

■ Survival

☐ Grieving/Adjustment

Energy is defined here as the force that allows people to be and to think and to do. Energy can be viewed as a circle (Reeves, 1999). Some people have bigger circles than others, but for everyone, energy is finite. Going past energy limits means needing more rest later. Many grieving people have the same amount of energy they always have had; it is just being used differently.

To illustrate how his or her energy is being used, ask the bereaved person to divide a circle, representing all of the energy he or she has into three pie-shaped pieces. One piece represents the energy they are using for survival, that is, for the activities that must be performed for life to go on. One piece is the energy used for life enhancement or self-care and the things that bring pleasure. The last piece, or remainder, is the energy going to grief. When grief is most intense, most of the available energy goes into grieving. This helps to explain why people feel exhausted or why their concentration and memory are poor.

In using this chart, it is important that people are thinking about their energy as separate from their time.

Figure 9.1. The Energy Circle.

Validate the grief work that people are doing. People need encouragement to trust that what they are experiencing has value and that it assists their grief process or healing.

> *"You've been remembering how things were between you and your father when you were a young child. He was a pretty strict disciplinarian, and you felt angry and ashamed when he punished you. Looking back, Earl, is there anything you can identify now that you learned from these experiences and from your father? How does this affect the way that you live your life?"*

Parkes and Weiss (1983) noted that

These consequences [of the loss of the conflicted relationship] include guilt and self-reproach, lack of sufficient positive memories to support continued feelings of worth, sadness, and anger that the relationship never was what the mourner might have wished it to be, a sense of hypocrisy for mourning what appears to have been such a negative relationship and surprise that the deceased is missed, and the loss of opportunity ever to resolve the conflicts. (cited in Rando, 1993, p. 172)

COMMON CLICHÉS ABOUT GRIEVING

Linn (1986) groups the common clichés about grieving into five categories. There are those that

1. Exhort people to be strong: "The person who died wouldn't want you to cry."
2. Want people to hurry up their grief: "Life goes on."
3. Increase guilt about how people are grieving: "You aren't counting your blessings."
4. Suggest that a religious explanation should be comforting: "God never gives you more than you can handle."
5. Discount and minimize grief: "I know just how you feel."

FOCUS ON: GRIEVING STYLES

It is important for counselors and others who provide bereavement support to have a working image of healthy grief. Assessments are based on this image and judgments about interventions and programs grow from it. There is a shadowy side to the image, however, and from that comes our expectations about how people should grieve. Ideas about gender differences, comfort or discomfort with certain expressions of grief, and beliefs about what is healthy or efficacious are just a few examples of this shadowy side. These biases will affect how care providers help bereaved people, who is supported and understood, and what is offered.

Do you believe, as Staudacher stated, "Simply put, there is only one way to grieve...Only by experiencing the necessary emotional effects of your loved one's death is it possible for you to eventually resolve it" (1991, p. 3)? Many people, including a number of grief counselors, believe that bereaved people must feel their grief and express it fully in order to heal; they should talk about how they feel, weep, rage, and share their fears. Certainly for some people, this way of moving through grief seems to be natural and effective. Some bereaved people, however, do not grieve in this emotional way, nor do they wish to. If this belief is accepted, then bereavement programs, especially support groups, will be designed primarily to facilitate emotional expression. Bereaved people who don't grieve this way may feel pressured to behave in a manner foreign to their usual ways of coping. Judgments about how well a person is doing in their grief will be based on expression of emotion alone.

Who are the people who do not fit into the expressive mode? Is this a matter of gender differences in grieving? Do you believe that men and women grieve

Table 9.1   Grief and depression

Aspect	Grief	Depression
Mood states	Range and variability of moods and feelings Quick shifts from sadness to normal state in the same day Variability in mood, activity, appetite, communication, sexual interest in the same week	Moods and feelings are low, more static, little variability Consistent sense of depletion, psychomotor retardation, anorexia, decreased sexual interest –OR– Compulsive communication, eating, or sexual behavior
Expression of anger	Capable of expression, internally or externally directed	Absence of externally directed anger, internally directed
Expression of sadness	Weeping	Difficulty weeping or controlling weeping
Self-concept	Guilt associated with aspects of the loss Experience the world as empty and meaningless Preoccupation with the loss	The loss confirms they are bad or worthless Focus on punitive thoughts, guilt has global aspect Preoccupation with self
Responsiveness	Periodic, want solitude but respond to warmth and involvement	Static, fear being alone or are unresponsive to others
Pleasure	Sporadic restriction, retain sense of humor	Restrict all pleasure, loss of sense of humor
Reactions of others	Others want to offer support	Others often feel irritated

The deep sadness of grief resembles depression and, in fact, bereaved people often say they feel depressed. A significant loss may trigger or exacerbate a clinical depression but most commonly, the depression felt in grief is directly related to their current situation. It is a response to the distress felt and the change experienced. This table differentiates grief and depression on a number of parameters.

Also, in grief, bereaved people's focus is on the person who died and the loss. Conversely, people who are depressed are more likely to be emotionally flat and focused on themselves. Caution should be exercised in deciding whether a bereaved person is depressed and professional advice sought in situations when concern about the person continues.

From Fleming, J.S. (1986). Psychological intervention with the bereaved. Presented at the Canadian National Palliative Care Conference, Calgary, Alberta, Canada; adapted by permission.

differently? As mentioned previously, socialization, social roles, and social expectations are different for men and women. These factors influence the grief experienced by the bereaved person, the response of the person's social circle, and the assessments of grieving by professionals. Much of the early literature on grief was based on studies of widows, which has led to criticism of this material as being specific to women. More recent efforts have described what men's grief may look like. It has been suggested that themes of men's grief include control of emotion, action, privacy, and a cognitive approach to issues (Moss, Rubenstein, & Moss, 1996–1997; Staudacher, 1991). Golden (1994) stated, "In general, men tend toward action as a primary mode in healing grief while using relating as secondary, and women are the opposite." Simply put, this means that men will do something about their grief, whereas women will share the grief with someone.

Men certainly seem to utilize bereavement support services less than women and may not-so-readily identify themselves or be identified by others as a bereaved person in need of follow-up after the death of a family member (Oliviere, Hargraves, & Monroe, 1998). Yet, it is apparent that men do benefit from support and contact during their bereavement (Tudiver, Permaul-Woods, Hilditch, Harmina, & Saini, 1995).

Table 9.2. Patterns of grief response

	Intuitive grieving	Instrumental grieving
Experience of grief	Feelings of intense inner pain and helplessness	Intellectual response to loss and challenge to adapt
	Inner cues viewed as feelings rather than thoughts	Ability to differentiate thoughts and feelings
	Inability to separate from feelings of others	Ability to maintain sense of control
Expression of grief	Outward expression that mirrors inner experience	Control of feelings and behavior with energy directed toward activity
	Need to share and discuss feelings while working through grief	Need to sit quietly, think, and plan activities
	Low physical energy and depression	High physical arousal, anxiety
Adaptive strategies	Feelings control actions, connections with other people	Need to express feelings in a controlled way through activity
	Time allowed for grief	Restoration of normal routines
	Slow adjustment	Rapid adjustment
	Need to find ways to fulfill responsibilities and handle problems	Planned activity used to channel energy, memorialize the person who died, and solve problems related to the loss

Source: Martin & Doka, 1993

Martin and Doka pointed out that "patterns of grieving are certainly influenced by gender, but are not determined by gender" (2000, p. 100). They proposed that patterns of grieving form a continuum from an intuitive grieving pattern to an instrumental grieving pattern. Intuitive grieving is very expressive and emotional, a pattern traditionally associated with women. Instrumental grieving is very cognitive and active, a pattern associated with men. Martin and Doka suggested that each of these patterns is found in both men and women.

Intuitive and instrumental grieving patterns are the extremes of the continuum (see Table 9.2). Most people fall somewhere in between, with characteristics of both patterns. One pattern is, however, likely to be predominant in a bereaved person's experience of his or her grief.

Bereavement counseling and support has traditionally addressed the need of people who fall toward the intuitive-grieving end of the spectrum. They appreciate support that attends to the need to express feelings and share experiences with others. Bereavement care providers typically use active listening to encourage people to talk about their grief reactions. Exploration of feelings helps these people express emotions as a form of catharsis. Support groups that focus on sharing and connecting with others will also suit the relational needs of intuitive grievers.

Bereaved people who are more instrumental in their grieving do not find traditional types of support as helpful. Their need is to discuss how to adapt to the changes that they face and what to do with their grief responses, apart from expressing the feelings. They may appreciate a chance to participate in groups that focus on activities such as walking and social interaction. Reading about grief, workbooks, or journal keeping may provide private ways to acknowledge the impact of the death and loss. Work, artistic projects, gardening, or creating some kind of memorial are all practical ways that help them to express the significance and meaning of the loss.

Often, the tendency to encourage and support intuitive grieving is evident in the larger community. There is, however, often a lack of understanding about different styles of grieving within bereaved families, as styles and needs vary among the family members. It is often very difficult for family members, who are vulnerable and hurting, to be patient and understanding with someone who has a different style in grieving.

Spiritual Questions

> Philip had long discussions with the priest about life and death, faith, and his future. A widowed friend told Philip that she had a vision of her husband after his death. This had been a great comfort to her, and Philip longed for some such consolation. Instead, he experienced vivid memories of the traumatic times in Kari's illness and recurring thoughts of her last day.

As bereaved people face the meaning of this death, they encounter suffering—that of the person who died and their own present suffering. Western society fosters a general sense that suffering is not supposed to happen. There may be little acceptance of suffering in bereaved people's beliefs or among those of their support network. People may rail against the unfairness of the suffering and death of a beloved friend or family member. They may wonder why they should love when loving ends only in pain. The direct experience of suffering may lead them to ask, "How can I bear this?" or "Why must I suffer?"

Bereavement is often a time of retreat or withdrawal from normal life or activities. People may find themselves cocooning, in a "physical and psychological movement inward from the outside world to a safe place that requires less activity, energy and engagement" (McGee, 1993, p. 114). They can feel very alone, separate, and on the fringes of life. The experience feels as if a membrane or invisible barrier exists between them and the rest of the world. They may feel as if they have lost their grip on what is real and doubt they will ever be able to go on living.

People struggle with terrible feelings of loneliness and emptiness. They often feel exhausted and filled with doubt about their ability to tolerate, or even survive, their loss. Some bereaved people experience deep despair and wish to die—or even contemplate suicide—as they cannot see meaning or purpose in their own lives. Questions such as "Who am I now?" or "Why am I here?" may surface.

Following the death, bereaved people long for the presence of the person who died. Some experience visitations from, or connections with, that person. Many include the person who died in the newly emerging life of their families. They recognize that there can be an ongoing relationship, changed but continuing, which helps them to bridge the gap between what was and what will be. For some, love may emerge as the very point and meaning of life. An excerpt from the poem, "The End," by P.K. Page (see page 346) captures some of these emotions.

> "The secret cause of all suffering is mortality itself, which is the prime condition of life. It cannot be denied if life is to be affirmed."
>
> –(Joseph Campbell, 1988, p. xiii)

Thus, bereaved people may experience the presence, in some form, of the person who died. These experiences may be called visitations, hallucinations, paranormal experiences, or after-death communications. A surprising number of bereaved people have these experiences in one form or another. Rando (1986) estimated it may be as high as 90%. Other, more cautious estimations are still impressive; Greeley (1987) found that two thirds of widows and two fifths of other bereaved people reported contact with a dead person. In Parkes' (1972) study, 15 of 22 widows reported feeling the presence of their deceased husbands. From these figures, it is apparent that this is a common experience, more common than is generally admitted.

Bereaved people may be hesitant to reveal these experiences because they expect judgment or skepticism from others. They do not wish to be considered crazy, abnormal, or maladjusted. They do not want their experiences dismissed as a product fabricated from a longing for the deceased person or as a ghost story (Parkes, 1972). For most bereaved people, these experiences are not only very real, but also very precious. Following such an experience, they often have a sense of comfort and peace that was previously lacking; they will say, "I know she is all right now" or "I know that he is still watching out for me and giving me strength."

LaGrand (1997) listed different types of contact that are experienced by bereaved people. These include

- *Postmortem presence* refers to an experience in which the person who died is seen.

  A mother whose daughter had died wished, "If I just knew that she was all right now, I wouldn't feel so bad." A few days later, as she was sitting on her couch, the mother heard a little clinking sound like a cup being stirred in a saucer. She turned to see her daughter sitting at the other end of the couch, cup in hand. The daughter smiled and said, "I am okay, Mom. I am really okay." The mother glanced away as she took a deep breath. When she turned back, her daughter was gone.

THE END (verses 2 & 3)

And one, composed of light, came back he said
to tell me it was not *not* everlasting there
as once he had assumed, that I was right.
Was he no proof? "Touch me." He said. I touched
and he was flesh, blood, hair—even as before.
It was the purest heartbreak.
"Tell me..." I said. Bemused, he shook his head.
"It's personal. When your turn comes you'll know.
Till then you cannot guess what you will think

Watching the pier as the ship sails away, or what it will seem like,

"nor can I possibly tell you." His voice was fading
and beneath the palms of my hands he suddenly vanished
as if he had never been—except for two things:
in the darkness I could see, and I was staring
at my fingers where they had touched him, staring
at my mouth, new, where he had kissed it; and
it was clear to me now there was nothing to fear
and no reason for anyone, here or anywhere
to suppose he will be drowned
when he's held by the sea's roar, motionless, there at the end.

—(P.K. Page, 1997, p. 240)

- *Intuitive experience* is one in which one or more people sense the presence of the person who died. Often, this is a sense that the person is watching over those who are left behind.

  Two young women decided to honor their friend who had died with a ritual act at the sea-shore. At the end of this ritual, they threw three flowers into the water to symbolize the friendship among the three of them. To their surprise and delight, one flower floated to sea, whereas the other two washed up on the shore. The two friends felt that this was a sign from the woman who had died that she was on a different journey now, but encouraging them in their own journeys here.

- *Auditory contacts* include sounds that are associated with the person (e.g., their actual voice, a conversation with them).

  A man whose wife had died saw her several times in the house in which they had lived for many years. At these times she did not speak to him. When he was driving on the highway, however, he would imagine talking to her and would, in his mind, hear her answers, her advice, and her encouragement.

- *Dreams* of the person who died may be vivid and have a particular significance for the dreamer.

A man whose secret lover had died had a vivid dream of her standing at the end of his bed. She could not, or would not, speak to him. He did not know what to make of this dream.

A daughter who had cared for her dying mother at home had a series of dreams after the mother's death. In the first dream, the mother was in her nightie and was very distressed because she didn't know where she was or what she was supposed to do. There was a hospital bed in the dream and the daughter helped to settle her mother into the bed. In the next dream, the mother was in bed and told the daughter that she was having visits from a great teacher and that soon she would be ready to move on. In the last dream, the mother was dressed in street clothes and was carrying a suitcase. She told her daughter joyfully that the teacher would be coming for her very soon but that she had wanted very much to say good-bye to her daughter and to express her love. The two women hugged and cried and yet felt happy and peaceful.

- *Symbols and signs* include the appearance or disappearance of some article or natural phenomenon at a particular time that is significant to the bereaved person.

A man who was very sad and despairing after his wife's death was sitting in his living room with the curtains mostly drawn. He cried out in his pain and said, "I don't think I can make it without you!" Just then, the sun broke through the clouds and a sunbeam came through the chink in the curtains. It fell on his face and shoulders. This light and warmth were the essence of his wife to him and he felt that she was with him, comforting and strengthening him.

In addition to those phenomena already listed, there are many other ways that people make a connection to the deceased. The presence of birds and animals may communicate some message or may be connected with the presence of the person who died, particularly when the animal behaves in an unusual way. A scent or smell associated with the deceased person may occur with no source of it to be found. In some instances, a third party will experience a presence or message and pass it along to the bereaved person.

Not all experiences of contact or visitation are pleasant or comforting. Some people react to such experiences with fear. The bereaved person may be upset if, for example, the person who died is seen covered with blood. People's interpretations of the presence are influenced by their ideas about what happens to a person after he or she dies. They may think that the person who died is not at rest if he or she is still in this world, and they may worry about what is holding him or her back. Sometimes, individuals experience fears arising from a belief that these experiences are an indication that they are crazy or that something is wrong with them.

With all of these experiences, each one very different and personal, many questions arise for bereavement care professionals. How should they consider these experiences? What responses and interventions are appropriate?

Bereavement care professionals must not discount those who have these experiences, or patronize those who do not but long for such contact. It is important that counselors be neither too scientific—dismissing these experiences out-of-hand—nor too eager, accepting them indiscriminately. Whatever personal beliefs the counselor may have, he or she should be open to talking about these experiences and inquiring into the bereaved person's explanation of and response to them. Bereavement care professionals find that bereaved people appreciate validation of the meaning of these experiences and respect for the value they have ascribed to them. Although they may not need an explanation, having someone listen breaks the silence. Many people are relieved to share these significant events in an atmosphere of interest and acceptance.

Life is so changed by loss. People are anxious about experiencing more losses and deaths, and often feel vulnerable. Faith and trust in the normal workings of the world and life may be shattered. The belief that for decent human beings things will work out disintegrates. Rando (1993) called this "relinquishing the old assumptive world," whereas others write of the need to relearn the world or reconstruct philosophical systems (Attig, 1996; Martin & Doka, 2000). Bereaved people struggle to integrate this death into their understanding of the world and their beliefs about life.

As people search for meaning in what has happened, they reexamine their personal beliefs and values. They look for a source of strength or faith to help them at this time of depletion. In the search for personal resources, people recall past successes and return to effective ways of coping. Some people will begin a spiritual or religious practice at this time or return to one that may have lapsed. A practice that quiets the mind or brings bereaved people into contact with nature can sustain them now. They find that such practices as a regular walk in the woods or along the shore, meditation, or prayer, can be a source of comfort. This can be a time of honoring a need for peace and quiet withdrawal to nurture and heal the spirit.

Interventions

These psychosocial interventions have been designed to specifically address the key consideration *spiritual questions*. There are several assessment questions that will help open up a discussion, followed by more focused comments or tips that will facilitate further exploration of the issues that frequently arise at this time; each tip is followed by a sample dialogue.

Assessment Questions

- In what ways has your sister's death affected your view of the world? Your personal beliefs and values? Your view of yourself?

- How has your father's death affected your thinking about relationships?

- What are your sources of strength and comfort? What spiritual, meditative, or religious practices are helpful to you at this time?

Be with people in their suffering. It helps to provide a safe environment in which to share the questions that arise.

> *"Since your mother died, you feel very alone and nothing seems important. How is this different from what you used to think and feel? What has changed for you or within you?"*

Assist people to create supportive practices for reflection and renewal. Being in nature provides a reminder of the natural cycles of life. Prayer and meditation help to quiet the mind and promote calm. These practices help people attend to the present moment and to themselves.

> *"You used to attend temple regularly but now don't go. Have you considered reconnecting with your faith community? How might you be able to fit prayers into your daily routine?"*

Ask directly about experiences of presence or visitations. Your openness and gentle interest will create opportunities for people to share and discuss their hopes and fears.

> *"I know that you miss your son terribly and just want to know that he is alright. Have you had any dreams about Gary, or any sense of his presence since his death?"*

OUR EXPERIENCE

Our goal at this transition is to offer support to bereaved people by providing a normative context for their experience and providing opportunities to express the deep emotions they feel. The purpose of this information is to enhance people's ability to understand their grief responses and to help them tolerate the intensity and extent of their reactions. We hope to help people engage their strengths and find compassion for themselves.

When we contact people at this time, we are inquiring about how people are adapting to the changes in their lives, their emotional ups and downs, and the quality of the support they are getting from others. We know that responses, concerns, and priorities change frequently. Bereaved people often ask how long grief takes and how to get through this painful time as quickly as possible. Our assurance that grief takes more time and energy than people generally anticipate helps to create a context for their grief. Our faith in grief as natural, important, and healing is a relief to family members who are concerned that they continue to be affected and feel worse rather than better.

This is a time when we receive requests for counseling services from people worried about themselves or another bereaved person. Our assessment of their grief status and difficulties helps us to identify their present concerns and issues. An individual or family history of loss identifies the strengths and struggles that result from their past experiences. Often education about what to expect, how to console and be consoled, and what help is available will be sufficient to help people soothe themselves or find what works for them. We advocate for respect and understanding of individual concerns and unique ways of grieving among family members. We model how to talk about grief and encourage open communication within families. Planning for realistic goals, appropriate services, and helpful interventions is based on the assessment and the desires of the individual or family.

Unexpected, repetitive, or intense reactions interfere with some people's ability to tolerate their grief or to function in their day-to-day lives. Through our willingness to hear the story of loss and to hear it again and again, we create opportunities for people to face their grief. We provide safety for the expression of intense emotions and bear witness to depths of feeling. We invite individuals to explore the loss, its meaning, and the impact it has on various aspects of their lives. We may teach new strategies for coping with emotion, reframe beliefs and thoughts, or assist with the creation of rituals for healing unfinished business. We are companions to grief when others may not be willing or able to tolerate the pain.

Our experience tells us that many bereaved people need to attend to their own personal well-being. The usual supports available to them from their family and social network may be altered following a death. Their habits of replenishing their energies and their ordinary patterns of behavior may be interrupted or changed in this time of stress. Our interest in and information about taking care of oneself presents an opportunity to discuss stresses and problems. We help them to figure out how to be, and even who to be, with all that has changed. We may problem solve with bereaved people about dealing with situations at work, advocating for pensions and benefits, or managing in social settings. Through discussion, these topics can be explored and encouragement can be offered.

Because, at this time, bereaved people often feel out of step with the usual interests of the world, we offer support groups in which they can meet other people in similar circumstances. We recognize that hearing others voice comparable thoughts and feelings will normalize grief more fully than all of our teaching. The

TEN THINGS TO KNOW ABOUT GRIEF

1. Global effect of loss: The death of someone very close can be a life-transforming event that affects all aspects of one's self and one's life. It can feel as if the world has been shattered.

2. Grief is a natural process: Grief is a normal part of life and a natural response to loss. It is the consequence of living and loving, of meaningful connections with others.

3. Individual differences in grieving styles: Grief is a unique result of personality, past history of loss, and the relationship with the person who died. Family members each grieve in their own way and on their own timetable. Some people will openly express emotions whereas others will master their thoughts and feelings and internalize their grief.

4. Children and grief: Children look to the important adults in their lives to learn how to grieve and will not talk about their thoughts and feelings of loss unless the adults do. Simple information about death and grief is helpful to them.

5. Social connections and support: All relationships are altered in some way after a major loss and it is normal to reassess, change, or end certain relationships. Because of awkwardness or their own feelings of grief, some friends and family members may not be able to provide the understanding and caring that is expected from them.

6. Experiences of grief: When people are actively grieving, their emotions, brain, and reactions seem unreliable. They may be feeling intense pain and emotions never felt before. Responses such as fatigue, forgetfulness, and irritability result from attention and energy being directed toward grief and adjustment to loss.

7. Fluctuations in the grief process: Feelings and responses vary at different times and phases of the grief process. The journey through grief is marked by unpredictable ups and downs.

8. Self-care and what helps: Getting information about grief, being gentle and patient with one's self, keeping a normal routine for health and social contact, and seeking professional help for concerns are things that help at this challenging time.

9. Time for grief: There are no timelines for grief; it takes as long as it takes. A loss continues to be part of life and there are always times when the person who died is thought about, grieved, and missed.

10. Grief as a spiritual journey of healing: Bereaved people must somehow go on and find meaning in the altered path before them. They may experience healing and personal growth as a result of the suffering endured and the lessons learned about what is truly of value.

connections that people make in groups create mutual understanding and permission to be as they are.

TEAM ISSUES

Being present to the expression of grief leaves bereavement counselors vulnerable to feel the pain of others. This sometimes triggers their own pain and makes them more aware of their own needs. When they are busy with their own feelings, it is difficult to continue to be open and responsive to bereaved people. Assessment skills and judgment may be impaired by projection. To remain compassionate and responsive people, bereavement care providers must be aware of and deal with the emotional and grief issues in their private lives. Also, it is essential that they consistently discharge the stress and pain of listening to heartrending accounts of grief.

As bereavement care providers meet individuals in emotional pain, they must be responsive to their need for relief and comfort, without imposing judgments about how this should be accomplished. It is critical to hold awareness that there is no right way to grieve. Certain clients may be relatively easier to work with because their style of expression matches that of the counselor. It is important to resist putting pressure on bereaved people to conform to a style of grieving that the professional thinks is helpful and, instead, explore what is natural and helpful for that person.

Another consideration is what the bereavement care provider brings to this work in terms of hidden perspectives and biases. Although they may strive to maintain awareness of how cultural, religious, philosophical, and familial background influences their work, the professional self is inseparable from the personal self. If team members are blind to aspects of their own personalities, there will be times when they will be caught off guard by an assumption about how things should work, or an unexpected personal reaction. It is important to respond openly and honestly to solicited and unsolicited feedback, and be willing to examine their biases.

In working with bereaved individuals, the care team endeavors to normalize grief without depersonalizing the unique, and extremely personal, nature of individual responses. At times, it can be easier to use a cookie-cutter approach rather than carefully attending to what people say. It is important to find a balance between being objective and informative about the common human experiences of grief and being sensitive and open to the individual pain, experience, and views of the person in front of them.

SUMMARY

A great deal happens for bereaved people in this phase. They experience many small transitions within this larger framework (see Table 9.3). The time spent in this phase can vary, but things will get worse before they get better. The numbness of early grief is wearing off and the support offered in the days and weeks immediately after the death are often withdrawn. Bereaved family members begin to adjust to living with grief as a central factor in their lives. Each person will have his or her own style in grieving and may experience a variety of volatile and distressing emotions. For many people, spiritual questions about value, meaning, and connection with a higher power are significant aspects of grief.

As bereaved people begin to adjust to the death and experience the pain of their loss, they are entering the depths of grief. They are in the midst of grief, at the center of the labyrinth. The way through the labyrinth is forward, taking many turns

Table 9.3. Phase 2: Adjusting to loss

Description	Transition and image	Grief task(s)
As the numbness subsides, bereaved people begin to deal with the emotional pain of grieving. The intensity of this may surprise and frighten them, but it is natural and can be resolved. The time needed for the relationship is affected by the quality of support, other losses, and peoples approach to life.	Grief deepens and is the focus of attention and energy. Bereaved people live their grief. Image: entering the depths	To acknowledge, experience, and work through feelings related to the loss To adjust to life without the person who died

Social	Physical	Emotional	Cognitive	Spiritual
Continued withdrawal and isolation Wanting company but unable to ask Rushing into new relationships Self-consciousness	Tight chest, sharp pangs, shortness of breath Digestive upsets Aimless activity, gnawing emptiness Changes in appetite or sleep patterns	Intense and conflicting emotions Anger, sadness, guilt, hopelessness Generalized anxiety Magnified fears for self, others	Sense of going crazy Memory problems Understanding and concentration poor Vivid dreams or nightmares	Sensing the presence of the person who died; visitations Continued lack of meaning or purpose Attempts to contact the person who died

and going back and forth over what seems like the same territory. Although people may fear they will never find their way to the end of this journey, there is no turning back. Persevering, moving forward is the surest route to healing and a restored sense of wholeness.

REFLECTIVE ACTIVITY

Literature provides us with a rich resource of what has been said, thought, experienced, and written about death, dying, and bereavement. Many pieces are available to bereavement care providers that can be used individually or in groups to stimulate thought and discussion and to encourage and speak to the heart of those with whom they work. Two sample pieces follow.

"Every one of us is called on, probably many times, to start a new life. A frightening diagnosis, a marriage, a move, loss of a job or a limb or a loved one, a graduation, bringing a new baby home . . . In my own worst seasons I've come back from the colorless world of despair by forcing myself to look hard, for a long time, at a single glorious thing: a flame of red geranium outside my bedroom window. And then another: my daughter in a yellow dress. And another: the perfect outline of a full, dark sphere behind the crescent moon. Until I learned to be in love with my life again. Like a stroke victim retraining new parts of the brain to grasp lost skills, I have taught myself joy, over and over again."

—(Barbara Kingsolver, 1995, pp. 15–16)

Who do the dead think they are!
Up and dying in the middle of the night
leaving themselves all over the house,
all over my books, all over my face?
How dare they sit in the front seat of my car,
invisible, not wearing their seat belts,
not holding up their end of the conversation,
as I drive down the highway
shaking my fist at the air all the way
to the office where they're not in.
The dead get by with everything.

—(Bill Holm, 1991, p. 78)

The following exercise is designed as a group exercise, for use in training sessions for professionals and volunteers, to facilitate discussion about experiences of grief.

Instructions

1. Have someone in the group read the poem or piece aloud.
2. Take 5 minutes to write a brief response to the poem or excerpt. It can be about any aspect of the piece that had an impact on you. You may want to ask yourself the following questions:
    *   What images, emotions, or experiences does this piece evoke?
    *   What issues does it prompt me to consider?
    *   Is there anything special about the way in which it is written (e.g., choice of words, perspective of the narrator) that strikes me?
3. Share and discuss some of your responses within the group.
4. Identify the themes that arose from the discussion. What did you learn?

RESOURCES

Bowman, T. (1999). Literary resources for bereavement. *The Hospice Journal, 14*(1).

Coloroso, B. (2000). *Through the rough times: Parenting with wit and wisdom in times of chaos and loss.* St. Catherines, Ontario, Canada: Lothian.

Forte, J., Barrett, A., & Campbell, M. (1996). Patterns of social interconnectedness and shared grief work: A symbolic interactionist perspective. *Social Work with Groups, 19*(1), 29–50.

Kushner, H.S. (1997). *When bad things happen to good people.* New York: Avon Books.

Staudacher, C. (1994). *A time to grieve: Meditations for healing after the death of a loved one.* San Francisco: Harper.

Stroebe, M.S. (1998). New directions in bereavement research: Exploration of gender differences. *Palliative Medicine, 12,* 5–12.

REFERENCES

Alexander, P. (Ed.). (1952). *William Shakespeare: The complete works.* New York: Random House.

Attig, T. (1996). *How we grieve: Relearning the world.* New York: Oxford University Press.

Attig, T. (2000). *The heart of grief: Death and the search for lasting love.* New York: Oxford University Press.

Flowers, B.S. (Ed.). (1988). *Joseph Campbell: The power of myth.* New York: Doubleday.

Golden, T. (1994). Different paths toward healing: The experience and healing of a man's grief [Booklet]. (Available from the author in Kensington, MA.)

Greeley, A. (1987). Mysticism goes mainstream. *American Health, 6,* 47–49.

Holm, B. (1991). *The dead get away with everything.* Minneapolis, MN: Milkweed Editions.

Kingsolver, B. (1995). *High tide in Tucson.* New York: HarperCollins.

LaGrand, L. (1997). *After-death communication: Final farewells.* St. Paul, MN: Llewellyn Publications.

Linn, E. (1986). *I know just how you feel.* Incline Village, NE: The Publisher's Mark.

Martin, T., & Doka, K. (2000). *Men don't cry... women do: Transcending gender stereotypes of grief.* Philadelphia: Brunner/Mazel.

McGee, P. (1993). *Movements in bereavement.* Unpublished doctoral dissertation, Ontario Institute for Studies in Education, University of Toronto.

Moss, S., Rubinstein, R., & Moss, M. (1996–1997). Middle-aged son's reaction to father's death. *Omega, 34*(4), 259–277.

Oliviere, D., Hargreaves, R., & Monroe, B. (1998). *Good practices in palliative care.* Aldershot, UK: Ashgate Publishing Ltd.

Page, P.K. (1997). The end. In *The hidden room.* Erin, Ontario, Canada: The Porcupine's Quill.

Parkes, C.M. (1972). *Bereavement: Studies of grief in adult life.* Harmondsworth, UK: Penguin Books Ltd.

Parkes, C.M., & Weiss, R. (1983). *Recovery from bereavement.* New York: Basic Books.

Rando, T. (1986). Lecture at British Columbia Hospice Palliative Care Association conference, Vancouver, British Columbia.

Rando, T. (1993). *Treatment of complicated mourning.* Champaign, IL: Research Press.

Reeves, N. (1999). *A path through loss: A guide to counting your healing and growth.* Victoria, British Columbia, Canada: Author.

Robinson, P., & Fleming, S. (1992). Depressive cognitive patterns in major depression and conjugal bereavement, *Omega, 25*(4), 291–305.

Staudacher, C. (1991). *Men and grief.* Oakland, CA: New Harbinger Publications.

Tudiver, F., Permaul-Woods, J., Hilditch, J., Harmina, J., & Saini, S. (1995). Do widowers use the health care system differently? *Canadian Family Physician, 41,* 392–400.

Victoria Hospice Society. (2001). *Ten things to know about grief* [Brochure]. Victoria, British Columbia, Canada: Author.

Worden, W. (1991). *Grief counseling and grief therapy: A handbook for the mental health practitioner.* New York: Springer Publishing.

DIFFICULT GRIEF
AND MULTIPLE LOSSES

In the literature on grief, there has been much discussion about defining and differentiating complicated grief or mourning from normal grief and whether complicated grief should be considered a *Diagnostic and Statistical Manual of Mental Disorders (DSM)* diagnostic category (Bonano & Kaltman, 2001). Here, we are not trying to define a complex syndrome or diagnosis. Rather, we are offering helpful information for counselors and other psychosocial care providers who work with bereaved people who are struggling with their grief. We wish to share what we have noticed in our experience with bereaved people in terms of the phases of grief and the underlying issues that influence their reactions. Bereaved people often ask us for counseling help when they experience unexpected, repetitive, or intense reactions that interfere with their ability to tolerate their grief or to function in their day-to-day lives. This is what we mean when we speak of difficult grief.

In hospice and palliative care, it is essential for counselors and others to have a way to situate difficult grief within the spectrum of normal grief. Bereaved people experience difficulty in grieving within the context of the normal grief process. In the model of grief that we use, we see that people may face problems at each of the three phases (i.e., when a death occurs, during the initial period of grief, as life goes on) (Cairns,

Johnson, & Wainwright, 1993). They are stuck in a particular place in their grief and unable to sufficiently resolve the issues that arise as a result of the loss; therefore, they cannot make the transition to the next phase of the process. The responses and reactions of people experiencing difficult grief are predictable and reasonable given what has happened in their lives. These difficulties usually arise in relation to the circumstances associated with the death or to unresolved loss issues.

The circumstances that might trigger difficult grief include a number of deaths that occurred closely together in time or a single death that was unexpected, untimely, traumatic, or violent. For example, the death of a child or a young parent seems untimely and is difficult. In palliative care, deaths following a sudden event, such as a bleed or a fall, can be unexpected and traumatic. Also, families in hospice and palliative care may be grieving other deaths that are traumatic and violent, for example, accident, suicide, or murder. It may be that other pressing responsibilities, such as another ill family member or a new and demanding job, add to the stress of the circumstances following the death. Having a challenging or complex relationship with the person who died, such as an unacknowledged lover or an abusive or estranged relationship can also precipitate difficult grief reactions in an individual.

When people are actively grieving, this can activate unresolved feelings and thoughts about past loss issues, including abandonment, death, trauma, and the losses associated with dysfunctional family patterns, such as drug or alcohol dependency and childhood abuse. If people have not been able to fully grieve earlier deaths, they may not have the personal resilience to face yet another loss.

Bereaved people may encounter difficulty in their grief only once, related to a particular issue, or they may find that each step of the way is painful and challenging. Often, people who are experiencing difficult grief feel unsupported and misunderstood. People in their support network may be critical, worried, or frightened about what they see.

It is helpful to describe difficult grief in relation to each of the phases or transitions of the grief process, rather than in isolation. The following overview includes suggestions for what helps people engage with and overcome their issues and difficulties within each phase, and what signals that they are moving forward in their grief process.

PHASE 1: WHEN A DEATH OCCURS

People experiencing difficult grief find themselves unable to accept the reality of the death or take care of the practical tasks required at this time. They are stuck in denial, disbelief, or panic and are unable to acknowledge, express, and experience their grief. The reasons for such responses might be that they have a need to protect themselves from overwhelmingly unpleasant information or to maintain some sense of control in the midst of the chaos caused by the death. They may be unable to begin grieving because they must first attend to some important, immediate responsibilities or because they do not have sufficient support.

What Helps

The goal here is that people begin to grieve their losses. The counselor will help people understand why they have been unable to acknowledge or accept what has occurred and explore ways they might express their grief.

- **Opening to grief.** Safety, support, and permission to grieve help bereaved people express their thoughts and feelings. Exploration of what stops them from grieving and opportunities to talk about the death and the person who died help bereaved people begin to feel.
- **Accepting the reality of the death.** Activities such as reviewing detailed information about the death, participating in memorial services or rituals, settling the estate, and sorting the belongings of the person who died bring the reality of the death into awareness.

When People Move Forward in Grief

- Grief is more apparent.
- A variety of feelings arise.
- The relationship with the person who died is reviewed.

PHASE 2: ADJUSTING TO LOSS

People experiencing difficult grief have powerful, persistent patterns to their grief reactions. They might feel that they are going around and around with some aspect of their grief, such as anger, guilt, confusion, or despair, and are unable to find any resolve or relief. They are distracted by grief and can focus on little else. The reasons for such responses include disturbing aspects of the death; inability to adjust to the demands of a new life situation; or the triggering of old, unresolved issues. Often, the people around those experiencing difficult grief are uncomfortable with these reactions and express concern.

What Helps

The goal here is to help people begin to resolve the issues that are keeping them locked in emotional chaos. The counselor will help people understand what is preventing them from dealing with these issues and develop strategies that will support exploration and expression of their emotions.

- **Resolving the pattern.** Exploration of when patterns of grief occur, what triggers them, and what helps to settle them provides a new perspective for people experiencing difficult grief. Worries about being "crazy" can be alleviated by normalizing responses. Highlighting the normal range of grief, complex circumstances, and personal history provide a context for understanding what is happening.

- **Managing the intensity or amount of grief.** Skilled support can provide opportunities for people to express the intensity of their grief and address the crises they experience. Through counseling, they can learn effective strategies to deal with reactions and safely discharge excess energy and emotion. Sharing with other bereaved people through mechanisms such as support groups, chat rooms, and message boards, provides an expressive outlet and the support of others in similar circumstances.

When People Move Forward in Grief

- Intense times occur less frequently and do not last as long.
- Thoughts and emotions become more tolerable.
- Energy for daily living returns.

PHASE 3: MENDING THE HEART

People experiencing difficult grief later in the grief process can feel isolated as family and friends become impatient with them or avoid talking to them about the person who died. Unable to see a future for themselves, people experiencing such grief remain focused on the loss. They can feel guilty about their own lives going on, or about participating in enjoyable activities. The reasons for difficulty might be a fear of the future without the person who died or something in their relationship with that person that feels unfinished. Some people may be unable to create a new routine in life because of poor health or a limited social network.

What Helps

The goal here is to help people shift their focus toward the future. The counselor will help people bring some closure to their grief and explore ways they can invest energy in new relationships, roles, and activities.

- **Facing the future.** Examining fears and worries about the future can help people choose small, realistic goals for moving forward. Imagining conversations with, or writing letters to, the person who died may assist people in reconciling aspects of their relationship with the person. Identifying people and community resources can help people begin to build a more supportive network of social connections.
- **Attending to self.** Information on the normal grief process can provide reasonable expectations for people and allow them to focus on their own needs and pleasures. Recalling both the good and the not-so-good memories can provide a more realistic view of the relationship with the person who died. Encouraging people to reach out to others may include suggesting that they reconnect with old friends or start new activities.

When People Move Forward in Grief

- The death and loss become integrated as part of personal history.
- Remembering and missing occur without threat to daily functioning.
- Interest in life is recovered.

MULTIPLE LOSSES

Sometimes, bereaved people experience difficult grief as a result of multiple losses. Circumstances and unresolved losses may come together in an overwhelming way when there are a significant number of unresolved losses from the past, a number of deaths occurring close together in time, or a single relationship that held so much meaning its end is catastrophic. Such a number of deaths and losses brings a multiplicity of grief reactions.

Because of the enormousness of change associated with what has happened, there is no constancy or solidity in the lives of people grieving multiple losses. Their former support system is often seriously depleted as a result of loss and death. They may experience a lack of connection to the way life used to be and suffer a loss of their sense of self. Their reactions may seem chaotic as one grief connects with another. Other people find it hard to comprehend the extent of their grief or to tolerate the intensity of the feelings.

It takes considerable time and energy to grieve multiple losses. There are times when these people seem self-centered as they focus on their loss of self and ignore their grief over the deaths that have occurred. Both the bereaved individuals and others may feel judgmental about their own lack of feeling. Some people indulge in harmful behaviors, such as increased risk-taking, inattention to safety, or drug and alcohol abuse.

What Helps

The goal here is to help people begin to redefine who they are and find manageable ways to cope with the complexity of grief. The counselor will help people identify and understand the impact of the multiple losses and develop strategies that will support them to work through their grief.

*   **Understanding the impact.** Identifying the losses and their significance provides a context for the depth of the grief, despair, or isolation experienced. People benefit from making time for grief and healing activities in their daily routine.

- **Renewing sense of self.** The focus on self reflects people's need to survive in a chaotic situation and is an important part of the process of beginning to grieve multiple losses. Care of the body, mind, and spirit rebuilds the strength necessary to engage grief. Remaining and new support people alike can provide meaningful connections and assistance.

- **Identifying themes in grief.** The connections among losses, such as the similarities in fact, thought, or feeling, are the themes of the grief process. Awareness of these themes helps to provide a sense of order in the face of chaos and provides more manageable pieces to focus on.

- **Pacing grief.** People grieving multiple losses can learn to balance times of expressing thoughts and emotions and times of controlling them. This creates some respite from the intensity of their grief. Acknowledging the losses and remembering those who have died helps to integrate the past with the present.

- **Getting support for grief.** People need sufficient support and safety to begin expressing the complexity and intensity of their grief. A counselor, bereavement support group, or trusted advisor can create an environment or relationship within which grief may be explored.

REFERENCES

Bonano, G.A., & Kaltman, S. (2001). The varieties of grief experience. *Clinical Psychological Review, 21*(5), 705–734.

Cairns, M., Johnson, A., & Wainwright, W. (1993). *Bereavement care: A plan for grief support.* Victoria, British Columbia, Canada: Victoria Hospice Society.

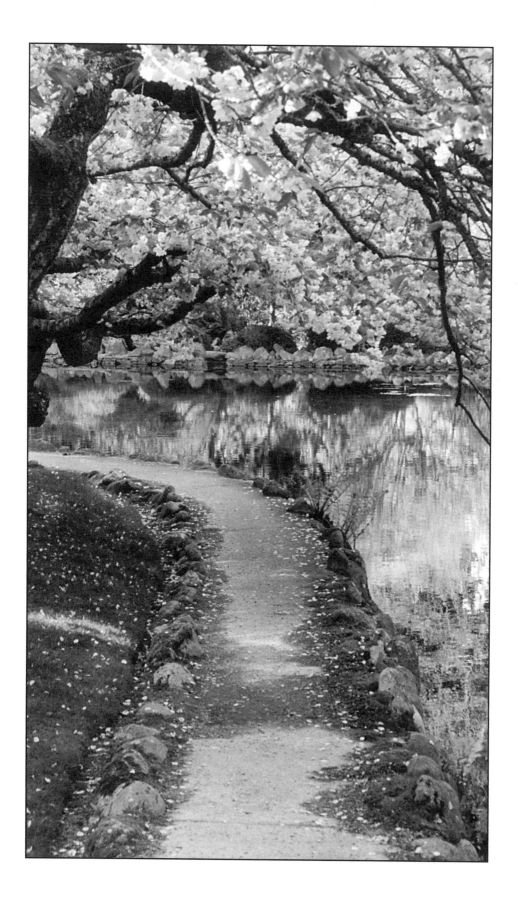

10

Reconnecting with the World

MENDING THE HEART

Phase 3

In the earlier transitions of grief, the person who died and the death itself are the reference points for everything in bereaved people's lives. The death and grief shape everything about them and life is, in some ways, small and focused. Now, at this transition, the death gradually becomes part of family history. People have adapted and adjusted in many ways to the changes in their lives and their families, and they continue to do so. The grieving process naturally moves people away from a focus on death and toward life. Having traveled to the center of the labyrinth, people are now EMERGING FROM THE PAIN of grief and beginning to re-enter the larger world. It is as if they stop looking at death's closed door and see the open door of life through which it is possible to go on. Other things become important as people begin to respond to the richer, fuller, busier mosaic of life.

Paradoxically, just as people feel themselves moving out of the depths of grief, they recognize THE ONGOING NATURE OF GRIEF. With a new perspective on life, people also find a new relationship with their grief. Although this important person will always be missed, people realize they are able to bear the loss and survive the periodic upsurges of grief. New endeavors or new relationships may bring an upsurge of feelings, as people miss the familiar support or comfort of the person who has died. Life transitions may be fraught with longing or aware-ness of the absence of that special person.

REMEMBERING now becomes an important task for bereaved people. For perhaps the first time, the possibility of forgetting occurs to them. Keeping some-one's memory alive becomes extremely important. Families want to foster memo-ries for children and grandchildren or create a way for those who did not know the person who died to have a sense of that person. Families are amazingly creative in the ways that they find to honor and remember. They consider the habits, thoughts, and values of the person who died, and, in this way, he or she continues to be part of the family.

Bereaved people find themselves altered by the magnitude of their experience of the death and grief and they have a changed sense of PERSONAL IDENTITY because of it. As they come to think about the world differently, learn new skills and behaviors, and adapt to the loss of the person who died, they become differ-ent people. Self-image also changes in response to this new reality. Family and friends are mending their hearts and emerging from grief, rather like a butterfly emerging from its chrysalis. The struggle to reenter life strengthens them. Many bereaved people are, eventually, able to identify personal growth that has occurred due to the loss and grief that they have survived.

MARJORIE

Marjorie is a 74-year-old aboriginal Canadian woman and a widow of 18 months. She has decided that she cannot afford to keep either her car or the small house where she lived with her husband, Harry, for 14 years. She wants to move back to the reservation to be closer to her extended family and her friends. She hopes to move into a house with her sister, brother-in-law, and aunt. Her daughter, Meg, is helping her with the move. Marjorie is looking forward to having a little extra cash, so that she can do a bit of traveling. Although Marjorie believes the move is a good thing, she is still nervous about this big change. She is extremely sad to be leaving the house and feels guilty about leaving Harry's prized garden behind. She hopes this is the right decision.

Harry died of advanced heart disease. He also had Alzheimer's dis-ease. Their son, Graeme, and daughter-in-law, Bonnie, helped Marjorie take care of Harry at home until he died. Their two daughters, Meg and Pippi, were estranged from their parents. Marjorie blamed Harry's advanc-ing Alzheimer's on the stress of this rift. Before Harry died, Pippi and Meg had wanted the family to discuss the fact that Harry had left the family for several years when the girls were quite young. This abandonment had never been discussed before and they had hoped that talking would result in some healing of the pain it caused. Marjorie and Harry had refused to talk about it, however.

> "Grief...is influenced, shaped, and determined by a constellation of factors that combine to render a mourner's response unique—as individual as a fingerprint."
>
> —(Rando, 1993, p. 29)

Since Harry's death, Marjorie has had contact with her daughters and some reconciliation has been achieved. Meg and her mother are able to talk relatively comfortably about current topics. Pippi still struggles with continuing anger at her father and mother. She is frustrated with Marjorie's ongoing denial of the effects of Harry's time away from them. Marjorie sometimes shows her own disappointment and hurt at being abandoned by her daughters when she most needed them. She rarely mentions Harry to her daughters, but she talks to her daughter-in-law, Bonnie, about how much she misses him. On the anniversary of Harry's death, they went to the cemetery and spent time remembering Harry's life. Next year they hope to dedicate a bench in his name.

Marjorie belongs to a healing circle on the reservation and finds the people there comforting. This group is the center of her social world. She has reconnected with her church and also participates in a women's singing group. She volunteers one afternoon a week at the school on the reservation, and she has returned to painting classes that she had given up when Harry's condition worsened. Now she has activities each day of the week.

KEY CONSIDERATIONS

Emerging from the Pain

Although Marjorie believes the move is a good thing, she hopes this is the right decision. She hopes to move into a house with her sister, brother-in-law, and aunt. Marjorie belongs to a healing circle on the reservation and finds the people there comforting. This group is the center of her social world. She has reconnected with her church and also participates in a women's singing group. She volunteers one afternoon a week at the school on the reservation, and she has returned to painting classes that she had given up when Harry's condition worsened.

When grief has been life's central or most-important issue, it is natural that bereaved people feel ambivalent about moving on. They may feel guilty about positive emotions and thoughts of the future; they do not want to ignore or forget the person who died. As people shift away from active grieving, self-judgment can arise about when this should happen. People ask themselves what the right amount of time to grieve is and whether they are ready to be over this loss. They worry that they may be shallow or uncaring if they let go of grief. Other people's comments suggest that, on the one hand, they should have achieved this point some months ago or, on the other hand, imply that it really is too soon to be feeling or behaving in this manner. It is challenging to move away from the role and behavior of a bereaved person.

Although people experience a certain amount of relief at feeling more normal and at having greater energy and interest for a variety of postponed or ignored activities, they are reluctant to let go of the person who died. So much advice is given about letting go, and confusion can plague bereaved people as they wonder what they are supposed to do. Well-meaning acquaintances exhort them, "You have to let him go and get on with your own life." Worden (1991) suggested that it is healthy to say good-bye, to wish for the person who died to be alive, and to fantasize that he or she might somehow return. Saying good-bye might also include gradually letting go of the central place the person had in the life of the family. Hogan said bereaved people "are gradually learning to let go of dwelling in the past with pain and hopelessness and dedicating energy to creating a new future that [has] hope and meaning" (1996, p. 57).

At some point after the death people discover that they are not so emotionally volatile or fragile. Despair and emptiness begin to lift. Individuals find that they no longer need to protect the emptiness and pain within, but are willing and able to risk looking at the new world that lies before them. Within families, people arrive at this place at different times making it challenging for them to help each other to move forward. Some of them may not yet be ready to do so. Some people find the renewed energy at this transition allows them to revisit regrets about earlier grief and to deal with some unresolved issues in a new way.

Many people emerge from the labyrinth to find that the world is different than it was prior to the death. Throughout the illness and death of a family member and the period of bereavement, social connections may have suffered and perhaps been lost. People must figure out how and where to begin the process of reconnecting. Some connections are not resumed. In their place, new relationships and new interests are sought.

The emergence from grief may be activated by a major positive change such as a move, a birth, or especially a new relationship. The excitement of the present

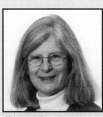

Christine Piercey is a
Victoria Hospice
counselor and a former
hospice physician with
an M.A. in transpersonal
psychology.

In My Own Voice
Must We Let Go of the
Departed?

Christine Piercey

"Deep inside the grief of the bereaved the dead are at work, making
themselves into religion and culture, imagining themselves into soul.
We are the afterworld in which our loved ones dwell."

–Greg Mogenson, 1992

The question of how bereaved people create a new relationship with
their deceased loved ones has interested me for some time now. Freudian
theoretical understanding of the tasks of grief includes the idea that one
must relinquish all connections to the dead in order to release emotional
energy to invest in other relationships or activities. In my experience of
facilitating grief support groups, however, I have been struck by the
strength of the feelings that arise around the ideas of "accepting" the
death of a loved one and "letting go" of that person. Most people resist
this letting go and find some way of staying connected with the one who
died, whether it be symbolically (e.g., "I imagine him as being in that
star up there"), physically through linking objects, or more literally in
an ongoing inner conversation. Fortunately, theory is catching up with
experience and more people are now beginning to understand that it is
possible to have an ongoing relationship with departed individuals and
to be well invested in life and connected with others.

Interpretation of "visits" from the dead, whether as dream, image,
vision, or sense of presence goes along with this transition. Freudian
theory referred to these as the illusions and hallucinations of a wishful
psychosis. We now recognize that continuing bonds with departed
loved ones can provide both support and comfort for bereaved people.
(Of interest is the fact that this shift in understanding parallels the
move from Newtonian science, which does not acknowledge what can-

not be explained, to quantum science, which postulates an essential interconnectedness of all phenomena.) At a time when overwhelming emotions leave many people feeling unhinged from their moorings to a concrete world, it is small wonder that visits from departed individuals may add to the fear of losing control, or the fear that others will label them crazy. Inquiring of bereaved people where they feel their loved one is now and if they feel connected with them will often lead to stories shared in hushed and conspiratorial tones. I think it is important to ask about this possibility, as it is a great relief for people to know that they are not falling into madness. This line of questioning can also lead into an exploration of the deeper layers of grief, a further working through of the relationship, and perhaps to making some sense of the loss. Death and loss very frequently challenge spiritual beliefs and our ideas of an orderly world ruled by justice. Each person will interpret visits from a departed person in a way that is congruent with his or her views. When interpretation is not possible, and the belief system is shattered, it can be a profoundly devastating and disorienting experience for the person.

North American culture prizes autonomy and rationality, so it is not surprising that these otherworldly experiences are often kept hidden and only revealed in a context that feels safe, respectful, and nonjudgmental. In palliative care circles, we are becoming more familiar with the communications of dying people that seem to suggest an in-between world or a journey from this dimension to another, portrayed in image and metaphor. Bereaved people are not always surrounded by a circle of caring people, nor do they always have access to an accepting witness. Yet they, at times, seem to have a greater access to other dimensions than those of us who are not dealing with crisis.

The emphasis we moderns place on rationality and autonomy was not always the case. A study of ancient, indigenous, and religious beliefs reveals a wealth of stories about life after death and the connection between the living and the dead. Indeed, a belief in life beyond death can be seen as archetypal. I am not, however, advocating that we should let go of either rationality or autonomy, but rather that those in bereavement might be better served if we find a path that also includes a place for nonrational experience and interconnectedness.

pushes grief into the background. There will be predictable and natural upsurges of grief, however, and they can be threatening to the new happiness. People may find it difficult to tolerate conflicting emotions of excitement and sadness at the same time and wonder if they are going backward in their grief.

Bereaved spouses face particular challenges as they return to social interactions. They may find their status as a single person unnerving. If they are dating, they may feel uncertain and awkward, especially if they have not dated since adolescence. The reactions of other family members to a widow or widower dating are sometimes less than encouraging or supportive. When a bereaved spouse finds a new partner, everyone in the family will be affected. Each person may have a different response, ranging from anger at the spouse for being disloyal to the person who died, to delight that this person, once again, has a partner to share in his or her life. Whatever their feelings, this change is another loss that must be grieved. Tolerance, humor, and patience can help to create balance between honoring the memory of the person who died and welcoming a positive new future.

When one parent has died in families with young children and teens, the surviving parent may have been very present at home and close to the children through the earlier phases of grief. When this parent begins to participate in his or her own outside activities and spend time with friends, it is a big adjustment for the children. They may have feelings of resentment and jealousy or fears of abandonment.

Interventions

These psychosocial interventions have been designed to specifically address the key consideration *emerging from the pain*. There are several assessment questions that will help open up a discussion, followed by more focused comments or tips that will facilitate further exploration of the issues that frequently arise at this time; each tip is followed by a sample dialogue.

Assessment Questions

- What changes in your grief are you aware of? How do you feel different now than just after your grandma died?

- Tell me about your socializing with family, old friends, and new friends. How would you describe the support you get from them?

- How would you describe your energy and interest in the future now?

Reframe "letting go." People appreciate both reassurance that letting go does not mean forgetting the person who died and permission to bring the person forward in a new way in the life of the family.

"You have received a lot of advice about letting Matthew go and getting on with your own life. What does "letting go" mean to you? You certainly won't ever forget him or want to stop talking about him with your husband and other children. But things are not the same as they were and can't be. Knowing he is not here, how could you find ways for Matthew to be part of your family's life?"

Normalize ambivalence as part of this transition. Explore any feelings of guilt. People may interpret their guilt and hesitation as indications that they are not yet ready to move forward. Knowing that it is normal to be unsure of how to reenter the world makes it safer to try out some new activity or go to a new place.

"You want to have some fun and relaxation after the long months of loneliness and despair. You think you might join a singles hiking group, but feel nervous about meeting new people. You and Sonny used to do everything together. It is natural to be hesitant. What might help you feel more comfortable on your first hike?"

Identify when a person is ready for change. This includes ways of dealing with other people's expectations about the person moving on. Talking openly about this can facilitate understanding and acceptance within the family.

"Brian's mother is shocked that you are developing this new relationship, but you feel you are ready for intimacy again. You really value her love and support and worry about losing your closeness with her. Could you talk with her about your needs and concerns? How might you do that?"

The Ongoing Nature of Grief

Although Marjorie believes the move is a good thing, she is still nervous about this big change. She is extremely sad to be leaving the house and feels guilty about leaving Harry's prized garden behind. She rarely mentions Harry to her daughters, but she talks to her daughter-in-law, Bonnie, about how much she misses him. On the anniversary of his death, they went to the cemetery and spent time remembering Harry's life.

Gradually, people learn that grief is an ongoing process. Although grief alters in its pace and duration as people move through this transition, it is nevertheless a continuing part of life. Fleming (1988) refered to "walls of grief," indicating that there are periods when grief is present and felt and periods when people feel normal. Over time, these "walls" or grief upsurges occur less frequently and for shorter periods, surfacing when significant life events and developmental stages trigger reactions. Rando refers to these as "subsequent temporary upsurges of grief" (1993, p. 64).

The first anniversary of the death is a significant time for all bereaved people. It may arrive while people are still very actively grieving. If people are at a later transition, however, they may be surprised by the strength of their grief reaction. As the date of the anniversary draws close, memories of what was happening at this time 1 year ago are poignant and powerful. The hopes, fears, sadness, and exhaustion of that time are vividly recalled. This reactivation of powerful feelings can seem like being right back at the beginning. Some bereaved people worry that they are relapsing or regressing in their grief. Most often, they find that these feelings subside again as the anniversary passes.

For some people, the second anniversary of the death is devastating. They find that the connection to events at the time of death is no longer so temporal. Much time has passed since the death and connections to it are less immediate. The bereaved person can be very aware of the gulf between the death and themselves and grieve that loss as well.

Many families plan to honor and remember the person on the anniversary of the death. Some people, however, choose to do as little as possible on this particular day, taking quiet contemplative time. Others dread the anniversary and may stay in bed for the day. In some religions and cultures, the anniversary, especially the first, is celebrated with special rituals for remembering the person who died and/or marking the end of the bereavement period for the family. When the anniversary coincides with another holiday or special family date (e.g., a birthday, a

LATE LOVE

He dies.
She dies.
And after great loneliness
Those who are left behind
Find each other,
Or redefine each other
From neighbor or old friend
To companion,
Intimate,
And, most amazingly,
Lover.

Their middle-aged children
Sulk,
Saying, without saying it,
This is unseemly.
Devote yourself
To good works,
Educational cruises,
Your grandchildren,
And do not abandon
Your lost mate,
Your past life,
Or us.

Those who are left behind
Turn to each other,
Their soft, used flesh
Renewed in a forgiving embrace.
And in their hearts
Such gratitude.
Such gratitude.

—(Judith Viorst, 2000, pp. 66–67)

wedding anniversary), the paradox of a day of celebration being a day of mourning can be difficult for everyone.

Holidays, and special family gatherings that are a part of these times, can take on a new and lasting sensitivity as the person who died continues to be missed. Families find various ways to alter and adapt their celebrations to acknowledge their loss. They may do something different on the first occurrence of a particular holiday, then return to usual practices or create new traditions to replace or augment the old.

When family members cannot share their ongoing grief, people feel isolated and alone. Throughout the grief process, shifts and changes happen in family patterns of relating. Although this is to be expected, it is very difficult to go through. Sometimes, family members have had radically different relationships with the person who died. Some family members may be missing the person deeply, whereas others experience less intense feelings of loss. When family members have unresolved issues with the person who died, it might take them longer to reach this transition and to emerge from grief. In such situations, it is difficult to talk about grief, and remembering can be painful or discouraged. The recurrent times of grief, both predictable and unforeseen, do not bring the family together or allow them to express love and support. In fact, some families split apart and never come back together. Then, each person in the family must find his or her own way or look for support and understanding outside the family.

Grief recurs for people as they reach new developmental stages. This is true for both families and individuals. Families revisit grief as significant life events change the dynamics within the family and the tasks for their particular family life-cycle stage. For example, when a child graduates from school, someone marries or remarries, a baby is born, someone retires, and so forth, the person who died is missed and mourned. That person is unable to participate in the growth and the changes that happen as the family develops and matures. Major changes that might have been shared with the deceased person will always include some sadness and longing. At each age or stage of individual or family development, bereaved people may see the past and understand the person who died in a new light (Rando, 1993).

Children's grief will recur not only in relation to significant events, but also as they reach new levels of cognitive development. Children have different needs and understandings associated with death at different ages and stages of their development. Each stage builds on the one before with an increasing awareness and understanding of the full implications of death. As bereaved children get older and approach developmental maturity, they need additional information and opportunities to learn about death.

Interventions

These psychosocial interventions have been designed to specifically address the key consideration *the ongoing nature of grief*. There are several assessment questions that will help open up a discussion, followed by more focused comments or tips that will facilitate further exploration of the issues that frequently arise at this time; each tip is followed by a sample dialogue.

Assessment Questions

- What are you planning for yourself or your family on the anniversary of your brother's death?

- Tell me about the rhythms of your grief now. How have they changed over the past months?

- Within your culture (or religion), what rituals or practices are related to the anniversary of a death or the period of bereavement?

- How are you feeling about your Dad not being at your graduation?

ANNIVERSARY STORY

Paul, a 6-year-old, was upset some months after his father's death. He lived with his aunt, Janet, who realized that the upcoming anniversary might be distressing him. They talked together and made a plan for the day. Janet and Paul looked at family photos first and remembered and talked about his dad. Paul then wrote a letter to his father that they put into a bottle along with a rose. They took this bottle to a special place where Paul had spent a lot of time with his dad. They threw the bottle into the sea and observed 2 minutes of silence. Paul's father was a Navy man and this act seemed appropriate to Janet and Paul as a closure to their day of remembering.

Encourage people to plan together as a family for holiday gatherings. Honest communication about what each person wants and needs allows families to create celebrations that are workable and satisfying.

> *"Last year at Thanksgiving you tried to do everything just the same as usual, but this year you don't think you can manage that. Yet, you are afraid to disappoint your children. How might you discuss your concerns with them? What traditions do you want to keep and what things would you like to change?"*

Normalize anniversary reactions. Explore emotions experienced at that time. Powerful memories can recreate the feelings of early grief and cause worry about progress in grieving.

> *"The anniversary of Martin's death is in a few days, and you said that you are having a difficult time again. People often remember what was happening a year ago and go over the events of that time in detail. What thoughts and feelings have been coming up for you?"*

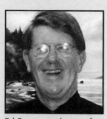

Ed Fougner, whose wife
died on the Victoria
Hospice in-patient unit,
wrote this letter to the
bereavement coordinator.

In My Own Voice
A Letter of Thanks and
Remembrance

Ed Fougner

All of the family, my children and grandchildren, were at my son's home this Thanksgiving weekend to mark this first anniversary of Aggie's death. We all thought it was going to be a sad occasion. Surprisingly, the weekend was anything but sad. Certainly there were some tears, but for the most part it was a celebration with a lot of reminiscing and a lot of laughter.

The grandchildren decorated a table that contained pictures, gifts, and mementos of/from their Nana. As well, we visited places we had gone as a family when we all lived in Victoria. I had prepared a biography of Aggie's and my life together from the time we first met until Aggie's death last year, and I presented the small document to each of my four children as a gift. We looked at old slides and shared stories and memories. It was a very rich experience, a wonderful weekend together.

My year has been difficult but manageable, I think, largely because of my hospice experience and because of the support and wise counsel I received from friends and neighbors. At first, I craved social contact; when I was with others, I was able to push my grief into the background. However, a good friend encouraged me to spend time by myself in order to begin to confront my feelings of grief. Being by myself was very hard, but it forced me to deal with the unpleasant memories and the emotions those memories evoked. As time goes on I find that I am crying less and smiling more as I remember our times together.

I have enrolled in a Hospice Volunteers Orientation Program here in Parksville, and I am enjoying meeting people, many of whom have also lost loved ones in the last year or so.

Identify the impact of other changes on people's experience of grief. Information about how new losses or new demands to adapt can reactivate feelings of grief helps people to understand their experience.

> *"Your wife died almost 2 years ago and you have been coping fairly well until the last few weeks. Your son, who has been living with you, has been offered a job in another city. How do you think this might be affecting your grief?"*

Explore any unresolved issues and identify resources and options for people to work on these. Longstanding issues may be beyond the scope of bereavement support and counseling.

> *"Alcoholism has been a part of your family's history. You have been 'dry' for many years, but find some old patterns of behavior persist. Kevin, would you like me to refer you to an agency that provides alcohol counseling?"*

Acknowledge that children and teens will miss the person who died for the rest of their lives. People may assume that children forget or that their grief ends.

> *"Martina, your mother died when you were a child. Now that you are a mother yourself, what can you learn from your memories and knowledge of her?"*

Remembering

Marjorie sometimes shows her own disappointment and hurt at being abandoned by her daughters when she most needed them. She rarely mentions Harry to her daughters, but she talks to her daughter-in-law, Bonnie, about how much she misses him. On the anniversary of his death, they went to the cemetery and spent time remembering Harry's life. Next year they hope to dedicate a bench in his name.

As time passes and grief changes, most bereaved people want ways to maintain a sense of connection and to keep the person in their lives. Happiness and hope no longer seem incompatible with remembering the person who died. A more realistic view of the person is available to the family now as they become aware of the good and challenging aspects of the person, the happy and sad memories, and the ways in which relationships were fulfilling or not (Rando, 1993).

New relationships evolve with the person who died as families adjust to the reality that the person is no longer alive, yet continues to be an important part of the family (Moules, 1998). Many bereaved families and individuals say that imagining what the person would say about the doings of the family, blessing him or her in prayers, or having a one-sided conversation with the person comforts them. Privacy or conflict in the family may lead some people to keep their connection to the person who died very quiet. In cases in which there has been a conflicted relationship with the person who died, remembering can continue to be fraught with hurt. Once the tenor of grief changes in this transition, these people may be able to slowly piece together some healing in connection to unhappy remembrances.

The ways that bereaved people find to memorialize, honor, and remember their loved ones are as varied as the people themselves. Books of family history, family trees, and collections of stories preserve memories for future times and generations. Photo montages fill walls, mantelpieces and albums, providing frequent opportunities to point out the person who died and to talk about family life at the various times depicted in the photos. Memorial gardens, public and private, are special places for contemplation or conversation. Grave sites are decorated and tended not only as a way to honor the person who died but also to give family members something concrete and positive to do. Cremation ashes are kept in urns, divided among family members, included in sculptures, scattered in special places, or given to the oceans. These ways of dealing with the ashes provide strong connections to the last physical remains, either keeping them close or establishing a place where the person who died can be visited. During these visits, conversations are held, internally or out loud, to keep the person who died up to date, to consult him or her for advice, or to remind the person that he or she is remembered and missed.

Often, the anniversary of the death will continue to be important as years pass, and it may be commemorated through some custom of remembrance. People may visit the gravesite or other special place, make an annual donation in memory of the person, or put a notice in the newspaper.

Outside the family, people find ways to inform new acquaintances and remind old friends that the person who died, however long ago, is still part of the family. Parents, for example, learn how to explain how many children they have, including the child who died. Others learn how to identify the missing and missed person, as in, "I have two siblings, an older brother and a younger sister who died."

Once beyond the early phases of grief, when comfort and consideration are offered, children may find it very hard to say, "My dad died" or "My grandma died." The world of children may include more stigmas attached to death. When a parent has died, children are acutely aware of the differences between the other children and them. They may feel vulnerable and fearful and prefer to not draw attention to the death. If the important adults in the children's lives continue to openly talk about the death, the children are more likely to find a way to acknowledge it among their peers.

Interventions

These psychosocial interventions have been designed to specifically address the key consideration *remembering*. There are several assessment questions that will help open up a discussion, followed by more focused comments or tips that will facilitate further exploration of the issues that frequently arise at this time; each tip is followed by a sample dialogue.

Assessment Questions

- Do you often talk about your wife? Tell me about this.

- In what ways are you and your family actively remembering your sister? How are you keeping the memories of her alive for your own children?

- How comfortable are you telling your friends that your mom died and that Suzie is your stepmom?

> "It has taken me a very long time to understand that love is more powerful that death, and to realize that Frank is still with me. Everyone must make their own way through loss and grief, but, if I could give advice to others...I'd urge them to be receptive to the connection that will always exist between them and their loved one. It's no longer of this world, no longer physical, but it's real, powerful, and transforming. My visceral recognition of that truth has, finally, made my life blossom. Death does not have to be the end."
>
> –(Ginny Stanford, 1998, p. 81)

Explore any ongoing relationship with the person who died. Your openness may allow bereaved people to acknowledge their connection to the person who died. As you normalize this behavior, people may be relieved of concerns about themselves.

> *"George, you wonder if I might think you are crazy because you still talk to your wife. In my experience, most people who have lost their spouse keep talking to them in some way. Tell me more about this connection."*

Encourage activities that help families to remember and honor the person who died. It is important to do this in ways that suit their particular needs or style.

> *"Francine, you're worried that your two small children will not remember their grandfather. You are a writer. How can you use your talents to help your children know who he was and how much he loved them?"*

SOME WAYS OF MEMORIALIZING

Shrines

- Personal and family shrines in the home
- Memorial sites on the Internet
- Grave markers
- Plants and gardens
- Memorial benches
- Memorial plaques
- Photo galleries or collages

Creative projects

- Scrap books of mementos
- Journals of thoughts and doings
- Memorial albums
- Poems
- Artwork expressing love and grief
- Memory quilts
- Paper made from the sympathy cards
- Gardens
- Favorite crafts or art forms of the person who died

Symbolic activities

- Funerals or memorial services
- Rituals of remembering
    - Candle lightings
    - Letters to the person who died
- Personal changes
- Political, social, or personal actions
    - Scholarships
    - Volunteer projects
    - Fundraising projects
    - Public speeches

Review how the anniversary and other significant dates are being commemorated. Your interest in these personal and family rituals or celebrations gives people reassurance that these are normal and healthy ways to remember their family member. Also, encourage flexibility in these so that they reflect the family's current concerns and wishes.

> *"Tarjeet, the second anniversary of your wife's death is coming up soon. Tell me what you did last year on the anniversary. Are you wanting to do any of those things again this year, or do you want to do something different?"*

Personal Identity

> Marjorie has decided that she cannot afford to keep either her car or the small house where she lived with her husband, Harry, for 14 years. She wants to move back to the reservation to be closer to her extended family and her friends. She hopes to move into a house with her sister, brother-in-law, and aunt. Marjorie is looking forward to having a little extra cash so that she can do a bit of traveling. She has reconnected with her church and also participates in a women's singing group, and she has returned to painting classes that she had given up when Harry's condition worsened.

When someone close dies, a particular role or relationship is lost. For example, when Harry died, his wife became a widow, his sister no longer had a brother to be sister to, his children had no father, his friend no longer functioned as Harry's friend. Bereaved people must each deal with the loss of the particular identity that they had in relation to the person who died. This may represent a loss of a significant portion of personal identity when the relationship was central and active. Initially, the role of bereaved person may fill the space within the identity, but it can later become an empty space.

Although a new relationship with the person who died evolves, bereaved people deal with the question "Who am I now?" as they reconnect with the world. An altered identity is being developed and decisions made about what to include or nurture in that identity. The attributes that were loved and valued by the person who died will likely be maintained (White, 1989). For some people, this is a time of vulnerability and uncertainty without the comfort and familiarity of the former persona. For others, this is a time of freedom and expansion as they realize that they can be whomever they want. Whether they no longer present themselves as a bereaved person or intentionally identify themselves as, for example, a widow or widower, people search for ways to show who they are now.

Life begins to fill up again, both externally and internally. New decisions can be made such as selling a house or making a career change. In the time since the death, most people have become used to making decisions alone or have found others to help them. They have a broader perspective now, one that includes the past and future and helps them to make good decisions. Personal resources and skills are recognized and utilized. The friends, family, or professionals who have been supportive in times of pain become sounding boards or encouragers of new endeavors. People who had a difficult relationship with the person who died may now seek referrals for professional help to deal with challenging issues, such as abuse or alcoholism. Others may identify areas of personal growth that they want to work on in the future. The skills that people learned to cope with grief and bereavement are now part of their personal repertoire, and most feel more confident and less vulnerable than they have felt since the death.

Bereaved people often come to a sense of discovery about themselves in the face of loss and death. They wish that this death had not happened but, having survived the devastation, they begin to appreciate their own strength and resiliency. They identify new values and attitudes and believe that they are better, more appreciative people for the experience of having known and been influenced by the person who died (Rando, 1993). They say that life is precious and that they are growing more compassionate toward themselves and others. In describing the changes and stages that they experience in bereavement, people mention recognizing personal growth as the final stage of grief (Hogan, Morse, & Tason, 1996).

Interventions

These psychosocial interventions have been designed to specifically address the key consideration *personal identity*. There are several assessment questions that will help open up a discussion, followed by more focused comments or tips that will facilitate further exploration of the issues that frequently arise at this time; each tip is followed by a sample dialogue.

Assessment Questions

- In what ways do you think you are different now than you were before your daughter died?

- How have your values and priorities changed over this time?

- Can you identify anything that you have gained through this experience of grieving for your partner?

- In what ways are you like your brother who died? How are you different?

Review grief and acknowledge progress and personal growth. This helps people to recognize how much their grief has changed and how different their experience is now. Your recognition of their strengths helps people to own them.

> "It usually comes down to the bereaved person finally realizing the rest of their life belongs to them."
>
> —John Tomczak,
> Victoria Hospice Society
> volunteer and bereaved person

> *"Karl, as I listen to you speak about your lack of progress in grieving right now, I'm remembering the first time that we talked. What can you remember about that time? And later, when you first went back to work? And now that you have been working full time for a while and are even anticipating a promotion?"*

Explore options and resources. Facilitate new decisions. Trepidation is natural as people try new things. Your acceptance and encouragement can help people to overcome fear or inertia or anxiety.

> *"You want to do a little traveling, something you couldn't do for the years of Nigel's illness. It's hard to think about going without him, but you think you could ask another widow you met a few months ago to travel with you. What sort of trip might you plan for a first time together?"*

Discuss plans and hopes for the future. Your interest normalizes the continuation of growth and change.

> *"Now that you are the sole support for your family, you are thinking about going back to school to upgrade your skills. It has been a while since you've been at school and you are wondering how you will manage. Who can you talk to for information about courses, costs, and financial assistance?"*

Encourage people in their positive identification with the person who died. This may help them to internalize the values and behaviors learned from the person who died, or to seek other positive relationships for nurturing.

> *"Sally, you have missed your coach a lot over the past months. She really believed in you and gave you lots of encouragement. Now that she's gone, how does that happen for you? Where do you get that faith and encouragement now?"*

OUR EXPERIENCE

Our goal at this time is to help people find a personal balance between connection with the person who died and freedom to move forward. The purpose is to support people as they emerge from the pain of their grief and begin to build a new life. At this transition, we support bereaved people in emerging from the labyrinth journey of grief. They are stepping out of the private, contained environment of grief and back into the mainstream of life. We see people who are puzzled by their mixed feelings in response to new joys and successes. Ambivalence and guilt can color this transition, as bereaved people are reluctant to move forward. They worry that they will forget or fail to honor the person who died, his or her importance, or the impact of the death. We strive to help bereaved people find ways of continuing to feel connected yet free to continue their life path.

Part of our work with families at this time is to review their grief process and acknowledge the progress that they have made. We notice that as people begin to appreciate their own progress, they find incentive to go forward in life. We give them permission to incorporate the death as part of their family history and their grief as a part of who they are now. We encourage them to build and rebuild a new life including a realistic place for the person who died to be remembered.

After the efforts and anguish of the grief journey, we are pleased to graduate bereaved families from our follow-up service. We identify skills and experiences that will influence the way they respond to life forever. Together, we discuss the strengths that have brought them through the crisis of death and the darkness of grief. We use the image of mending the heart. When the heart is broken, loving care and attention can restore its vitality and strength. Although the repair may show, we know that scar tissue is stronger than normal tissue. As we bring our relationship with a bereaved family or individual to a close, we often have a sense of satisfaction as we see them find their wings.

When the picture is not so positive, we help people to identify issues and problems that remain. We encourage them to seek the help that they want or need. We may help them reconcile themselves to life as it is and to themselves as fallible human beings, worthy of care and respect.

TEAM ISSUES

It can be easy for the bereavement team to feel impatient with, or have judgments about, people who are not "getting on with it" after what, in their opinion, seems sufficient time. They may want certain people to be adjusting better than they are and to be ready to move on from needing their support. Judgments may be influenced by their personal, social, and cultural expectations of how long and in what manner people should grieve.

As bereavement follow-up draws to an end, team members may find they are attached to certain families or individuals and be reluctant to help them reclaim their independence. They need to remember that closure of the relationship between the bereaved person and the care provider is one goal of bereavement support. It is important to be mindful of professional boundaries. Good supervision is imperative to help volunteers and health care providers to know when their job is done.

When the parameters of bereavement programs do not match the human experience or need of bereaved individuals, the team can feel frustrated and stressed by this dissonance. Program policy and limited resources often restrict the ability to address the ongoing concerns encountered. A lack of alternative community resources will increase the team's obligation to respond. It is difficult to balance the needs of the many bereaved people and make decisions about how best to address the multiple concerns that exist.

SUMMARY

This transition may come upon people gradually or they may have an epiphany that changes the nature of their grief. These moments, though hard to describe, shift the person's experience of his or her grief (see Table 10.1). Perhaps it is a visitation from the person who died or an awakening to beauty and peace in the natural world and in the cycles of life. Somehow, the loss slips from being a very present concern into an event that becomes part of the past. There is a recognition that life goes on and has been going on even while grief was a present and constant companion. Moules suggested that bereaved people are now "developing a relationship with grief that is potentially lifelong, but liveable" (1998, p. 142) and that includes comfort and creativity as well as sorrow.

The grieving process naturally moves people forward toward life. In many ways, people have adapted and adjusted to the changes in their lives and their families, and they will continue to do so. As people emerge from the pain of active grieving, they may be aware that they are mending their hearts. Many bereaved people come to feel they are deeper, more caring people for having experienced significant loss and grief.

Bereaved people slowly re-enter the world from the center of the labyrinth, the center of their grief. Grief is like any significant journey: the traveler is changed by experiences along the way and the once familiar world is different upon their return.

Table 10.1.   Phase 3: Mending the heart

Description	Transition and image	Grief task(s)
As grief becomes more resolved, bereaved people have the energy and desire to reconnect with the world. Their loss begins to be seen in perspective as part of their past experience.	Grief lightens and bereaved people live with ongoing grief as a part of their life. Image: mending the heart	To re-invest energy in activities and relationships To create an appropriate relationship with the person who died

Social	Physical	Emotional	Cognitive	Spiritual
More interest in daily affairs of others Ability to reach out and meet others Energy for social relationships Desire for independence resurfaces	Physical symptoms subside Sleep pattern and appetite return to normal Gut-wrenching emptiness lightens	Emotions are less intense Feeling of coming out of the fog More peace and happiness Some guilt about how life goes on	Perspective about death increases Able to remember with less pain Memory and concentration improve Dreams and nightmares decrease	Connection with religious and/or spiritual beliefs Life has new meaning/purpose Acceptance that death is a part of life

REFLECTIVE ACTIVITY

This exercise can be used to help health care providers, volunteers, and others focus on a past situation that had a lasting impact on them. This could be an event that was profound or difficult, or that feels unfinished. It is an opportunity for people to revisit powerful memories, to process their reactions to the situation, and, possibly, to reframe them.

This is a group exercise. It is helpful if someone reads the instructions step-by-step to the group so that the participants can stay centered in the process of remembering and writing.

Suggest that people stay open to expressing their thoughts and feelings without censoring them or trying to make them poetic. People often have self-judgments about their creative abilities and may need encouragement to participate in the exercise. Each instruction is a line in the poem. Pace the instructions, allowing people sufficient time to complete each line before moving on to the next. It's important that they write each line without judging, editing, or reviewing, and read what they have written only when they have finished.

Sample Poem: **Mother and Son**

> Mother and son so alike.
> Their big hands clasped,
> Her wrists too frail.
> Their longing for her life is distilled into a small hope for time.
> My aching heart
> knows it is not enough,
> It is not enough.

1. Take a moment to remember an event from your work, something that has stayed with you, for whatever reasons. It may have touched your heart, scared you, or felt unfinished. Name this memory or event. Write down the name.

2. Recall one image, mental picture, or specific memory associated with the event. Write it down.

3. Recall another image and write it down.

4. Recall another image and write it down also.

5. Keeping the images in mind, develop a simile (a comparison using *like* or *as*) or a metaphor. You might want to begin this line with the word "Like ..." and describe how you were feeling.

6. Describe a physical sensation (smell, sound, texture, and so forth).

7. Include a new awareness or insight. Let it come to you now as you remember this event.

8. Write a concluding sentence.

In pairs, have each person read his or her poem out loud to a partner, or have the partner read the poem to the author. Debrief thoughts and feelings related to the exercise and the memories that arose in doing it. If people are willing, have them read their poems to the larger group.

This exercise can be used privately to work through responses to the work, to patients and families, to colleagues, and to past issues illuminated by present experience. Read the poem aloud to yourself. Decide if you wish/need to share or debrief with someone.

RESOURCES

Attig, T. (2000). *The heart of grief: Death and the search for lasting love.* New York: Oxford University Press.

Grollman, E. (1977). *Living when a loved one has died.* Boston: Beacon Press.

Kallenberg, K. (1992). Three years later: Grief, view of life, and personal crisis after death of a family member. *Journal of Palliative Care, 8*(4), 13–19.

Shapiro, E. (1994). *Grief as a family process: A developmental approach to clinical practice.* New York: Guilford Press.

Wylie, B.J. (1997). *Beginnings: A book for widows* (4th ed.). Toronto: McClelland and Stewart.

REFERENCES

Fleming, S. (1986). *Psychological intervention with the bereaved.* Keynote presentation at Canadian Hospice Palliative Care Association national conference, Calgary, Alberta.

Hogan, N., Morse, J., & Tason, M. (1996). Toward an experiential theory of bereavement. *Omega, 33*(1), 43–65.

Holiday hope: Remembering loved ones during special times of the year. (1998). Minneapolis, MN: Fairview Press.

Mogenson, G. (1992). *Death, value, and meaning series: Greeting the angels: An imaginal view of the mourning process.* Amityville, NY: Baywood Publishing.

Moules, N. (1998). Legitimizing grief: Challenging beliefs that constrain. *Journal of Family Nursing, 4*(2), 142–166.

Rando, T. (1993). *Treatment of complicated mourning.* Champaign, IL: Research Press.

Viorst, J. (2000). *Suddenly sixty and other shocks of later life.* New York: Simon & Schuster.

White, M. (1989). *Saying hello again: The incorporation of the lost relationship in the resolution of grief.* In M. White, *Selected papers.* Adelaide, Australia: Dulwich Center.

Worden, W. (1991). *Grief counseling and grief therapy: A handbook for the mental health practitioner.* New York: Springer Publishing.

THE LAST WORD

"The initial mystery that attends each journey is: how did the traveler reach his starting point in the first place?"

—Louise Bogan

The path through life-threatening illness, dying, and bereavement is the universal journey, one that encompasses our bodies, our minds, our psyches, and our souls. Those of us who work with dying and bereaved people can only know each individual's journey from the outside, for every journey is as unique as the person involved. It is difficult to speak in general terms of people's experiences with illness, dying, and bereavement because these experiences include a wide spectrum of individual, cultural, and social differences.

For health care providers, knowing when and how to intervene with both purpose and sensitivity is an ongoing challenge and privilege. It is our experience that recognizing and understanding the psychosocial transitions that many people experience makes the personal and professional work of providing care easier. This awareness of the patterns in the physical changes that impending death brings as well as the emotional, intellectual, and spiritual transitions along the way helps us act as guides on the journey.

Though this book had three primary writers, its true voice lies in the clinical and practical wisdom of many. The inspiration and stimulation of our colleagues, the patients and families we've known, as well as other writers, teachers, and mentors, has given us the confidence to carefully examine and illustrate our practice. Writing this book has allowed us to think openly and critically about what we actually do and why we do it. We found a renewed focus on the values inherent in our role as guides to patients and families:

- **An understanding of holistic care.** This includes not only the emotional, social, physical, intellectual, and spiritual aspects of the patient and family but of ourselves also. We recognize that helping others to journey, with dignity and authenticity, requires meaningful self-reflection for both the traveler and the guide.

- **An appreciation and respect for the strength of the team.** As on any journey, each guide, each traveler, has something essential to contribute. We work attentively with our fellow professionals and with those who undertake the journey to be sure each unique contribution is heard and supported.

- **The awareness that knowledge is power.** We continually strive to hone our knowledge and expertise. We share information with colleagues, patients, and families in ways that are reassuring, validating, and empowering.

We hope that this book supports those who work with patients and families to comprehend and convey the complexities of the journey and its transitions in a deeper and better way. We hope that it helps readers to improve their abilities to guide travelers who must move along the pathway of serious illness, dying, and bereavement.

Index

Page references followed by *f, t,* and *sb* indicate figures, tables, and sidebars, respectively.